Table of Contents

THE MODERN NUTRITIONAL DISEASES

heart disease
stroke
type-2 diabetes
obesity
cancer

and how to prevent them

2nd Edition

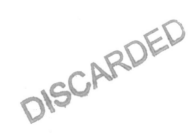

Alice Ottoboni, Ph.D.
Fred Ottoboni, M.P.H., Ph.D.

Vincente Books
Fernley, NV 89408
vbi@775.net

ISBN 0-915241-05-6
EAN 9780915241057
Library of Congress Control Number: 2013930402

Vincente Books
Fernley NV, 89408
vbi@775.net

CreateSpace Independent Publishing Platform
North Charleston, South Carolina

Printed in the United States of America

Chapter Nine
Essential Fatty Acids and Eicosanoids   **177**

Figures and Tables

Preface

America is in a very difficult situation. Current costs of medical care to cope with our large epidemics of chronic diseases threaten the economic stability of the nation. These diseases include heart disease, strokes, diabetes, cancers, obesity, Alzheimer's disease, plus a number of others. Medical care costs will continue to rise because these diseases are affecting younger and younger age groups. Importantly, all of these diseases, appropriately labeled modern nutritional diseases, have the same provable cause: chronic inflammation brought about by a national dietary policy that was created a half-century ago for the purpose of preventing heart attacks.

This book carries two overarching messages. One is that millions of Americans are slowly dying from one or more or the many chronic diseases that have been foisted on them, their parents, and their children by the many-decades-old official nutrition policy of their own government. These diseases are not the products of some unknown disruption of life processes. The truth that they are nutritionally based is revealed by the nutritional biochemistry and physiology presented within the pages of this book.

The second overarching message is that the modern nutritional diseases are preventable. America needs a national disease prevention program based on sound, hard science. Health care, as it is practiced today consists of medical care alone. Effective preventive programs do not exist. Medical care, namely early detection and treatment, is vitally important, but it is very costly because it addresses one patient at a time and depends on costly drugs and medical procedures.

The science and practice of scientific disease prevention has a history of low cost and reliable effectiveness because it eliminates causes using methods that protect whole communities, not just individuals. Many years ago, prevention was a common practice; causes were discovered, preventive methods were developed, and programs were put in place. For example, about a century ago, a prevention program eliminated goiters and cretinism throughout the country. This was accomplished at almost no cost by adding an iodide (salt of iodine) to table salt.

This book, using sound science, explains how the official American government dietary policy is responsible for distorted biochemical processes that underlie America's great and growing epidemics of chronic inflammatory diseases. The hope is that readers who have the determination and self-discipline to accept responsibility for their own health will be encouraged to start their own personal prevention program.

The information in this book should help you feel better, live longer, avoid the modern nutritional diseases, and be happier and more active as you grow older. The ideal outcome is to keep all systems functioning well until that point when everything wears out and fails all at once, like the fabled one-hoss shay. How tragic it is, for example, to have a sound body and mind capable of functioning efficiently for twenty or more years stilled by a heart attack or stroke.

The One Hoss Shay:

This delightful poem was introduced by Oliver Wendell Holmes with the thought that a superior being should be able to construct any machine in such a way that no one of its component parts would wear out before any other. To illustrate the concept, he wrote of a deacon who decided to build such a machine – a one-hoss shay. Holmes continues:

There is a practical lesson to be got out of the story. Observation shows us in what point any particular mechanism is most likely to give way. In a wagon, for instance, the weak point is where the axle enters the hub or nave. When the wagon breaks down, three times out of four, I think, it is at this point that the accident occurs. The workman should see to it that this part should never give way; then find the next vulnerable place, and so on, until he arrives logically at the perfect result obtained by the deacon.

> Have you heard of the wonderful one-hoss-shay
> That was built in such a logical way
> It ran a hundred years to a day,
> And then, of a sudden, it –ah, but stay
> I'll tell you what happened without delay—

The poem goes on to describe the building of the one-hoss shay in such a manner and with such careful workmanship that all of its structures would wear out at exactly the same time. The shay was driven hard for a hundred years and then, the poem continues, suddenly fell apart, and there was…

> The poor old chaise in a heap or mound,
> As if it had been to the mill and ground!
> You see, of course, if you're not a dunce,
> How it went to pieces all at once, –
> All at once and nothing first, -- Just as bubbles
>   do when they burst.

> End of the wonderful one horse shay.
> Logic is logic. That's all I say.

Notes for the Reader

As your read through this book, you will find that some difficult-to-remember facts, background materials, and explanations are presented more than once. These repetitions help chapters stand alone, which makes it easier for the book to be used as a reference document. We expect that the book will be perused a section here and a section there, at different times, depending on the needs of the reader. Thus we repeated points we considered important, not only to stress them but also to assure that they would not be missed in random reading.

You will find that references are numbered sequentially and listed in numerical order at the end of each chapter. We used this convention, rather than grouping all the references by chapter at the end of the book, because we found in our research it is the most convenient way to find citations. If information referred to is from a book or other long document, the page number on which the information can be found is given after the reference number (e.g. 27, p. 241). An "ff" following a page number indicates that the information referred to covers more than one page. When more than one reference is given to an item, the reference numbers are separated by a semicolon.

As you read through the book, remember – it is your book. If or when you come to a thought or idea that especially interests you or one that you want to remember, mark the passage or write in the margin. The book was designed with wide margins specifically for that purpose. Use a yellow highlighter or any writing tool you prefer. The margins can also be use to make notes about your own thoughts or to record questions you might want to research further on your own. Mark and use the book as you will.

Finally, please remember that neither of us is a physician. Our contribution through this book is based not on degrees in medicine, but on education in biological and health sciences and experience in the field of public health and disease prevention. Our backgrounds enable us to review the conflicting articles, books, and recommendations regarding health, nutrition, and aging and identify what is right and useful, what is wrong and useless, and, in some cases, even what is harmful.

Part One

The Problem

You can ignore reality, but you cannot ignore the consequences of reality.
Attributed to Ayn Rand

The goal of Part One is to set the stage for an investigation of why long-known chronic diseases that were merely a few troublesome statistics a hundred years ago have evolved to their current prominence as major epidemics that now threaten the solvency of our nation.

The true causes of the nutritional diseases discussed in this book have been the subject of controversy since the 1950s, when heart disease began to be recognized as a major problem. For many years, the position of the American government, nutrition academia, and the medical establishment has been that our current epidemics of chronic debilitating diseases are caused by a diet that contains too much red meat, saturated animal fat and cholesterol, and an insufficiency of vegetable seed oils, vegetables, and grain-based carbohydrate foods.

Over the years, a few physicians and scientists have argued to no avail that the government-sponsored diet is the problem and that a diet resembling that on which the human genome evolved would prevent or at least reduce the risk of these diseases. The truth of this argument is well documented in the scientific literature. Its acceptance is vital to public health.

To set the stage for consideration of the problem, Part One reviews the evolution of the human diet from its beginnings in prehistoric times to the modern day American dietary regimen (Chapter One); the concurrent fast increase to epidemic proportions in the incidence of old diseases combined with the advent of new, hitherto unknown afflictions (Chapter Two); and the pseudoscience, intermingled with political management, that gave birth to an official U. S. Government nutrition policy (Chapter Three).

Chapter One

The Evolutionary Diet versus the Modern Diet

To be ignorant of what occurred before you were born is to remain always a child. For what is the worth of human life, unless it is woven into the life of our ancestors by the records of history. **Marcus Tullius Cicero, 106-43 BC, Roman statesman and orator.**

Every human being alive today is the most recent offspring in a string of survivors that go all the way back to the beginning of life – not just human life, but life itself (1). The inescapable fact is that all living organisms are beautifully designed systems based almost totally on self-regulating biochemical reactions. Every creature living today is the product of its biochemistry, and this biochemistry is the product of countless numbers of biochemical trials and errors throughout the eons. Human biochemical systems were fashioned by the diet of the ancestral species of the human family as they evolved from their first appearance on earth through the Paleolithic period.

The diet of the Paleolithic period was the evolutionary diet of the human species. It was central to the development of the physical and mental characteristics that transformed the ancient primate into the modern-day human. Because the pace of biologic evolution is so extremely slow, there has not been time for the genetic changes that would be necessary to accommodate major modifications in the composition of the evolutionary diet to occur. The genetic constitution that dictates the nutritional requirements of modern-day humans is the same as the genetic constitution of their hunter/gatherer ancestors (2; 3, p.38 ff).

The Paleolithic Diet

The Paleolithic diet describes the food habits and composition of the ancestors of early man during the Paleolithic period, which began several million years ago during the Pleistocene geologic epoch. The name Paleolithic, literally meaning "ancient stone," was given to this period because it was the time during which primitive man developed and used stone and bone tools. It should be noted the even though the Paleolithic period long predates current existence, descriptions of the Paleolithic diet and way of life are not based on fantasy or conjecture but rather on compelling archeological findings and a voluminous fossil record (2).

THE FIRST HUMANS

The human journey began about 4,000,000 or more years ago with the appearance of the first ape-like creatures that walked upright. The first of these bipedal creatures with sufficient brain capacity to be classed as human in the genus *Homo* (*Homo habilis*) appeared approximately 2,000,000 years ago. Anatomically modern humans (*Homo sapiens*) are thought to have arisen sometime between 90,000 and 40,000 years ago (3, p. 20 ff).

During the millennia prior to the appearance of *Homo sapiens*, human ancestors developed the instincts that were the foundation for their societal structure; the banding together in small groups to serve common needs and goals (4, p.11). These bands, usually related by blood or marriage, were small enough to travel as a unit but large enough to provide for simple division of labor. The band served its members in many ways: with mutual aid and comfort; protection from dangers; and cooperation in hunting and food gathering.

HUNTER-GATHERERS: The archeological record indicates that human ancestors were hunter-gatherers. It also shows that human ancestors of 2,000,000 years ago were considerably smaller than were those that succeeded them. They ate whatever they could find, mainly small animals, insects, eggs, nuts, fruits, berries, and green plants. The only sweet available to them was honey. Their progeny became physically larger and stronger and their tools more refined through succeeding generations, which enabled them to hunt larger animals. This made meat a more prominent component of the diet than previously had been possible (3). Extensive reviews of quantitative dietary studies suggest that meat may have provided 65 to 68 percent of calories of the hunter-gatherer diet (5).

SCAVENGERS: Despite the increased capability to hunt, the killing of large animals probably contributed less to the meat supply than did the scavenging of carcasses that had been killed by other predators. Scavenging was a much more energy efficient method of obtaining meat and other valuable animal parts such as bones and skins. Scavenging was easier than killing and safer because it permitted transport of a carcass to a central, more secure, area where desired parts could be removed. Because of scavenging, the Paleolithic diet was expanded to include brains and bone marrow, which were obtained by using hammer stones to break the skulls and long bones of scavenged carcasses (6).

BRAIN VOLUME

What is most interesting about the addition of brains and marrow to the Paleolithic diet is that these parts of large animals were a particularly rich source of both essential fatty acids (see Chapters Eight and Nine) required for brain development, namely docosahexaenoic acid (DHA) and arachidonic acid (AA). Work by Williams and Crawford indicates that a coastal environment where evolving humans had access to both fish and land animals would also provide the DHA and AA required for brain development (7). It is estimated that over the hundreds of thousands of years prior to the beginning of farming, evolving humans became nutritionally dependent on diets rich in DHA and AA. The addition of DHA and AA to the Paleolithic diet was accompanied by a slow but steady increase in human brain volume (8).

The fossil record shows that the earliest human ancestors had a brain volume of from 375 to 550 cc (cubic centimeters). The first *Homo* species to be recognized, *Homo habilis*, had a brain volume of about 500 to 800 cc, which increased to 775 to 1225 cc in the later *Homo erectus* and to 1350 cc in the first modern humans (*Homo sapiens*). Regardless of what specific evolutionary factors were responsible for the increase in the size of the human brain, it could not have occurred without an increased intake of the preformed essential fatty acids DHA and AA that are major components of brain tissue. Thus, there is good reason to believe that the current large human brain size is the product of the essential fatty acids provided by the Paleolithic diet (9).

The critical importance of DHA in the human diet is underscored by the fact that recent analyses of modern-day cranial capacity show that it has declined by 11 percent in the last 35,000 years. Almost all of this 11 percent decline (8 percent) has occurred since the advent of farming 10,000 years ago (10), which was accompanied by a significant increase in consumption of carbohydrates (grains) and a decrease in consumption of animal foods in general and DHA in particular.

LIFE SPAN

Paleolithic man had a significantly shorter life span at birth than does modern man (3, p.4ff). The most common causes of death were microbial diseases, complications of childbirth, and trauma. There is no evidence that he suffered from any of the chronic diseases that plague today's populations, and his teeth were remarkable free of dental caries. The nutritional practices responsible for the modern nutritional diseases were nonexistent in Paleolithic times. The argument that early humans did not live sufficiently long enough to develop degenerative diseases is not borne out by the fossil record; many who survived childhood lived well into and through the age of vulnerability for such disorders.

Transition from Paleolithic Diet to Modern Diet

The onset of farming about ten thousand years ago gradually changed the human diet. Although certain aspects of the hunter/gatherer lifestyle still persist today in remote regions of the earth, it became impractical in areas beset by population pressures. By the end of the Paleolithic period, sometime before 10,000 BC, the original small bands of early humans had become large bands or tribes as a result of a slow and gradual increase in population. This not only made them less mobile but also increased the amount of land they required to provide an adequate food supply. These conditions helped usher in the Age of Agriculture (3, p.24ff).

FARMING

Groups who were fortunate enough to live in fertile valleys and who adopted a farming lifestyle were freed from dependence on nature for provision of their sustenance. They grew their own grain and bred their own animals. The gradual growth of community living

brought increasingly complex social customs and greatly increased the consumption of carbohydrates in the form of grain and grain products.

ANCIENT EGYPTIAN SOCIETY

A harbinger of the current-day modern nutritional diseases can be found in the records
of archeologists and paleopathologists who studied a highly successful Egyptian farming
society that lived in the Nile Valley from about 2500 BC to 395 AD (11, p.394ff). Two
circumstances provided an extraordinary wealth of material that enabled the researchers to
draw a highly detailed and accurate picture of diet composition and health status of these
early farmers. One, the Egyptians were expert in mummification and applied the practice
through all social strata, and two, they left a meticulous and voluminous written record on
papyrus describing all aspects of life of the time.

Many thousands of ancient remains were studied in such detail by paleopathologists that
not only blood type and body characteristics but also the presence of bacterial or parasitic
infections, other diseases, and cause of death could be determined. These studies reveal
that the early Egyptians did not have the same robust health that was characteristic of their
hunter/gatherer predecessors. The early farmers tended to be short and obese with brittle
bones, severe dental problems and gum disease. The records show clearly that cardiovascular diseases occurred extensively throughout ancient Egypt.

The diet of the early Egyptian farmers was primarily whole grain bread, cereals, fresh
fruits, some vegetables, honey, goat's milk, and some fish and poultry but almost no red
meat. It was a low-fat, high-carbohydrate diet akin to that recommended by the government-sponsored Food Guide Pyramid described later in this chapter.

Like the ancient Egyptians, modern-day humans have not yet had time to evolve (change
genetically) to be able to thrive on the present-day high-carbohydrate diets. On an evolutionary time scale, ten thousand years is not enough time to influence significantly our
evolutionary biochemistry (9; 12). Humans today live in a nutritional environment that is
far different from that of the prehistoric period during which their genetic composition was
selected (13). In short, genes today are very similar to those of prehistoric ancestors and,
thus, they are not programmed to provide strong, disease-free bodies and minds on today's
high-carbohydrate, low-protein, low-animal-fat, and low-omega-3 essential fatty acid diet.

THE CONTRIBUTION OF WESTON A. PRICE

Supporting evidence for this conclusion is provided by dietary studies done in the 1930s by
Weston A. Price (14). Price's studies compared the health and, in particular, the prevalence
of dental caries in isolated ethnic groups who were still living on their primitive diets with
matched groups of the same stocks who were routinely consuming "white man's" food.
The groups examined lived in the Swiss Alps, the Outer Hebrides Islands, Alaska, Northern
Canada, Australia, Africa, and the Pacific Islands. Without exception, the groups living on
their primitive diets were far healthier than their counterparts, as measured by dental car-

ies, brain function, physical stature, birth defects, and immunity to diseases, particularly tuberculosis. Price also noted that personality disturbances and unsocial traits were far less common in primitive diets groups (14, p.1ff).

The diets of the groups consuming white man's food were approximately uniform throughout the world, consisting of refined flour and its products, polished rice, sugar, jams, canned goods, and vegetable fats and oils. Very little fresh meat, fish, vegetables, or dairy products were included in these diets. Of particular interest were the uniformly high numbers of dental caries and cranial, facial, and dental arch deformities among the groups that had adopted the western diet. High rates of tuberculosis in the latter were also common, even when special clinics and medical care were available.

The diets of the primitive groups varied in their details, but were quite uniform when viewed in terms of their dietary macronutrients. All of these diets regularly included protein and fat from fish, shellfish, animal meat, animal organs and entrails, bone marrow, insects, and/or dairy products. Carbohydrate was always in the form of fruit, vegetables, or unprocessed grain. The diets of these primitive groups contained no sugar, refined grain, or vegetable fats or oils. The isolated Swiss groups had lived for centuries on a diet of only dairy products, cheese, rye seeds, and meat from dairy cows and goats.

Hebrides Islanders lived almost exclusively on fish, shellfish, fish heads, porridge made from whole oats, and locally grown vegetables. These individuals had essentially no cavities, no cranial or other bone deformities, and no tuberculosis. People of exactly the same ethnic stock who lived on the same island but ate white man's food had high rates of tuberculosis and rampant tooth decay. Many had lost all their teeth by age 30. The average height of the men had decreased by several inches as compared to those on the primitive diets. The pattern throughout the rest of the world was approximately the same; those eating their traditional primitive foods were healthy, and those eating white man's food were unhealthy.

Among his research activities, Price operated a dental clinic in a poor neighborhood of Cleveland, Ohio, during the period of the Great Depression. The grade school children in this neighborhood had numerous large cavities that penetrated into the pulp tissues of their permanent teeth. Temporary fillings were necessary to control the pain caused by the exposed pulp tissue. Price described the regular diets of these children as consisting primarily of highly sweetened strong coffee, white bread, vegetable fat, pancakes made of white flour and eaten with syrup, and donuts fried in vegetable fat.

In a careful clinical study of three of these depression-era grade school children, Price found that he could control their dental caries with a special diet formulated to be nutritionally similar to the native diets that he had been studying. Under his direction, the three children were given a special noontime meal at a local mission, every day except Sunday, for a six-month period. These meals began with a small amount of tomato or orange juice and one teaspoon of a mixture of high quality butter and cod liver oil. Following this, they were fed a rich stew made from fish or from meat, bone marrow, and animal organs, plus carrots and a few other vegetables. Also included in these meals was freshly ground whole-grain wheat bread with butter, two glasses of fresh whole milk, and cooked fruit with no sugar added.

Regular chemical analysis of saliva of these children revealed that, after five months, a change consistent with cessation of tooth decay had occurred. Dental examinations and x-rays showed that a new dentine layer was growing over and reincasing the exposed tooth pulp. Price concluded that this feeding program had clinically controlled the dental caries of the children in the study group. Interestingly, during the study period, schoolteachers reported that one child in the study group had improved from the poorest to one of the best in the class in ability to learn (14, p. 288ff).

ACTIVATOR X: Price concluded that the key factor in native diets and the diet he designed for the schoolchildren was the unswerving balance among proteins, fats derived from animal sources, and carbohydrates, plus vitamins and minerals derived from vegetables, fruits, and unprocessed grains. This combination supplied both the energy and the essential nutrients required for the healthy growth and maintenance of body tissue. During his many years of research, Price actively sought to identify the food component responsible for the beneficial effects conferred by native foods but not by white man's food. He considered that this food component, which he labeled Activator X, was an especially powerful essential nutrient.

Price found from chemical analyses of many foods evidence of Activator X in fish, cod liver oil, animal organs, dairy cream, and butter. He was never able to identify the specific chemical involved because of the laboratory limitations of the time, except that he was able to rule out vitamins A and D. However, because this nutrient was soluble in fat, he spoke of it as a fat-soluble activator. Particularly rich sources of this activator were cod liver oil, and the very yellow butter from cows eating fresh grass.

The health benefits attributed to Price's fat-soluble Activator X mirror those of cod liver oil, which made cod liver oil an effective folk remedy centuries ago. In the 1950s, Johanna Budwig, a German physician, referred to oils found fish and flax as very delicate, highly unsaturated, health-promoting oils (15). In recent years, the fragile chemicals in these oils have been identified as omega-3 and omega-6 essential fatty acids. The similarity in health benefits between Activator X and the omega-3 essential fatty acids (EFA) lend strong support to a conclusion that Price's Activator X was an omega-3 EFA. Recently, an alternative hypothesis that suggests that Dr. Price's Activator X was vitamin K and not an essential fatty acid has appeared in the scientific literature. The data accompanying the paper suggests that the characteristics of Activator X closely correspond to those of vitamin K (16).

The Modern Diet

The diet of modern humans bears little resemblance to that of prehistoric man. In just the last hundred years, five significant changes have occurred in the average American diet

(17). Calorie intake has increased. The use of sugars and other sweeteners has about doubled. The per capita use of starch from grain and potatoes has increased by 40 percent or more. Egg use has dropped significantly. And Americans are now eating about 40 pounds per year of brand new fats and oils (vegetable seed oils) that have never before been a part of the human diet. How did all this happen?

BEGINNING OF CHANGE

Sometime before 1900, the American food supply and diet began a long, gradual change. The family farm was disappearing, and an agricultural industry based on mechanization and higher efficiency was emerging. These changes, along with better transportation and new methods of food storage and preservation, reduced the costs of American agricultural products and made them more widely available throughout the country. More than ample supplies of grains made products manufactured from refined wheat flour (white flour), such as bread, sweet bakery products, and pasta, available to everyone in America at very affordable prices.

THE NEW SUGARS

Sugar was also becoming a low-cost product. Before 1900, sugar was a luxury item made from sugar cane or from maple syrup. The sugar beet was long known in Europe. A few sugar beet factories came into operation prior to WWI, but the general use of beet sugar did not come about until WWII. Rapid development of the sugar beet industry increased the availability of sugar and greatly reduced its cost. Later, new processes capable of deriving sugar from corn (as corn syrup) added to the supplies.

The commercial demand for more intensely sweet products combined with the fact that fructose has a more sweet taste than either glucose or sucrose (a dimer of glucose plus fructose) led to the development of high fructose corn syrup. These advancements made sweet products of all kinds widely available and affordable to virtually every American.

After World War II, public acceptance of commercial food products made from sugar and from refined wheat flour grew rapidly. Sliced bread and sweet products such as pies, cakes, donuts, sweet rolls and sticky buns, cookies, and fancy desserts enjoyed a growing demand. Candy manufacturing and soft drink production grew into major businesses that reached every family and corner of the country. This great expansion of the baking and commercial soft drink industries has resulted in a very large increase in the dietary use of carbohydrates in the form of both sugars and starches.

THE NEW EDIBLE OILS AND FATS

New sources of edible oils and fats were also developed in the early 1900s. Prior to that time, the major dietary sources of fats and oils were butter, lard (pork fat), tallow (beef fat), coconut oil, and olive oil. Other sources were meats, fish, nuts, and various whole grains. Fats and oils derived from vegetable seeds, such as cotton, corn, soybean, or safflower, were not widely sold because the oils extracted from these seeds became rancid during storage. Also, unprocessed vegetable seed oils were not suitable for frying because they smoked at very high temperatures.

A new chemical process called hydrogenation solved these problems. Mild hydrogenation altered the chemical composition of the vegetable oils so that the processed oils did not become rancid in storage and did not smoke at frying temperatures. An additional advantage of this process was that more intensive hydrogenation would convert the liquid vegetable oils into semisolid and solid fat products. These very low cost vegetable fats were sold as deep frying oils, vegetable shortening, and margarine. It is important to note that the hydrogenation process destroys the more highly unsaturated oils that are present in the raw oils, which happen to be omega-3 EFAs.

Today, these vegetable-based fats and oils have displaced the traditional fats and oils and hold the major share of the market in this country for edible fats and oils. In neighborhood markets and other commercial outlets, these fats and oils are found as vegetable oils, salad oils, polyunsaturated fats and oils, partially hydrogenated vegetable oils, vegetable shortening, or margarine.

CALORIE INTAKE

One unforeseen result of the new American diet has been that total per capita calorie intake has increased steadily during the last 30 or more years. According to the 2001-2002 United States Department of Agriculture's (USDA) publication *What Do American's Eat* (18), calorie intake by Americans in the year 2000 was just under 2,700 calories per person per day, an increase of about 530 calories per day or 24.5 percent between 1970 and 2000. This reflected higher consumption of all three macronutrients, carbohydrates, fat, and protein.

According to this official government publication, more calories, along with reductions in average physical activity, are behind the tremendous increase in obesity among adults, adolescents, and children in America. Sixty-two percent of adult Americans were overweight in 2000. This represents an increase of 46 percent since 1980. Twenty-seven percent of these overweigh adults were classified as obese because they were 30 pounds or more above their healthy weight. This obesity rate is twice what it was in 1960. Of great concern is that the upward trend in obesity is also occurring among American children.

USE OF CARBOHYDRATES

Consumption of carbohydrates in the form of both sugar and starch has increased significantly in the last hundred years. The average use of sweeteners such as sugar in 1900 is estimated to have been about 88 pounds per person per year. According to the USDA, per capita consumption of caloric sweeteners, namely sugar and corn sweeteners, including high-fructose corn syrup, grew from 110 pounds per person in 1950 to 152 pounds in 2000, an increase of about 42 pounds per person (18).

In the year 2000, carbonated sodas and other beverages provided more than a fifth of the added sugars (22 percent) in the American diet. This compares with 16 percent in 1970.

Sugar and corn sweeteners are used today as almost universal food additives in common foods such as hot dogs, canned fruits and vegetables, salad dressings, fruit drinks, bread and most bakery products, dry cereals, flavored yogurt, salad dressings, mayonnaise, and some peanut butters (18).

The per capita average use of grains (wheat, corn, and rice) increased from 138 to 200 pounds per year, about 45%, over the 30-year period 1970 to 2000. Most of this grain is refined before its use to make bread, bakery items, pasta, pizza, tortillas, and breakfast cereals. Consumption of ready-to-eat cereal has grown at the expense of eggs, which formerly were a common breakfast item. Egg use has steadily declined from an average of 374 per person per year in 1950, to 250 in 2000 (18).

The consumption of potatoes approximately doubled between 1970 and 1996. This large increase in potato consumption was due to the great growth in demand for potato chips and French fried potatoes. More recent data suggests that, when chips and fries are excluded, growth in potato use has not increased significantly. Per capita consumption of fruits and vegetables since the 1970s has increased about 20 percent. Total fruit use (processed and fresh) was up by 12 percent and total vegetable use by 23 percent (18).

COMPARISON WITH PALEOLITHIC DIET: The carbohydrate component of the typical American diet is estimated to be 51.8 percent of daily calories, which is considerably lower than the 60 percent recommendation of official government policy as published in *Dietary Guidelines for Americans* (DGA) (19). Cordain et al. estimate that the carbohydrate component of the Paleolithic diet was between 22 and 40 percent of calories (20). Thus, the carbohydrate component of the modern American diet is far in excess of that for which the human body was genetically programmed.

It is important to note that carbohydrates in the modern American diet are essentially all high glycemic sugars and starches (see Chapter Six), while most of the carbohydrates in the primitive diet were low glycemic plant varieties. As will be discussed in later chapters, this dissimilarity is an important underlying cause of the current epidemics of chronic inflammatory diseases.

USE OF PROTEINS

Total meat consumption (meat, poultry, and fish) increased to 195 pounds per person in the year 2000. This is 57 pounds above the average annual consumption in the 1950s. Red meat use was up by 7 pounds, poultry use increased by 46 pounds, and fish and shellfish use grew by 4 pounds. Despite the increase in per capita consumption of total meat in 2000, the proportion of fat from meat, poultry, and fish declined from 33 percent in the 1950s to 24 percent in 2000. As mentioned earlier, annual egg use has steadily declined from an average of 374 per person per year in 1950, to 250 in 2000.

Consumption of beverage milk declined from an annual average of 36 gallons per person in the 1950s to less than 23 gallons in 2000. Consumption of soft drinks, fruit drinks and other sweet drinks appears to be displacing beverage milk in the diet. The trend in beverage milk is toward lower-fat milk. That trend continues. Whole milk represented 92 percent of all beverage milk (plain, flavored, and buttermilk) sold in the 1950s, but its share was only 36 percent in 2000 (18). Average annual use of cheese, not including cottage cheese, increased 287 percent between the 1950s and 2000 and from 7.7 pounds per person to 29.8 pounds. The use of cottage cheese dropped from about 4 pounds per year per person to 2.6 pounds (18).

COMPARISON WITH PALEOLITHIC DIET: The current protein intake, calculated to be 15.4 percent of daily calories (20), is at the upper limit of the 10 to 15 percent recommended by the DGA (19). However, the DGA added a proscription against red meat plus a warning not to exceed twice the recommended percentages. It is estimated that the protein content of the Paleolithic diet was between 19 and 40 percent of calories (20), twice that in the DGA. Interestingly, with regard to the DGA proscription, it should be noted that the protein in the Paleolithic diet included the red muscle meat of animals.

Analysis of plant/animal subsistence ratios indicated that, wherever it was ecologically possible, early hunter-gatherers obtained from 45 to 65 percent of calories from animal foods (21). They ate not only muscle meat but also all other edible parts such as organs, brains, and marrow. Clearly, the modern human consumes significantly less protein, including red muscle meat, than did the ancestors from whom he evolved. Sears makes the case, based on sound data, that the optimum dietary intake of protein is about 30 percent of daily calories (22).

USE OF FATS AND OILS

Before 1900, the production and dietary use of fats and oils derived from vegetable seeds was essentially zero. By 1970, consumption of fats and oils from vegetable seeds had risen to 49 pounds per person per year. By the year 2000, consumption amounted to 66.5 pounds per person per year and represented more than 89 percent of the added fats and oils in the American diet.

Much of this increase in use of vegetable fats and oils went into the production of salad and cooking oils and margarine to take the place of butter, vegetable shortening to replace lard in cookies, cakes, and pastries, and frying fats to replace tallow for deep fried foods of all kinds, including potato chips and French fries. The consumption of butter, lard, and tallow decreased significantly between 1950 and 2000. The use of butter decreased from 9.0 to 4.6 pounds per person per year. Lard and tallow decreased from 10.5 to 6.0 pounds per person per year (18).

The nutritional qualities of the new fats and oils are different from those of the traditional fats and oils they replaced. The new fats and oils were not only resistant to heat and rancidity but also were good-tasting, low-cost substitutes for traditional fats and oils, such as butter, lard, olive oil, and tropical oils. Significantly, as a result of these substitutions, alpha-linolenic acid, an omega-3 EFA, virtually disappeared from the American diet, and dietary intake of linoleic acid, an omega-6 EFA, rose to record levels. In addition, large amounts of fatty acids known as *trans* fats were introduced into the human diet for the first time in evolutionary history.

COMPARISON WITH PALEOLITHIC DIET: The fat content of the modern diet is estimated to be 32.8 percent (20), slightly more than the 30 percent maximum recommended by the DGA (19). The fat component the Paleolithic diet was largely provided by wild animal foods. The percentage of fat in food animals, including fish, varied with species and size of animal and season of year. It ranged from 2.5 to 20 percent, with the lowest percent occurring at the beginning of the grazing season and the highest at the end. From these data, it is estimated that hunter-gatherers on a plant/animal subsistence ratio of 35/65 would have a dietary fat intake of from 23 to 58 percent of daily calories (21).

Early humans apparently prized the fatty parts of animals. When scavenging a large animal kill for food, fat depots and organs would be selected first, with lean muscle meat taken if needed. Prehistoric humans must have had an intuitive sense for the tremendous importance of dietary fat. It was essential for the prevention of a condition known as "rabbit starvation," which was described by early American explorers. It occurred in humans who, for extended periods, had only fat-depleted lean meat of wild animals as their sole source of food. Symptoms of rabbit starvation included nausea, followed by diarrhea, and ultimately death if untreated. It is cured by the addition of carbohydrate or fatty foods to the diet (21). Rabbit starvation apparently does not exist as a clinical entity today; however, its potential suggests that it is appropriate to warn dieters who eliminate sugars and starches from their daily fare to make sure that they do not also eliminate fats. The diet *must* provide energy from one or the other.

A feature of the Paleolithic diet that would be unacceptable to the modern-day nutrition establishment was its high level of animal fat and its accompanying cholesterol. It is estimated that the daily intake of cholesterol and saturated fat by Paleolithic humans was about 520 milligrams (3), which is considerably higher than the official recommendation of a maximum daily intake of 300 milligrams or less (19).

Among the differences between the Paleolithic and modern-day diets, perhaps the one that has the most significance for today's epidemics of modern nutritional diseases is the ratio of omega-6 to omega-3 EFAs (23). In Paleolithic times, the intake of these two EFA families was approximately equal, whereas today the modern diet contains at least 10-times more omega-6 EFA than omega-3. As will be amply documented as this book progresses, the introduction and widespread use of vegetable seed oils and the hydrogenation process have had several profoundly negative effects on human nutrition and health. Both the lopsided ratio of omega-6 to omega-3 fatty acids and the new, man-made *trans* fats adversely affect basic human biochemical processes.

Official U. S. Government Nutrition Policy

The official entry of politics into the field of nutrition occurred in 1977 with the publication of *Dietary Goals for the United States. Dietary Goals* signaled government approval of the low-fat, high-carbohydrate diet that had been promoted by the medical and nutrition establishments since the mid-1950s as a heart-healthy diet. *Dietary Goals* was the product of Senator George McGovern and his Senate Select Committee on Nutrition and Human Needs.

Senator McGovern, an unapologetic advocate for the low-fat, high-carbohydrate diet, was not swayed by considerable credible testimony that implicated sugar and starch as the likely underlying cause of the then-growing attack rates of heart disease. The USDA was chosen to be the lead agency in drafting the official dietary guidelines. The Human Nutrition Center was created within the USDA to oversee the project (24).

The USDA hailed *Dietary Goals* as a new direction for dietary guidance with the observation that it shifted the focus from choosing food components that contained healthful nutrients to avoiding intakes of food components linked to chronic disease. The USDA Human Nutrition Center began its task of formalizing the role of food components as risk factors for cardiovascular and other chronic diseases with particular emphasis on dietary fats and cholesterol. The official federal nutrition policy was written jointly by the USDA and DHHS (Department of Health and Human Services). The first edition of *Nutrition and Your Health: Dietary Guidelines for Americans* was issued in 1980 (25).

The goal of this official policy is stated to be education of the public in healthful nutrition. The policy was formulated by nutritional scientists who were selected from government and academia. The policy decreed that healthful nutrition was a diet low in fat (less than 30 percent of daily calories and restricted in animal fat), moderate in protein (16 to 20 percent of daily calories), and high in carbohydrates (50 to 60 percent of daily calories). It provides a wealth of detailed information on how to implement the so-called heart-healthy diet (26).

Personal eating preferences and habits, although often prescribed by social customs or religious dictates, had never before in recorded history been the subject of governmental action. Sound science was vanquished by political pressures when the U.S. federal government adopted its official policy prescribing what the American public should put on its dinner table.

DIETARY RECOMMENDATIONS PRE-1977

Prior to World War II, the only agency that had any interest in or responsibility for food production or consumption was the USDA. In 1894, it published what might be considered the first dietary recommendations. It simply described the basic food groups (protein, carbohydrate, and fat) and advised that a variety of foods from all three groups be consumed in adequate quantity. Research was begun on identifying the nutrient composition of a wide variety of foods. Little was mentioned about minerals or vitamins because so little was known about what they were or what they did (25).

The period during and after World War II was a very active one for the USDA. In addition to responsibilities relating to the nutrition requirements of the military, analytic work on food composition continued unabated. The food composition database, which was begun in 1891 and continues to the present, has been an invaluable resource for nutrition research and practice. Currently, the database contains detailed information on the composition of thousands of foods (27).

After the World War II, the USDA became occupied with the new and flourishing field of research into the functions and requirements for trace minerals and the newly discovered vitamins. The USDA published the first set of recommended intakes for essential nutrients, known as Recommended Daily Allowances (RDAs), which were set by the Food and Nutrition Board of the National Academy of Sciences. These original RDAs were for calories, protein, iron, calcium, vitamin A, vitamin D, ascorbic acid (vitamin C), thiamin, riboflavin, and niacin (25).

THE FOOD GUIDE PYRAMID: A number of years after the DGA was introduced in 1980, the USDA and DHHS became concerned that the DGA recommendations were too complicated for consumers to understand. This was because the growing incidence of cardiovascular diseases, which the DGA was designed specifically to address, had not reversed or even leveled off in the years since introduction of the DGA. It was concluded that consumers must not have been getting the message and therefore were failing to meet the DGA guidelines. For that reason it was decided that some sort of a simple graphic was needed to help explain the DGA guidelines.

It appears that the American public actually had gotten the message and was following the guidelines. Over the period from 1971 to 2000 (28), dietary carbohydrate consumption increased from 43.9 to 50.3 percent; total fat decreased from 36.5 to 32.8 percent; saturated fat dropped from 13.3 to 10.9 percent; and protein fell slightly from 16.7 to 15.3 percent of total daily calories. The growing incidence of cardiovascular diseases is testimony to the fact that it was not the public but the message that was at fault.

The possibility that the DGA itself might be responsible for the disturbing cardiovascular disease statistics apparently was never considered. Thus, in 1988, development of the Food Guide Pyramid was begun in an effort to design an "appealing illustration that would convey in a memorable way the key message" of the governmental dietary recommendations (26). It was unveiled to the public in 1992 (25).

MYPYRAMID: (Note: During the process of verification of Internet references after this manuscript was completed, it was discovered that references to the name *MyPyramid* had been unobtrusively renamed *My Plate*).

Many changes have taken place in *Dietary Goals* since 1977. Unfortunately, all of these changes have been changes in style only. In the 2005 revision, an elegant three-dimensional graphic known as MyPyramid replaced the memorable Food Guide Pyramid. The accompanying recommendations, called *Dietary Guidelines for Americans,* were greatly expanded, increased in detail, and highly individualized. But, there were essentially no changes in substance.

MyPyramid was released to the public on April 19, 2005 (29). The pyramid icon underwent significant alterations but no changes were made in the basic low-fat, high-carbohydrate dietary recommendations of the DGA; the latter despite lack of progress in slowing the incidence of cardiovascular diseases. The three-dimensional MyPyramid that replaced the Food Guide Pyramid was much more complicated in that was composed of a series of pyramids individualized for sex, age group, and activity level. Therefore, the MyPyramid icon was not just one pyramid but actually 48 different pyramids. There are two pyramids for gender, eight for different age levels, and three for activity levels.

The answer to the question of whether MyPyramid, the current icon of the revised DGA, corrects the serious nutritional defects of its predecessor is an unequivocal "No." The only clue, albeit an unacknowledged one, to the fact that the DGA has failed its mandate in preventing obesity and chronic disease is the addition of a third dimension to the pyramid icon. The third dimension is physical activity, a nonfood component that is considered essential for the DGA to be fully effective. This stairway represents Exercise, which was hailed as the key to the anticipated success of the 2005 dietary guidelines (28). Exercise, in many cases, is considered either a useless or a harmful method for treating or preventing obesity or heart disease (30, p.90).

THE 2010 DGA REVISION

In 2011, as work began on revising this book, the 2010 revision of the *Dietary Guidelines for Americans* was already a year overdue. However, many documents containing recommendations that were expected to become incorporated in the *2010 Dietary Guidelines for Americans* have been available on the Internet (31; 32; 33).

A review of the proposed revisions for the 2010 DGA revealed that the recommendations were either the same or, in a few instances, more restrictive than those in the 2005 DGA. For example, the 2010 DGA continues to recommend a total fat intake of no more than 20 to 35 percent of calories; however, it adds the dire admonition that there is no small amount of saturated fatty acid intake that does not incrementally increase CVD risk (33). The document continues with the unequivocal and unsettling statement: "Dietary fatty acids and cholesterol are major determinants of two major causes of morbidity and mortality, namely CVD and T2D [type-2 diabetes]." The document concludes with the admission that there is no way to avoid saturated fatty acids in the diet (33).

Thus, the low-fat dogma that the McGovern committee made official nutrition policy decades ago has finally presented the Dietary Guidelines Committee with an insoluble dilemma: It has decreed that: 1.) Saturated fatty acids and cholesterol are major determinants of heart disease and diabetes; 2.) Any amount in the diet can cause disease, AND; 3.) There is no way that saturated fatty or cholesterol can be eliminated from the diet!

References

1.) Dawkins R. *River Out of Eden; a Darwinian View of Life*. New York, NY: Basic Books, 1995.

2.) Readers interested in further information on paleolithic diets will find the subject extensively covered on the Internet: http://www.paleodiet.com/ Accessed Sept. 2, 2012.

3.) Eaton, SB, et al. *The Paleolithic Prescription*. New York, NY: Harper & Row, 1988.

4.) Hayek FA. *The Fatal Conceit: The Errors of Socialism*. Chicago, IL: The University of Chicago Press, 1988.

5.) Cordain L, et al. The paradoxical nature of hunter-gatherer diets: meat-based, yet non-atherogenic. *European Journal of Clinical Nutrition*. 2002; 56: Suppl. 1 S42-52.

6.) Johnson AW, Earle TK. *The Evolution of Human Societies, 2nd Edition: From Foraging Groups to Agrarian State*. Palo Alto, CA: Stanford University Press, 2000.

7.) Williams G, Crawford MA. Comparison of the fatty acid component in structural lipids from dolphins, zebra and giraffe: possible evolutionary implications. *J. Zool. London*. 1987; 213: 673–684.

8.) Crawford MA, Sinclair AJ. Nutritional influences in the evolution of the mammalian brain. *In*: Elliot K, Knight J (editors). *Lipids, Malnutrition and Developing Brain*. A Ciba Foundation Symposium. Elsevier, Amsterdam. 1972; 267–292.

9.) Crawford MA. The role of dietary fatty acids in biology: their place in the evolution of the human brain. *Nutrition Reviews*. 1992; 50(4): 3-11.

10.) Ruff CB, et al. Body mass and encephalization in Pleistocene Homo. *Nature*. 1997; 387: 173-176.

11.) Eades MR, Eades MD. *Protein Power, Paperback Edition*. New York, NY: Bantam Books, 1999.

12.) Diamond J. *Guns, Germs, and Steel*. New York, NY: Norton & Co, Inc., 1998.

13.) Simopoulos, AP. Evolutionary aspects of the diet, the omega-6/omega-3 ration and genetic variation: nutritional implications for chronic diseases. Biomedical Pharmacotherapy. 2006; 60(9): 502-7.

14.) Price, Weston A. *Nutrition and Physical Degeneration*. Los Angeles, CA: Keats Publishing, 1998.

15.) Budwig J. *Flax Oil as a True Aid against Arthritis, Heart Infarction, Cancer, and Other Diseases*. Vancouver, BC, Canada: Apple Publishing Company Ltd, 1994.

16.) Masterjohn C. On the trail of the elusive X-factor. *Wise Traditions*. 2007; 8(1): 14-32.

17.) U.S. Department of Agriculture. *What do Americans Eat*? Agriculture Fact Book, 1998.

18.) U.S. Department of Agriculture. *What do Americans Eat*? Agriculture Fact Book, Profiling Food Consumption in America, 2001-2002. For caloric use of carbohydrates, proteins, and fats.

19.) http://www.cnpp.usda.gov/ Accessed Sept. 2, 2012.

20.) Cordain L, et al. Origins and evolution of the Western diet: health implications for the 21st Century. *American Journal of Clinical Nutrition*. 2005; 81: 341-354.

21.) Cordain L, et al. Plant-animal subsistence ratios and macronutrient energy estimations in worldwide hunter-gatherer diets. *American Journal of Clinical Nutrition*. 2000; 71: 682-692.

22.) Sears B. *Enter the Zone*. New York, NY; Regan Books/Harper Collins: 1995.

23.) Simopoulos AP. Evolutionary aspects of diet, essential fatty acids and cardiovascular disease. *European Heart Journal*. 2001; 3 (Supplement D): D8-D21.

24.) Taubes Gary. *Good Calories, Bad Calories*. New York, NY: Alfred Knopf, 2007.

25.) http://en.wikipedia.org/wiki/History_of_USDA_nutrition_guides/ Accessed Sept. 2, 2012.

26.) http://health.gov/dietaryguidelines/ Accessed Sept. 3, 2012.

27.) http://fnic.nal.usda.gov/food-composition/usda-nutrient-data-laboratory/ Accessed Sept 3, 2012.

28.) Trends in intake of energy and macronutrients – United States, 1971-2000. *Morbidity and Mortality*

Weekly Report. February 06, 2004; 53(04):80-82.

29.) http://www.mypyramid.gov/ Accessed Sept 3, 2012.

30.) Schwarzbein D, DeVille N. *The Schwarzbein Principle.* Deerfield Beach, FL; Health Communications, Inc: 1999.

31.) Report of the Dietary Guidelines Advisory Committee on the Dietary Guidelines for Americans, 2010. http://www.cnpp.usda.gov/dgas2010-dgacreport.htm/ Accessed Sept. 3, 2012.

32.) http://www.cnpp.usda.gov/publications/dietaryguidelines/2010/dgac/report/d-5-carbohydrates.pdf / Accessed Sept. 3, 2012.

33.) http://www.cnpp.usda.gov/Publications/DietaryGuidelines/2010/DGAC/Report/D-3 FattyAcidsCholesterol.pdf/ Accessed Sept 3, 2012.

Chapter Two

The Chronic Disease Epidemics

...plagues and pestilences are not acts of God or natural hazards; they are of mankind's own making. Disease is a social development no less than the medicine that combats it. **Roy Porter (1, p. 15).**

At the present time, the United States is in the midst of major epidemics of heart disease, stroke, cancer, adult-onset diabetes, and obesity that threaten to bankrupt our health care system. The cost to U.S. taxpayers for health care related to obesity alone is estimated to have been approximately 75 billion dollars in 2003 (2). This health crisis is of such a magnitude that it has become a matter of concern not only for physicians and other health scientists but also for officials in the highest levels of government (3).

Heart disease, stroke, cancer, adult-onset diabetes, and obesity are not new diseases but old diseases that over the last century have grown to epidemic proportions. The incidence of these diseases began to increase in about 1900. Today, they are major causes of disability and premature death. Importantly, Alzheimer's disease has followed this example. It was known, but it was of very low incidence up until about a half-century ago. Now it is a burgeoning health problem.

The expression "epidemic" was traditionally used to describe widely diffused and rapidly spreading diseases of infectious origin. Today, chronic diseases, which were formally thought to be only peculiarities of old age, are increasing rapidly in incidence and attacking ever-younger age groups. The fact that the attack rates of these diseases meet all of the criteria for an epidemic except that of "infectious origin" requires that the definition of "epidemic" become more inclusive.

Heart disease, stroke, cancer, type-2 diabetes, obesity, and now Alzheimer's disease, are much more common today than they were a century ago. The trend lines for new cases of these chronic, debilitating diseases have moved generally upwards from the early 1900s to the present time. Porter, a medical historian, mentions that coronary heart disease (CHD) was relatively rare before 1892 but 20 years later was responsible for slightly more than 10 percent of all deaths in advanced nations (1, p. 580). The mortality rate for CHD was responsible for 25 percent of all deaths in the year 2010 (4). By the year 2030, it is estimated that 40 percent of US adults will have some form of CVD (5). The direct medical costs for all CVD are expected to rise from a current 273 billion dollars annually to 470 billion in 2020 and 818 billion in 2030 (5).

Taken together, heart disease, stroke, cancer, and adult-onset diabetes currently account for 56 percent of all the deaths in the United States (4). These diseases not only showed increases in the older age groups but they were also occurring in younger adults and, after about 1980, in children.

The Impact of Life Span

An often-stated justification for America's current high death rates caused by chronic inflammatory diseases is as follows: Now that the infectious diseases that were major causes of death in past years have all but disappeared, it is only logical for people to die from other causes. The fallacy in this point of view is that it fails to consider a critical medical question, namely should a decline in the occurrence one group of diseases require, or even justify, the increasing occurrence of a different group of diseases? If people living a hundred years ago did not suffer high disease and fatality rates due to infectious diseases, should they now, of necessity, die of cardiovascular diseases or cancer? And conversely, if people living today had the same diets as their grandparents, would they be suffering the current epidemics of heart disease, stroke, cancer, type-2 diabetes, and obesity? These are questions worthy of very serious reflection.

Cardiovascular Disease

Cardiovascular disease (CVD) includes the diseases that affect the heart and blood vessels of the body, namely high blood pressure, coronary heart disease, stroke, and congestive heart failure. Currently, an estimated 80 million Americans, one in three, have one or more types of CVD, and CVD accounted for about 35 percent of all deaths in 2005. Except for the impact of the flu epidemic in 1918, CVD has been the leading cause of death since the year 1900, when there were about 50,000 deaths due to this cause. Total CVD deaths increased to approximately one million per year in 1970, and then gradually declined to 870,000 deaths in 2005 (6).

Despite this drop in mortality, incidence rates (new cases) of cardiovascular disease have continued to increase. Statistical data show that the decline in deaths after 1970 is largely the result of fewer deaths due to atherosclerotic heart disease. These deaths are being prevented by cardiovascular surgery, more use of prescription drugs, smoking cessation, and increased vitamin supplementation, particularly with vitamins B_6, B_{12}, and folic acid, (6,). Surgery has been particularly important. Over the past decade, inpatient cardiovascular surgery and procedures increased 30 percent from 5,444,000 in 1996 to 7,191,000 annually in 2006. These procedures included cardiac catheterizations, percutaneous coronary interventions, coronary artery bypass surgeries, and heart transplants (6).

The underlying medical causes of most cases of heart disease and stroke are arteriosclerosis and atherosclerosis. Arteriosclerosis is a condition in arterial blood vessels marked by loss of elasticity and hardening that is observed as toughened areas that often contain calcium deposits called plaque. Atherosclerosis is an advanced form of arteriosclerosis characterized by deposits of cholesterol, fats, and blood clots within the plaques of the artery walls (6). The generally recognized symptoms of atherosclerosis are high blood pressure (hypertension) and elevated blood cholesterol levels (hypercholesterolemia).

Atherosclerotic deposits make the inner diameter of arteries smaller. This narrowed diameter increases the resistance to blood flow and decreases the volume of blood that can flow through the affected arteries. When this happens in the major arteries that supply blood to the heart, it is called coronary atherosclerosis, coronary heart disease, or coronary artery disease. Heart attacks occur when blood flow to the heart is severely restricted or stopped.

HEART DISEASE

Diseases of the heart are considered the leading cause of death in United States, totaling more than 743,000 in 2005. This category includes two different forms of heart disease, specifically atherosclerotic heart problems, which are primarily myocardial infarctions, and heart failure, also known as congestive heart failure. Myocardial infarctions and related atherosclerotic heart problems were responsible for 451,000 deaths in 2005, and, as mentioned earlier, have been trending downward for about a decade mainly due to increasing use of sophisticated medical procedures.

STROKE

Like heart disease, most cases of stroke are related to atherosclerosis. Three forms of stroke may occur. In the most common form, a loose blood clot plugs an artery and cuts off the blood supply to a part of the brain. In the second form, clogged arteries caused by a buildup of fatty deposits close and shut off the blood supply to a part of the brain. In the third form, high blood pressure causes a blood vessel in the brain to burst. Stroke is the third leading cause of death in the United States. More than 158,000 stroke deaths were reported in 2004, and about 5.8 million adults over age 20 were living with the effects of stroke (6).

CONGESTIVE HEART FAILURE

Fatalities from congestive heart failure have increased steadily from 50,000 in the 1960's to 292,000 in 2005 (5). Total deaths from this cause are expected to continue growing. Hospital admissions and hospital discharges for nonfatal cases of congestive heart failure rose from 877, 000 in 1996 to 1,106, 000 in 2006 (5). According to the American Heart Association (AHA), the specific cause of this disease is not known. Hypertension is reported as the most common risk factor for congestive heart failure, and among women with coronary heart disease, diabetes is the strongest risk factor for this disease (6).

Reliable scientific studies are not in agreement with the position of the AHA. These studies show that patients with congestive heart failure have measurable deficiencies of coenzyme Q_{10} in both the blood and heart muscle and that Q_{10} is necessary to sustain the viability of the heart muscle. It is also known that Q_{10} is a natural nutrient produced by the body; that human biosynthesis of Q_{10} declines with age; that cholesterol-lowering drugs, commonly referred to as statins, block the biosyntheses of Q_{10}; and that heart muscle weakness and heart failure develops after years of treatment with statin drugs. Daily supplementation with Q_{10}, which is now widely available as a nutritional supplement, will both prevent and reverse the disease (7; 8; 9; 10).

Deaths from congestive heart failure have steadily increased from approximately 50,000 in 1960, when statins were introduced, to nearly 300,000 in 2005. During this same period, sales of statin drugs increased from zero to the best-selling drug in America. The enormous utilization of this drug is illustrated by the fact that prescriptions for its purchase averaged 13.1 million per month in the period June through December 2006 (11).

Utilizing its leadership position, the National Heart, Lung, and Blood Institute (NHLBI) may have inadvertently contributed to this new epidemic by encouraging the use of cholesterol-lowering drugs. In 1985, the NHLBI launched its National Cholesterol Education Program designed to reduce blood cholesterol levels on a nationwide scale based on the premise that high cholesterol levels were a cause of heart disease.

For approximately 30 years, the NHLBI has carried on an aggressive and authoritative educational activity aimed at persuading physicians and the general public to believe that high blood cholesterol levels are risky, that cholesterol levels should be checked routinely, and that the heart healthy diet and cholesterol-lowering drugs (statins) should be used to reduce blood cholesterol.

A 2009 report from the NHLBI, announced that significant strides have been made toward their nationwide goal. Average total cholesterol levels in the U.S. adult population have dropped from 213 in 1978 to 203 mg/deciliter currently (12). However, the statistics on diseases of the heart, cited above, indicate that lowering cholesterol levels on a nationwide scale has been of no benefit.

Overweight and Obesity

In the last half-century, overweight and obesity have become huge public health problems. About 61 percent of all adults in the United States, about 130 million individuals, are overweight or obese. Over the period of 1960 to 2004, overweight increased from 45 to 66 percent among adults age 20 to 74. During this same time period, the prevalence of obesity grew from 13.3 to 32.1 percent, with most of this rise occurring since 1980. Less than one-third of American adults are at a healthy weight (13).

Along with the statistics for adults, the numbers of overweight and obese children and adolescents are also growing. A 1998 report from the University of Colorado Health Sciences Center, said that more than 25 percent of American children were overweight or obese. This figure was almost double that from 16 years earlier (14) and has continued to rise.

Between 1988-94 and 2003-2004, childhood obesity, increased from 7.2 to 13.9 percent among 2-5 year olds, increased from 11 to 19 percent among 6-11 year olds, and increased from 11 to 17% among adolescents aged 12-19 (15).

This number has not changed significantly over the past decade. Research is showing that 60 percent of overweight five- to ten-year-olds have at least one risk factor for heart disease, including hyperlipidemia (fatty substances in the blood), elevated blood pressure, or high insulin levels (16). Worldwide, among the developed nations, obesity among children is also very high and growing (17).

The statistics for obesity and its forerunner overweight are included here because these two conditions are powerful risk factors for many of the modern nutritional diseases, specifically hypertension, lipid disorders (high blood cholesterol and triglycerides), adult onset diabetes, coronary heart disease, stroke, gallbladder disease, osteoarthritis, sleep apnea and other respiratory problems, certain cancers (18), and Alzheimer's disease and cognitive decline (19). About 70% of obese adolescents grow up to become obese adults and face a high risk of onset of these diseases while still relatively young (20; 21). Obesity in adolescence has been shown to be accompanied by earlier medical problems, earlier disabilities, and earlier deaths.

It is interesting to note that, as recommended by official nutrition policy, there is evidence that fat intake among children in the United States has been dropping over the last three decades. During this same period, USDA surveys have found an increase of 118% in the consumption of carbonated drinks and a 23% decline in beverage milk (20).

THE BODY MASS INDEX (BMI)

The BMI, the official measure of overweight and obesity, will be covered more fully in Chapter Twelve. The BMI is an excellent tool in the planning and implementation of a healthful diet and lifestyle. It is sufficient to say here that, for adults 19 years and older, overweight is defined as a BMI of 25 through 29, obesity is defined as a BMI of 30 or greater, and extremely obese is a BMI of 40 or more.

It is important to note here that the definitions of childhood overweight and obesity have been changed and are now different from adult values (22). The BMI commonly used for children up to 18 years is modified as follows: Obesity is a BMI at or above the 95th percentile of the BMI for the age group, and overweight is a BMI between the 85th and 95th percentile for the age group. Recently, the definition of childhood obesity has replaced "obesity" with "overweight" and "overweight" with "at risk for overweight."

Diabetes

There are two forms of diabetes, type-1 and type-2. Type-1 diabetes is not common; only about 15,000 people per year are diagnosed with this form of the disease (6). Type-1 diabetes tends to occur in childhood and is the result of a defective pancreas that is unable to produce insulin. For this reason, victims of type-1 diabetes cannot metabolize glucose and suffer from high glucose blood levels that, in decades past, were often fatal. Today, insulin is available by prescription, and its daily use allows type-1 diabetic patients to live near-normal lives. For this reason, type-1 diabetes is also referred to as insulin-dependent diabetes.

Type-2 diabetes, which is also known as adult-onset diabetes or non-insulin-dependent diabetes, is a different disease. Type-2 diabetes generally occurs in people who are over age 45 and overweight; however, it has begun to present itself in younger age groups. The symptoms of type-2 diabetes are similar to those of type-1 diabetes, namely high levels of glucose in the blood and urine. However, the pancreas in early type-2 diabetes, unlike type-1, is not defective and produces insulin normally. Nevertheless, as the disease progresses, the pancreas eventually weakens and may fail to produce insulin. Type-2 diabetics are often obese, whereas type-1 are usually normal or below normal.

Type-2 diabetes is large and growing health problem in the United States. In 1999, it was the seventh ranking cause of death and was responsible for about 70,000 deaths annually (4). Seven years later in 2006, it was the sixth leading cause of death with 75,119 fatalities (23). Importantly, type-2 diabetes increases the risk of heart attack and stroke two to four times (6), and is the leading cause of new cases of blindness, fatal kidney disease, and lower extremity amputations (24). More recently, type-2 diabetes has been linked to increased risk of Alzheimer's disease and decline in cognitive function (19).

In 2006, the prevalence of physician-diagnosed type-2 diabetes (among adults 20 years or older) was 17 million or about 7.7 percent of the adult population. During this same year in 2006, the prevalence of undiagnosed diabetes was 6.4 million, or about 2.9 percent of the adult population; and the prevalence of pre-diabetes was approximately 57 million or 25.9 percent of the adult population. Additionally, the prevalence of type-2 diabetes in people under the age of 20 in 2006 was approximately 200,000 and increasing (5).

Altogether, these numbers indicate that 75 million people, or 36 percent of the American population, were living with some stage of type-2 diabetes in 2006. A study published in 2009 (25), concluded that the diabetic population will at least double in the next 25 years and that the majority of cases will be associated with obesity. Without major changes in public or private strategies, this large diabetic population, with its associated medical costs, will add a significant strain to America's already overburdened health care system.

Cancer

Cancer is the second leading cause of death in the United States with 559,888 deaths reported in 2006 (26). About 1.3 million new cases of cancer and 562,000 fatalities are expected in 2009 (27). These figures do not include more than one million cases annually of basal and squamous cell skin cancers (28). Lung cancer death rates have peaked and are now declining due to reduced cigarette use and improved treatments.

The top five cancer sites in America have not changed in recent years. They are prostate cancer, female breast cancer, lung cancer, colorectal (colon) cancer, and uterine cancer (29). Of this group, colorectal cancer in younger age groups is a growing problem. Although incidence rates of colon cancer, when averaged over all age groups, has been declining due to early detection and timely treatment made possible by colonoscopies, incidence rates in individuals in the 20-49 age group have been increasing by about 1.5% per year since 1995. Causes of these cancers appear to be the increasing rates of obesity and type-2 diabetes, both of which are known risk factors for colorectal cancer (30).

THE IMPACT OF SMOKING

Before leaving the subjects of cancer and cardiovascular diseases, it is important to say a few words about the impact of smoking on the statistical summaries of the numbers and causes of death that are routinely published in the United States. Population studies have clearly shown that smoking is associated with poor health in general and a higher death rate from all causes (31, p. 214). Smoking is also known to cause a number of specific medical conditions. These include: hoarseness, smoker's cough, chronic bronchitis, and emphysema; accelerated atherosclerosis which manifests itself primarily as high blood pressure and heart disease; and cancers, principally of the lung, but also of the mouth, tongue, throat, and possibly kidney (32).

In terms of long-term health and survival, there are two distinct populations in the United States, smokers and non-smokers. One group is healthier and lives longer than the other. However, the national statistical summaries that show death rates according to causes, such as heart disease and cancer, do not distinguish between smokers and non-smokers. The national statistics are averages for the entire population, which includes both smokers and non-smokers.

An average smoker dies about 8 years sooner than does a non-smoker. The major cause of this decreased life expectancy is accelerated heart disease. A second important cause of decreased life expectancy is lung cancer, 90 percent of which is the result of cigarette smoking. The risks of all of the diseases associated with smoking increase with the number of cigarettes smoked per day. As an example, one-pack-per-day smokers are twice as likely to get lung cancer as are non-smokers, and the risk to smokers who use two packs per day is three times that of non-smokers (31, p. 214). The national smoking-cessation program has been effective. Since 1965, the number of smokers has dropped by about half, from 42 percent to 24 percent of the population over 18 years of age (33).

Despite the aggressive national smoking-cessation campaign that has and is preventing significant numbers of cases of heart disease and lung cancer, heart disease remains the number one cause of death in America. Cancers from all causes, although having leveled off primarily as a result of the reduction in lung cancer, remain the number two cause of death in this country. The lesson to remember from these statistics is that smoking, while important, is not the only cause of heart disease and cancer. In short, important causes other than smoking underlie America's epidemics of both heart disease and cancer.

Mental Disorders

A number of disorders of mental processes that were unheard of or uncommon prior to World War II are now becoming serious causes of concern for the medical community. These diseases range across all age groups from behavioral disorders in childhood to disabling dementias in older adults. Some are diagnosable by specific medical tests, but others can be identified only by psychiatric tests based on behavioral and cognitive abilities. Many of these disorders, especially those that afflict children, also cause great distress to family members as well as to the patients themselves. Mental disorders, from mere mood swings to severe mental disabilities, can occur at any age. It is important for family members to bring any change in mood or attitude that seems extreme or persists for more than a few days to the attention of the health care provider.

In the year 2004, about 58 million individuals or 26 percent of Americans, age 18 and older, suffered from a diagnosable mental disorder. The impact of mental illness on health and productivity is very large and accounts for about 15 percent of the total costs of all diseases in the country (34). Current data shows that the attack rates (new cases) of some mental disorders, such as Alzheimer's disease, attention deficit-hyperactivity disorder, autism, and violent-aggressive behavior have been growing for a number of years.

ATTENTION DEFICIT-HYPERACTIVITY DISORDER

Over the past three decades in the United States, behavioral and learning disorders have emerged as major chronic conditions affecting the development of school-aged children and adolescents (35). The most commonly diagnosed among these disorders is Attention Deficit-Hyperactivity Disorder (ADHD). In 2006, an estimated 4.5 million school children had this affliction and about 2.5 million were receiving prescription medications to control its symptoms. Boys are more likely to acquire the disease than girls; about 9.5 percent of boys and 5.9 percent of girls have been diagnosed with ADHD (36).

ADHD children present difficult behavioral problems and perform poorly in school because of their inability to focus on school tasks or to sit still during the school day. Symptoms include inattention, inability to concentrate, failure to listen, hyperactivity, impulsiveness, disruptive behavior, sleep problems, and poor learning ability. ADHD often persists into adulthood. Worst case outcomes are school failure, delinquency, inability to hold a job, and encounters with the law. There is no known cure for ADHD, but its symptoms are to some extent controlled by medication and psychotherapy (37).

AUTISM SPECTRUM DISORDER

Autism spectrum disorder (ASD), commonly called autism, occurs in children beginning at about age two. These disorders are characterized by varying degrees of lack of ability in communication, social interactions, and restricted, repetitive and stereotyped patterns of behavior. ASD symptoms are first noticed as changes in a baby's behavior, such as sudden silence, becoming withdrawn, indifferent to attention by parents. As adolescents, these children are generally unmotivated and do not do well in school. Some adults are able to hold a job, but social problems can make this difficult. Others with more severe ASD may not be able work at all. Medications are used to treat behavioral issues, such as aggression, self-injury, and tantrums (38).

A government survey in 2007, found that attack rates of ASD have been growing since at least the 1980's. This report estimated that somewhere between one in 150 to one in 500 children has ASD and that the risk of ASD is three to four times higher in males than in females (38). Another study reported in 2009 that ASD rates had increased by 57% from 2002 to 2006, and that the prevalence of ASD in eight-year olds had increased to an average of one in 110 children. This amounts to one case of ASD in 70 boys and one case in 315 girls (39).

DEPRESSION

Studies suggest that the trend in the overall rate of depression is growing. The age at which depression first occurs is dropping, with incidences among late teenagers and early adults increasing (40). Most people experience feelings of depression at some time in their lives, such as those associated with loss of a loved one or with failure in some important endeavor. However, such episodes are usually not severe enough to fit the criteria for clinical depression, which is a biological disorder of the brain (41, p. 105).

Approximately 20 million American adults or about 9 percent of the U.S. population age 18 and older have some form of clinical depression. These include major depressive disorder and mild depressive disorder (42). Major depressive disorder affects approximately 14.8 million American adults and is the leading cause of disability in the U.S. for ages 15-44. Mild depressive disorder affects approximately 3.3 million adults or 1.5 percent of the U.S. population age 18 and older. The median age of onset for both forms of these depressive disorders is about 30 years of age (42). Alcohol and substance abuse or dependence may occur at the same time as depression. The coexistence of depression and substance abuse is common in the U.S. population. What fraction of these depressive disorders is related to diet is not known (43).

POSTPARTUM DEPRESSION: In recent years, shocking headlines have brought postpartum depression (PPD) to public attention. Approximately 12 percent of new mothers report being moderately depressed and 6 percent report being very depressed (44). It is difficult to comprehend that a depression could be so severe as to drive a woman to kill her own child. Although such episodes are rare, they are rendered even more tragic when one learns that PPD is strongly linked to a maternal nutritional deficiency of an essential omega-3 fatty acid (41).

The prevalence of PPD varies geographically, ranging from 11.7 percent in Maine to 20.4 percent in New Mexico, with younger, less educated, and poorer women being more likely to report PPD (45). In addition to disturbing the emotional well being of mothers, even mild postpartum depression can damage marital relationships, interfere with mother-infant bonding, and affect infant behavior.

LATE-ONSET DEPRESSION: Late-onset depression represents a large fraction of the cases of depression among older adults. It is defined as depression that occurs for the first time after age 60 (46). Such depression often coexists with chronic diseases such as heart disease, stroke, cancer, diabetes, Parkinson's disease, thyroid problems, and multiple sclerosis (43). Because most of these chronic diseases are caused by the modern American diet, it is reasonable to believe that dietary change would not only prevent these chronic diseases, but also late-onset depression.

SENILE DEPRESSION: According to Fries (47, p. 112), depression is the greatest enemy of the senior mind. He points out that depression is not an essential part of aging and should always be considered a problem of sufficient importance to be brought the attention of a health care provider because it can be serious or life-threatening.

It is estimated that 8 to 20 percent of older adults suffer some degree of depression. Symptoms include depressed mood, feelings of dejection, loss of concentration, feelings of sadness, hopelessness, or worthlessness, loss of interest, sleep disturbances, and recurrent thoughts of death or suicide. A four-year study of 1,286 community-dwelling persons aged 71 years and older showed that physical performance declined approximately twice as fast in depressed individuals as it did in normal individuals (48).

ANTIDEPRESSANT DRUG USE: A shocking statistic, revealed recently at a Society for Women's Health Research in Washington DC, requires special mention. In 2010, an analysis of the pharmacy records of more than two million patients found that 26 percent of the women took drugs to treat depression, anxiety, or attention deficit disorder (49). This was an increase from 22 percent in 2001. These statistics are notably higher than those for men; 15 percent of men took these medications in 2010, up from 12 percent.

The reason why more than a quarter of the women who take medications of any kind take antidepressants, which must be a mirror the entire adult female population, is not known. However, the possibility that women may be more likely than men to seek mental health care or that they might be more vulnerable than men to depression or anxiety are suggested. The relationship between essential fatty acid intake and depression (41) is not mentioned as a possible factor in causation of these tragic statistics.

BIPOLAR DISORDER

Bipolar disorder, formerly referred to as manic-depressive illness, is characterized by mood swings between periods of high, impulsive, and sometimes dangerous euphoria to episodes of deep, even suicidal, depression. The median age of onset for bipolar disorder is 25 years and it affects approximately 5.7 million American adults, or about 2.6 percent of the U.S. population age 18 and older (42). A review of the diagnostic criteria for bipolar disorder (41, p. 129ff) reveals the complexity of the illness. It is a serious and disabling brain disease that requires psychiatric treatment.

SCHIZOPHRENIA

Schizophrenia affects men and women with equal frequency. Like bipolar disorder, schizophrenia has a long history in psychiatric literature. Its original name was "dementia praecox," meaning "early mind," probably because symptoms usually appear during or shortly after adolescence. Schizophrenia, which literally means a schism between thought (ability to correctly judge the real world) and perception (illusions and hallucination), is not a rare disease. It is the most common of the serious mental illnesses, accounting for approximately 24 percent of all admissions to mental hospitals in the United States (50; 51).

SENILE DEMENTIAS

Mental disorders associated with aging are commonly grouped under the headings of senile mental disorders or senile dementias. Among these disorders only two, Alzheimer's disease and dementias caused by strokes, have been traced to actual physical changes in the brain that can be identified by pathologists. All of the other mental disorders associated with aging, including depression, anxiety disorders, memory loss, and confusion, have not been related thus far to physical changes or lesions in the brain. As a result of the lack of physical changes in the brain, the majority of these latter mental disorders can be diagnosed only on the basis of their outward symptoms, such as changes in cognition, emotional status, and/or behavior.

The victims of all the senile mental disorders show a range of nervous, psychiatric, behavioral, and personality problems that are difficult to diagnose accurately. Symptoms, particularly at first, are vague and overlap one another. In their early stages, all of these disorders tend not to be treated or taken seriously because patients, and their doctors, consider them a normal part of growing old (47). As these disorders become more severe, changes in behavior and mental performance become sufficiently pronounced so that more specific diagnoses are possible to make.

ALZHEIMER'S DISEASE: The cause of Alzheimer's disease is not known, but the brain damage associated with this form of senile dementia is visible microscopically as a tangled mass of abnormal brain tissue. National statistics show that Alzheimer's disease is a growing problem in the United States. Prior to 1998, this disease was not included on the list of ten leading causes of death for any age group (52, Table 33). In 1998, Alzheimer's disease appeared as the ninth leading cause of death among Americans 65 years and older when more than 22,000 deaths from this cause were reported. Six years later, in 2004, it was listed as the nation's seventh leading cause of death (53). It is likely that statistics for Alzheimer's deaths are underestimated because Alzheimer's patients often suffer coexisting diseases that could be listed as cause of death (54).

The incidence of Alzheimer's disease is projected to skyrocket in the next 40 years, tripling from the current 4.5 million cases to more than 13 million (55). This projection has caused great consternation on the part of health policy experts and legislators who recognize that such an increase could further cripple the seriously overburdened health care system. Apparently the only solution being considered is to urge Congress to greatly increase government funding of research for Alzheimer-modifying drugs with no thought for funding of research into causes and prevention of the disease.

DEMENTIAS CAUSED BY STROKES: Stroke is the result of brain damage that occurs when blood vessels in the brain either plug or break. Both events cause brain damage. Major strokes result in sufficient brain damage to cause obvious muscle paralysis and deterioration in mental performance. However, very small strokes, often not recognized by the victims or their doctors, are probably responsible for a large proportion of the cases of senile mental deterioration (frequently termed senility) occurring today.

The total number of individuals in America with brain damage and behavioral changes caused by these small strokes is not known. There are several reasons for this. The victim either does not notice the small amount of mental and physical degradation that accompanies these small strokes or may assume that the effects of the stroke, even though noticeable, are a normal part of growing old. The result has been that such cases are not reported, not counted, and are not part of the national statistics. Despite the fact that most small strokes are not reported, the number of cases of mental deterioration caused by small and unrecognized strokes is thought to be very large.

A recent study of 3,660 people over 65 years of age showed that 28 percent of those with no known history of stroke had brain damage consistent with small strokes, based on cranial magnetic resonance imaging (MRI) (55). MRI technology makes it possible for doctors to see and identify small areas of brain damage that were formerly invisible. What is clear from this study is that a significant fraction of people over 65 years old who were under the impression that they had never had a stroke actually did have very small, unrecognized strokes. Testing of this study group showed that the stroke-caused brain damage seen by MRI was associated with dysfunction, especially of cognition (memory, judgment, and reasoning) and with some dysfunction of the lower extremities (56). When extrapolated to the whole population of older adults, this study suggests that a very large number of people over 65, perhaps as much as 20 to 30 percent, have some brain damage and mental deterioration as the result of one or more unrecognized strokes.

A report on mental health by the Surgeon General of the United States supports this contention (46). It indicates that much of the late-onset depression (depression that occurs for the first time after age 60) may be the result of vascular damage that does not cause a discernible stroke. This report cites data suggesting that, even in the absence of clear stroke, disorders that cause vascular damage, such as hypertension, heart disease, and type-2 diabetes, may induce brain damage leading to depression.

ANXIETY DISORDERS

Anxiety disorders include panic disorder, obsessive-compulsive disorder, post-traumatic stress disorder, generalized anxiety disorder, and social phobia. Approximately 40 million Americans ages 18 and older, have an anxiety disorder. Anxiety disorders frequently co-occur with depressive disorders or substance abuse and approximately three-quarters of the victims will have their first episode by age 21 (42).

Anxiety disorders affect about 10 percent of older adults. The usual symptoms of anxiety are: worry and nervous tension; persistent fear of some activity or object that leads to a compelling desire to avoid that activity or object; persistent intrusion of unwanted thoughts accompanied by ritualistic actions; and sudden overwhelming fear or panic that produces hysterical behavior. The causes of these symptoms are not understood; however, treatment with prescription drugs is sometimes effective. The problem with these drugs is that they cause side effects such as memory loss, confusion, and depression, all of which add to the mental symptoms already being experienced by the patient (46).

HOSTILITY, VIOLENCE, AND SELF-HARM

The news media has made us well aware with almost daily stories of mass shooting sprees that many assumedly normal citizens are exceeding their limits of self-control. Violent and aggressive behavior resulting in criminal acts is on the increase and our jails are so overcrowded that many prisoners must be released before the end of their terms. Violent and aggressive behaviors are significant threats to public health (57). Further, self-harm, which is violence turned inward toward one's own being, is a major cause of morbidity worldwide (58).

It is easy to accept that chronic diseases may have a nutritional link, but the idea that psychiatric disorders and especially criminal acts could also result from dietary abuses is inconceivable. However, data are emerging that indicate criminal and other antisocial behaviors may be due in part to nutritional deficiencies, particularly of omega-3 fatty acids (59). The concept that some individuals may not be completely responsible for their criminal acts is contrary to the fundamental societal ethic that holds people responsible for their acts against society. As heretical as the notion may be that some offenders may not be able to help themselves, there are considerable data confirming that a brain whose biochemistry is disturbed by bad nutrition is a brain that may foster aberrant behavior. The research of Hibbeln and colleagues provides a wealth of information on the relationship between nutrition and pathologies of the brain (60).

SUICIDE: In 2006, 33,300 people died by suicide in the U.S. More than 90 percent of people who kill themselves have a diagnosable mental disorder, most commonly a depressive disorder or a substance abuse disorder. Four times as many men as women die by suicide and the highest rates in the U.S. are in white men over age 85 (42).

References

1.)   Porter R. The Greatest Benefit to Mankind. New York, NY: W. W. Norton & Company, Inc., 1997.

2.)   Taxpayers Foot More Than Half of Obesity-Related Medical Bills. The Wall Street Journal. Thursday, January 22, 2004; D2.

3.)   To Save Lives, OMB Urges Revising Dietary Guidelines. Press Release 2003-13. Executive Office of the President, Office of Management and Budget, Washington, DC, 20503. May 28, 2003.

4.)   http://www.cdc.gov/nchs/fastats/deaths.htm/ Accessed Sept. 4, 2012.

5.)   Heidenreich PA, et al. Forecasting the future of cardiovascular disease in the United States: A policy statement from the American Heart Association. *Circulation.* 2011; 123: 00-00. http://circ.ahajournals.org/ Accessed Sept. 4, 2012.

6.)   *American Heart Association, Heart Disease and Stroke Statistics At-A-Glance, 2009 Update.* American Heart Association; 2009. http://www.americanheart.org/statistics/ Accessed Sept. 4, 2012.

7.)   Silver MA, et al. Effect of atorvastatin on left ventricular diastolic function and ability of coenzyme Q_{10} to reverse that dysfunction. *American Journal of Cardiology.* 2004; 94(10):1306-10.

8.)   Langsjoen PH. Alleviating congestive heart failure with coenzyme Q_{10}. *Life Extension Magazine,* February 2008. http://www.lef.org/magazine/mag2008/feb2008_Alleviating-Congestive-Heart-Failure-With-Coenzyme-Q_{10}_01.htm/

9.)   Molyneux SL et al. Coenzyme Q_{10}: an independent predictor of mortality in chronic heart failure. *Journal of the American College of Cardiology.* 2008 Oct 28; 52 (18): 1435-41.

10.)   Beltowski J, et al. Adverse effects of statins. *Current Drug Safety.* 2009; 4(3): 1-19.

11.)   Consumer Reports, Consumers Union. February 2007. The Statin Drugs Prescription and Price Trends (October 2005 to December 2006. http://www.consumerreports.org/health/resources/pdf/best- buy-drugs/Statins-RxTrend-FINAL-Feb2007.pdf/ Accessed Sept. 4, 2012.

12.)   National Heart, Lung, and Blood Institute, National Cholesterol Education Program, Program Description, October, 2009. http://www.nhlbi.nih.gov/about/ncep/ncep_pd.htm/ Accessed Sept. 4, 2012. Weight-control Information Network (WIN), Statistics related to overweight and obesity. National

13.)   Institute of Diabetes and Digestive and Kidney Diseases. May, 2007. http://www.win.niddk.nih.gov/ Accessed Sept. 4, 2012.

14.)   http://www.cnn.com/ (from CNN News report: Americans Fatter than Ever. May 28, 1998).

15.)   *Prevalence of Overweight among Children and Adolescents: United States, 2003-2004.* National Center for Health Statistics, Hyattsville, MD 20782.

16.)   http://www.libraryindex.com/pages/1207/Diet-Nutrition-Weight-Issues-among-Children-Adolescents-HEALTH-RISKS-CONSEQUENCES.html/ Accessed Sept. 4, 2012.

17.)   Flodmark CE, et al. New insights into the field of children and adolescents' obesitya: the European perspective. *International Journal of Obesity.* 2004; 28: 1189.

18.)   National Institutes of Health/National Heart, Lung, and Blood Institute Communications Office. First Federal Obesity Guidelines. Released June 17, 1998.

19.)   Arvanitakis Z, et al. Diabetes Mellitus and risk of Alzheimer Disease and decline in cognitive function. Archives of Neurology. 2004; 61: 661-666.

20.)   Dehgan M, et al. Childhood obesity, prevalence and prevention. *Nutrition Journal.* 2005; 4: 24.

21.)   Belluck P. Child obesity seen as warning of heart disease. *New York Times.* November 12, 2008.

22.)   http://www.cdc.gov/obesity/childhood/basics.html/ Accessed Sept. 25, 2012,

23.)   National Center for Health Statistics. National Vital Statistics Report, Deaths: Final Data for 2006. April 17, 2009; 57(14).

24.)   http://www.cdc.gov/Features/DiabetesFactSheet/

25.)   Huang ES, et al. Projecting the future diabetes population size and related costs for the U.S. Diabetes Care. 2009; 32(12): 2225-2229.

26.) Centers for Disease Control and Prevention. http://www.cdc.gov/nchs/fastats/deaths.htm/ Accessed Sept. 25, 2012.

27.) http://www.cancer.gov/newscenter/newsfromnci/2012/ReportNationRelease2012/ Accessed Sept. 25, 2012.

28.) American Cancer Society. Cancer Facts & Figures 2008. Atlanta: American Cancer Society. 2008. http://www.cancer.org/acs/groups/content/@nho/documents/document/2008cafffinalsecuredpdf.pdf/ Accessed Sept. 25, 2012.

29.) Centers for Disease Control and Prevention. http://www.cdc.gov/Features/datastatistics.html/ Accessed Sept. 25, 2012.

30.) Siegel RL, et al. Increase in colorectal cancer among young men and women in the United States. Cancer Epidemiology Biomarkers Prevention. 2009; 18(6).

31.) Pauling, Linus. How to Live Longer and Feel Better. New York, NY; W. H. Freeman and Co., 1986.

32.) Fries JF, Vickery DM. Take Care of Yourself, 4th Ed. Reading, MA: Addison-Wesley Pub Co, 1989.

33.) Health, United States, 2000. Table 59, Current cigarette smoking by persons 18 years of age and over, according to sex, race, and age: United States, 1980 and 1998. DHHS Pub. No. 00-1232, National Center for Health Statistics.

34.) Kessler RC, et al. The individual-level and societal-level effects of mental disorders on earnings in the United States: Results from the National Comorbidity Survey Replication. *American Journal of Psychiatry,* published online ahead of print May 7, 2008

35.) Pastor PN, Reuben CA. Diagnosed attention deficit hyperactivity disorder and learning disability:

36.) United States, 2004–2006. National Center for Health Statistics. Vital Health Statistics. 2008; 10: 237. Centers for Disease Control and Prevention, Attention Deficit Hyperactivity Disorder (ADHD), Data and Statistics in the United States. http://www.cdc.gov/ncbddd/adhd/data.html/ Accessed Sept. 25, 2012.

37.) National Institute of Mental Health, Department of Health and Human Services, Attention Deficit Hyperactivity Disorder (ADHD), NIH Publication No. 08-3572, Revised 2008. NIH National Institute of Mental Health, NIH Publication.

38.) http://www.nichd.nih.gov/health/topics/asd.cfm

39.) Morbidity and Mortality Weekly Report December 18, 2009. Prevalence of Autism Disorders, Autism and Developmental Disabilities Monitoring Network, United States, 2006.

40.) Klerman GL, Weissman MM. Increasing rates of depression. Journal of the American Medical Association. 1989; 261(15): 2229-2235.

41.) Stoll AL. The Omega-3 Connection. New York, NY: A Fireside Book, Simon & Schuster. 2001.

42.) http://www.nimh.nih.gov/health/publications/the-numbers-count-mental-disorders-in-america/index.shtml/ Accessed Sept. 25, 2012.

43.) National Institute of Mental Health. Women and Depression: Discovering Hope. Science Writing, Press & Dissemination Branch 6001 Executive Boulevard Room 8184, MSC 9663 Bethesda, MD 20892-9663. http://www.nimh.nih.gov/ Accessed Sept. 25, 2012.

44.) http://www.cdc.gov/reproductivehealth/Depression/Publications.htm/ Accessed Sept. 25, 2012.

45.) Prevalence of self-reported postpartum depressive symptoms. Morbidity and Mortality Weekly Report. 2008; 57(14): 361-6.

46.) http://www.surgeongeneral.gov/library/mentalhealth/ (report titled: Mental Health: A Report of the Surgeon General; Older Americans; Chapter 5: Depression in Older Adults). Accessed Sept. 25, 2012.

47.) Fries F. Aging Well. A Guide for Successful Seniors. Reading, MA: Addison-Wesley Publishing Company, Inc., 1989.

48.) Penninx BD, et al. Depressive symptoms and physical decline in community dwelling older persons. Journal of the American Medical Association. 1998; 279(21): 1720-1726.

49.) Foster HD. What Really Causes Schizophrenia? Victoria, BC, Canada: Trafford Publishing, 2003.

50.) Hoffer A. Orthomolecular Treatment for Schizophrenia. Lincolnwood, IL: Keats, NTC/ ContemporaryPublishing Group, 1999.

51.) Leading causes of death according to age, U.S., 1980 and 1998. National Center for Health Statistics, U.S. Dept. Health and Human Services. Health, United States, DHHS Pub. No. 00-1232, July 2000.

52.) Alzheimer's Disease, Newt Notes. Center for Health Transformation. October, 2006. http://www.med.upenn.edu/cndr/documents/AlzheimersStudyGroup.pdf/ Accessed Sept. 25, 2012.

53.) http://www.spacedoc.com/alzheimers_statins.htm/ Accessed Sept. 25, 2012.

54.) Sullivan MG. Now is the time to prepare for the onslaught of Alzheimer's disease. Caring for the Aged. 2007; 8(8): 12. http://www.caringfortheages.com/ Accessed Sept. 25, 2012.

55.) Longstreth WT. Brain abnormalities in the elderly: frequency and predictors in the United States. Journal of Neural Transmission: Supplement. 1998; 53: 9-16.

56.) Hibbeln JR, et al. Omega-3 fatty acid deficiencies in neurodevelopment, aggression, and autonomic-dysregulation: Opportunities for intervention. International Review of Psychiatry. 2006; 18(2): 107

57.) Hallahan B, et al. Omega-3 fatty acid supplementation in patients with recurrent self-harm. British Journal of Psychiatry. 2007; 190: 118-122.

58.) Iribarren C, et al. Dietary intake of n-3, n-6 fatty acids and fish: relationship with hostility in young adults--the CARDIA study. European Journal of Clinical Nutrition. 2004;58(1):24-31. 59.)

59.) http://www.guardian.co.uk/food/Story/0,,1924088.00html/

60.) Hibbeln JR. National Institute on Alcohol Abuse and Alcoholism, 31 Center Drive (31/1B58), Bethesda, MD20892. Email: jhibbeln@niaaa.nih.gov/

Chapter Three

The Association between Diet and Disease

When you see water running uphill, look for a pump. **Anon.**

If one compares the national statistics on food consumption patterns with the attack rates of the modern nutritional diseases, it becomes obvious that there is a relationship between the two. Prior to World War I, the average American diet changed very little and the occurrence of chronic diseases, which were normally associated with the aging process, remained fairly static. But major changes in agricultural and food manufacturing industries that occurred at the turn of the 20th Century, as described in Chapter One, brought a long and gradual change in diet composition. During the same period, the incidence of several chronic diseases began a slow and steady climb.

This increase in incidence was first noted in the death rates for cardiovascular diseases, which had been rising steadily since the early 1900s. By the end of World War II, the ever-increasing number of cases of heart disease became a matter of serious concern to the medical community. This marked the beginning of a period of very active research relating to the causes of heart disease and stroke. About this same time, in 1948, with the support of the federal government, a very large, long-term, and now multigenerational project labeled the Framingham Heart Study was initiated to study the causes, common factors, or characteristics that contribute to heart disease and stroke (1).

The Heart-Healthy Diet

Numerous epidemiological studies conducted throughout the world over the next two decades led to the thesis that animal fat and cholesterol were the major dietary risk factors for cardiovascular diseases. By the late 1950s, despite the weakness of supporting data and considerable evidence to the contrary, the thesis became fashionable with the medical and nutrition communities. They promoted their thesis as a low-fat, high-carbohydrate, heart-healthy diet. In 1977, political wisdom dictated that this heart healthy diet should be national health policy. Ostensibly aimed at reversing growing rates of heart disease, the policy was formulated by the

Senate Select Committee on Nutrition and Human Needs and recommendations for dietary changes were adopted. As described in Chapter One, the dietary recommendations were formalized and presented to the public in the first edition of the *Dietary Guidelines for Americans* (DGA) in 1980.

It is now many decades later. A large fraction of the population has been eating the heart- healthy diet for more than 40 years. By now, it should be having a positive effect; people should be healthier. Disease rates should be dropping. But this is not the case; for example, it has been estimated that cases of Alzheimer's disease alone will skyrocket in the next 40 years tripling from 4.5 million now to more than 13 million (2). These health statistics are serious facts that translate to enormous numbers of individual cases of illness and premature death. The modern nutritional diseases have now grown to epidemic proportions. The trend lines for these diseases are still rising. Except for lung cancer, which has been falling due to the drop in cigarette smoking, the rates of all other cancers have not diminished.

How could it be that a government presumably dedicated to the health and well being of its citizenry foist on it a diet that nutritional biochemistry predicts would foster chronic disabilities? Numerous papers and books have chronicled the sequence of events in the decades between the time when chronic diseases were common only among the aged to the present day when they attack all ages and threaten to bankrupt our country. It is a story rife with contentious arguments about the causes of heart disease set in a professional atmosphere that early on became unreceptive to any scientists who challenged the validity of the low-fat, high-carbohydrate diet.

The most recent and most complete history of these events is detailed by Taubes in a book that should be required reading for all members of the medical and nutrition communities (3). One passage in particular epitomizes the frustration of the scientists who recognized the fallacies in the heart-healthy diet and argued vigorously against its implementation as official government policy. Philip Handler, then-President of the National Academy of Sciences, testified in the early 1980s before the House Agriculture Subcommittee on Domestic Marketing:

> What right has the federal government to propose that the American people conduct a vast nutritional experiment, with themselves as subjects, on the strength of so little evidence that it will do them any good?…The dilemma so posed is not a scientific question; it is a question of ethics, morals, politics. Those who argue either position strongly are expressing their values; they are not making scientific judgments (3, p. 51).

Dr. Handler expressed a deeply felt concern often in the minds of scientists who decry the interjection of political pseudoscientific manipulation into matters of science that impact the lives of people.

The Demonization of Dietary Fat

The demonization of dietary fat was a necessary prelude to the success of the low-fat diet. Shortly after World War II, while traveling in Italy, nutrition pioneer Ancel Keys and his wife Margaret discovered the diet of the region to be very pleasing to the palate. The cuisine was ample in pastas, cheeses, fruits, vegetables, olive oil, and wine. They named this culinary plan the Mediterranean diet. The Keys had long believed that animal fats and cholesterol were unhealthful dietary components and, as such, were probable contributors to the increase in cases of heart disease. Thus, they believed their Mediterranean diet would be a healthful one that would be protective against heart disease. This began their long quest to obtain statistics on deaths from heart disease and fat consumption from countries that had such statistics. They found strong associations between the two in six countries (4).

THE LIPID HYPOTHESIS

The Keys' research developed a strong following and led Keys to formulate the lipid (diet/heart) hypothesis for the etiology of heart disease. Meanwhile, the Framingham study had enrolled a large number of families whose diets, lifestyles, and environments were being studied and their medical and laboratory findings routinely recorded (1). Data from laboratory analyses were beginning to show a positive association between blood cholesterol levels and incidence of heart attacks. These associations gave strong support to Keys' lipid hypothesis with the result that he and his colleagues became more widely publicized and popular. Keys was a major player in convincing those who governed national dietary policy fifty or more years ago to direct a whole nation, using a flawed road map, down an unhealthful dietary path. The role of Ancel Keys was observed and neatly described by Taubes:

> Ancel Keys deserves the lion's share of credit for convincing us that cholesterol levels predict heart disease and that dietary fat is a killer…Keys's abilities as a scientist are arguable—he was more often wrong than right—but his force of will was indomitable (3, p.16).

The nutrition community enthusiastically adopted the lipid hypothesis, and clinical and epidemiological research in the field proliferated. The lipid hypothesis, sometimes called the cholesterol hypothesis, was accepted as fact by the medical community and, in 1956, representatives of the American Heart Association (AHA) presented the hypothesis to the public on national television. The public was informed that the cause of coronary heart disease was butter, lard, beef, and eggs. The diet recommended by AHA was labeled the Prudent Diet (5). It replaced traditional foods with vegetable seed oils, margarine, chicken, bread, and cereals. High-fat, high-cholesterol diets were accepted as the cause of cardiovascular disease and stroke.

DISSENTING VOICES: The condemnation of dietary fat was not without its critics. From the very beginning there were many dissenting voices despite the apparent solidarity displayed by the medical and nutrition communities about the dangers of dietary fat. In 1956, for example, the AHA program that introduced the Prudent Diet included an interview with the eminent cardiologist Dr. Paul Dudley White (5):

> When pressed to support the Prudent Diet, Dr. White replied: 'See here, I began my practice as a cardiologist in 1921 and I never saw an MI patent until 1928. Back in the MI free days before 1920, the fats were butter and lard and I think that we would all benefit from the kind of diet that we had at a time when no one had ever heard the word corn oil.'

Numerous articles critical of the lipid hypothesis appeared in nutrition journals. In 1969, William Kannel, a principle investigator of the Framingham Study, published a paper saying that it was difficult to pinpoint exactly what was responsible for high cholesterol levels found in the Framingham Study. In his paper, Kannel mentioned that there was a large nutritional overload of saturated fat, cholesterol, and refined carbohydrates in the average diet of the general public in the United States. He further pointed out that this overload influenced metabolic energy balances and was probably somehow related to high cholesterol levels (6).

KREHL'S REVIEW: An extensive review article was published in 1977 by Willard A. Krehl that summarized the diet/heart disease research up through the early 1970's. It covered the period in which the new low-fat, high-carbohydrate dietary policy was developed, adopted, and widely advertised as a preventive measure for heart disease and stroke (7). According to this article, a broad range of possible causes for cardiovascular disease had been studied. Krehl noted that the major risk factors for atherosclerotic coronary heart disease and stroke that had been identified before 1976 were high cholesterol levels, high blood pressure, and cigarette smoking. Other possible risk factors mentioned were glucose intolerance (unstable blood glucose levels), electrocardiographic abnormalities, elevated uric acid levels, and lack of exercise. Krehl reported that, at that time, obesity was considered a possible risk factor because of its association with the major risk factors, mainly high blood pressure and high cholesterol levels (7).

The research studies on the impact of diet on cardiovascular disease that were included in Krehl's review confirmed that the information available at the time concerning the impact of diet on cardiovascular disease did not produce a clear picture of cause and effect. Epidemiological studies among human populations showed that atherosclerotic cardiovascular diseases occurred at higher rates in affluent societies and among the higher socioeconomic classes. These studies associated the high disease rates with "luxious food" consumption, excessive caloric intake, sweets, sedentary lifestyles, and stress.

Krehl's review included papers that reported contradictory findings: One paper said sugar played no significant role in the causation of hypertension, heart disease, and atherosclerosis in humans; another paper implicated sugar as the major dietary cause of coronary heart disease. In the latter paper, Yudkin found that men with myocardial infarction or peripheral artery disease consumed twice as much sugar as did controls (8). Despite these contradictions, at the end of his article, Krehl embraced the official policy with the conclusion that a review of the scientific literature strongly supported the concept that diet and particularly saturated fat and/or cholesterol are significant contributors to the mortality of atherosclerotic coronary heart disease.

THE VERITAS SOCIETY: George V. Mann, one of the original directors of the Framingham Study, found that much of the data generated by the study "showed no relation between dietary makeup [fat/cholesterol content] and coronary heart disease." (9, p. 209). In 1962, Dr. Mann began to challenge publicly the diet/heart hypothesis and became a "kind of pariah" in biomedical and nutrition academia (9, p. 212).

As a result of concern about the unquestioned acceptance of the fallacious diet/heart hypothesis, Dr. Mann and a group of fellow scientists formed the Veritas Society "in order to focus our objections and call for a return to scientific and informational honesty." (10, p. 11). In November 1991, the society convened an international group of distinguished physicians and scientists in Washington, DC, to present the latest clinical, epidemiological, and laboratory data that demonstrate the lack of scientific basis for the diet/heart hypothesis. The proceedings of the meeting were published in 1993 (10). Dr. Mann states in the preface to the meeting that the public would be surprised to learn how many scientists disagree with the diet/heart hypothesis. He added:

> For 50 years an increasingly specious, pseudoscientific dogma has been growing in the Western world. This hypothesis originally proposed that coronary heart disease, the main cause of death here, is caused by the kind and amount of fat in our diets. That hypothesis was based upon fragile and selected data. The hypothesis has now been tested in dozens of clinical trials costing hundreds of millions of dollars. ...The evidence consistently says, 'No—this is not a sound hypothesis.' (10).

Scientific Missteps

An in-depth examination of the body of literature on which the government-supported diet/heart hypothesis was founded reveals many serious flaws in experimental design and data evaluation. Without evidence to the contrary, it should be assumed that these errors were due to lack of scientific knowledge or judgment rather than malfeasance on the part of the investigators. The fact that nutritional science was in its infancy fifty years ago may excuse some of the errors apparent in many of the earlier research efforts, but such a defense cannot be used today for the scientific missteps that are still occurring in research into the relationship between diet and disease.

SCIENTIFIC KNOWLEDGE OR JUDGMENT

The experimental shortcomings are varied and include incomplete or misdirected literature search, experimental design obviously calculated to produce desired results, and the prevalence of myths such as dietary-fat-makes-body-fat. The first two failings relate to skill and expertise of investigators in experimental methods and design. Unfortunately, the latter failing reflects a profound lack of knowledge of nutritional biochemistry and physiology. Although errors occurred in all types of studies that form the database for the hypothesis, they occur most commonly in epidemiological studies.

FLAWED EPIDEMIOLOGY

Starting with the research of Ancel Keys, the rationale for his lipid hypothesis came primarily from epidemiological studies. Unfortunately, the epidemiological competence of numerous investigators leaves much to be desired. A common fallacy in many of these studies is that if a statistical association is found between a dietary component and disease, the dietary component is assumed to be the cause or, in more contemporary terminology, a "risk factor" for the disease rather than merely an association. This is not epidemiology or even ethical science despite its current acceptance as such.

Rigorous epidemiology requires that any association found by statistical methods be proven by hard science before cause/effect can be assigned. In the case of diet/disease associations, nutritional biochemistry, well-controlled clinical studies, and/or human feeding studies would provide the hard science. Most of the investigations of the diet/heart connection that claim to be epidemiological studies are, in fact, no more than studies of associations revealed by complex statistical analyses.

EXCLUSION OF VARIABLES: Many of the diet/disease epidemiological studies, both from old studies and contemporary, contain serious defects in design one of which is not including all relevant variables. For example, in numerous studies, only fat consumption of participants was recorded to the exclusion of all other diet components. To their credit, a few of the early day scientists reported that people who consumed high levels of saturated fat also consumed high levels of sugar. They implicated sugar as the major dietary cause of coronary heart disease with convincing data correlating it to sugar consumption, but their data were ignored. However, by that time, the direction of research was firmly controlled by proponents of the lipid hypothesis, which already had been expanded to include dietary cholesterol as a cause.

The most flawed of the studies that supported the lipid hypothesis appear to be those of Ancel Keys. Although Keys' first paper presented data from six countries that had statistics on heart attack deaths and fat consumption, there were actually over twenty that had such statistics available at the time. An interesting question is why did Keys exclude the latter data? The fact is that the countries excluded did not show the same association between fat consumption and deaths from heart attacks. In a thoughtful analysis in *The Cholesterol Myths*, Ravnskov clearly revealed that if Keys had included data from all 22 countries, statistical support for

Keys' hypothesis would have been weak. Based on a thorough review of all relevant scientific literature, Ravnskov demonstrated that the lipid-cholesterol hypothesis is a fallacy (11).

Taubes' description of this fundamental flaw in Keys' research (3, p.18) recalled a personal experience that one of us (FO) had as a student in the School of Public Health, University of California, Berkeley, in 1962. Drs Stallone and Yerushalmy taught the epidemiology classes in the Master's program. During the semester, they presented papers they had found in the literature that were excellent examples of bad epidemiology – examples of how not to do an epidemiological study. Keys' paper introducing the remarkable relationship between dietary fat and coronary heart disease (4), which had been critiqued by Dr. Yerushalmy several years earlier (12), was held up in class as an example of a study containing multiple violations of good epidemiological research: it did not include all available pertinent data; it selected data that supported its thesis; and it claimed a cause-effect relationship for a mere association.

FAULTY PREMISES: Another design flaw is the use of a faulty premise as a study objective. A recent example is the Women's Health Initiative (WHI) Controlled Dietary Modification Trial (13). It was designed, in accordance with the prevailing opinions of international experts, to study the benefits of a low-fat diet on disease prevention. Its failure to do so relegates it to the host of large, long-term prospective studies, conducted through the decades since World War II, that have failed to provide a statistical association between dietary fat and chronic disease, positively or negatively, despite a tremendous expenditure of time and money.

There cannot be a cause/effect relationship in the absence of a statistical association; repeated attempts to find one are an immoral waste of resources when the premise that there is one is wrong. The Harvard School of Public Health (HSPH) Department of Nutrition wrote in response to the findings of the WHI study:

> The dietary fat reduction arm of the WHI was controversial from the beginning. Members of the HSPH Department of Nutrition argued that the hypothesis that a reduction in total fat would have major health benefits was not supported by existing data….long-term follow-up studies have found little relation between the percentage of calories from fat and risks of breast cancer, colon cancer, or coronary heart disease (14).

Unfortunately, this acknowledgment that the premise of the WHI study was ill-advised does not mean that the HSPH Department of Nutrition, world-renown nutrition authority largely responsible for the DGA, has abandoned the lipid hypothesis. To the contrary, it has merely refined it to mean "saturated" fat, not "total" fat (15, p.56 ff).

CONFUSION BETWEEN CAUSE AND EFFECT: A common failing in many current epidemiology studies is that, when an association is found, the investigators do not seem to know which the is "cause" and which the "effect." Even though such a failing does not occur in diet/disease research, because of the obvious relationship between diet and disease, it is important for health professionals to recognize its existence.

Vacations Make One Healthy: A number of years ago, a study was publicized that demonstrated this obvious confusion in the minds of its investigators. The *Wall Street Journal*, along with a number of other highly-regarded popular publications, reported the dire warning that for your health's sake, do not cancel a vacation if you have a choice:

> A growing body of research links long-term vacation habits and health. A 14-year study of 12,866 men, published last year in the journal Psychosomatic Medicine, found annual vacations sharply reduced the risk of death among middle-aged men. Similarly, a 20-year study of middle-aged women by the Centers for Disease Control found a link between lack of vacations and higher risk of heart attack and death. 'Vacationing may be good for your health,' concludes the first study (16).

Despite considerable anecdotal evidence that vacations are beneficial to one's health and well being, the above studies do not prove that regular vacationing prolongs life. They only show an association between health and recreational travel. But which is the cause and which the effect? Are people healthy because they take vacations or do they take vacations because they are healthy? People who are in ill health or who just do not feel well are not wont to go on cruises or engage in other vacation travel.

It not only takes reasonable good health to vacation, it also takes money. Thus, people who regularly take vacations are a select group; they tend not only to be more active physically than the general population but also wealthier. Thus, the data from the above studies provide no more validity to the conclusion that vacationing is good for health than they do to the conclusions that healthy people take more vacations than sick people or that wealthy people take more vacations than poor people.

Activity Reduces Risk of Alzheimer's Disease: In recent months, the relationship between Alzheimer's disease (AD) and physical activity has become a popular subject for epidemiological investigation. Among the latest of these is a study of 716 participants from a memory and aging project (17). Their average age was 82 years and all were dementia-free at the onset of the study. Their total daily physical activity was measured continuously for a period of 10 days. The mean length of activity was 3.3 hours per day; intensity of exercise was also measured. Participants were then followed for four years with annual structured clinical examinations and cognitive tests.

At the end of four years, 71 of the participants had developed clinical (AD). Participants who were the least active physically were more than twice as likely to develop (AD); those in the bottom 10 percent of intensity of activity were almost three times as likely. Accordingly, this study, like all its predecessors, found that physical activity and/or mental exercise lowered the chances that a person will develop AD. As the study reports, this is only an association – not proof of cause/effect; however, the message was that activity reduces AD risk.

Apparently, in this and other studies of the relationship between physical activity and AD, there is no recognition that, despite the outward similarity of participants, nutritional forces are probably unknowingly working within those destined to become victims of AD that make them different from other participants with regard to the study parameters. These future victims of AD may just not have the same get-up-and-go attitudes of their peers. Thus, the study's implied conclusion that people with a higher level of total physical activity have a reduced risk of AD is no more valid than a conclusion that people with a higher risk of AD have a reduced level of total physical activity.

The findings are commendable; everyone, regardless of health status, should be encouraged to be active and participate in life to the fullest. But are these studies giving false hope to the elderly? Are they diverting the elderly away from learning about nutritional preventive measures for AD that also offer a possibility for a reversal of early AD? (See A Personal Prevention Program – Chapter Eleven).

FLAWED EXPERIMENTAL ANIMAL STUDIES: The almost exclusive purpose of animal experimentation is to obtain data that is applicable for humans. Thus, in designing an animal experiment, it is critical to choose an animal model whose response will be as similar as possible to that of the human. Early animal experiments designed to test the lipid hypothesis erred in selecting an inappropriate test animal, the rabbit.

Studies conducted in 1954 reported that feeding of saturated fat and cholesterol to rabbits caused the formation of fatty deposits in their arteries (5). The rabbit is the wrong animal model for such a study because rabbits are obligate vegetarians. They would be expected to become ill on a diet containing high levels of saturated fat and cholesterol, which are animal products. A comprehensive review by Stehbens confirms that animals vary tremendously in their sensitivity to dietary cholesterol (18). Rabbits show increases in serum cholesterol up to 3,000 percent, monkeys 20 percent, and humans essentially no increase at all when cholesterol is added to the diet.

Recalcitrant Nutrition Policy Makers

The story of the origin and evolution of dietary recommendations that were formalized in the DGA and designed to provide healthful nutrition for all Americans tells the tale of an official governmental policy based on a foundation of seriously flawed epidemiological studies. Despite the large volume of solid data in the scientific literature implicating carbohydrates and/or an imbalance of essential fatty acids in the etiology of the chronic diseases, the makers of the American health policy are reluctant to change their long-held views that dietary fat, or now more precisely saturated fat, is the culprit.

CURRENTLY ACCEPTABLE DATA

The governmental and nutritional scientists charged with assuring the accuracy and adequacy of the DGA not only have embraced the original flawed science on which it was based but also have continued to accept new data from studies that are equally defective. An example of the quality of research that is acceptable to today's nutrition community is a paper recently published in the *Archives of Internal Medicine* entitled "Meat Intake and Mortality" (19). This paper concludes that the risk of overall mortality, cardiovascular disease mortality, and cancer mortality increases with increasing consumption of red and/ or processed meats. The inverse was found for white meats, with all mortalities decreasing with increasing consumption of white meats.

If this paper were permitted to slip silently into the dusty recesses of medical archives, it would be worth little more than passing mention as another example of pseudoscience. But, unfortunately, it has received widespread acceptance in radio, television, and print media with frightening headlines such as "Want to live longer? Cut back on red meat" (20) and "Study finds eating red meat contributes to risk of early death" (21). The harm that the publicizing of such fallacious allegations can do to a trusting public is inestimable. Thus, "Meat Intake and Mortality" must be exposed for what it is, namely an unnecessarily alarming report containing indefensible conclusions.

"Meat Intake and Mortality" is a sophisticated statistical exercise that fails the test of epidemiological competence. Because of a basic design flaw, it cannot possibly produce useful or meaningful results. The principal design flaw in this study is the exclusion of a critically important variable, the participants' consumption of high-glycemic carbohydrates (sugar and starch). Sugar and starch are major constituents of the average American diet. The study report states that participants answered a 124-item food frequency questionnaire about alcohol consumption, vitamin use, fruit consumption, vegetable consumption, and about consumption of all types and forms of red meat, white meat, processed meat, and fish. If participants were asked about bread and cereal consumption, sugar and dessert consumption, or daily intake of soft drinks, the paper makes no mention of the fact. The paper is totally silent on the sugar and starch components of the participants' diets.

The concept that high-glycemic carbohydrates play a role in the etiology of cardiovascular and other chronic diseases is not some arcane notion to which nutritional science is not privy. In the mid-nineteenth century, Banting's *Letter on Corpulence* (3) received wide public attention. In the early twentieth century, parents commonly warned children that eating too much candy would give them "sugar diabetes." During the years just prior to the promulgation of the DGA, John Yudkin's papers showing a strong association between sugar intake and coronary heart disease were published. Thus, it is fair to say that any modern-day diet/health study that excludes high-glycemic carbohydrate intake is about as intelligent and illuminating as totally ignoring the role of exposure to sunlight in a study investigating the cause of sunburn.

The observation that eminent nutritional scientists who are responsible for the validity of recommendations of the DGA are accepting of scientific incompetence in their peers is confirmed by public comments lauding the findings of "Meat Intake and Mortality." Barry M. Popkin, professor of global nutrition at the University of North Carolina is quoted as saying:

> …this would be the Rolls Royce of studies on this topic. The uniqueness of this study is its size and the length of follow-up. This is a slam-dunk to say that, 'Yes, indeed, if you want to be healthy and live longer, consume less red and processed meat'(21).

Despite acceptance by a reputable journal, there seems to be a hint that the authors felt a need to justify the paper's validity. The subtitle "A prospective study of over half a million people" is unusual in its prominent mention of the size of the study population. Unfortunately, size cannot remedy lack of substance. The most efficient pump in existence cannot bring up water from a well that is dry.

The tragic aspect of this study is not its design failings, but rather that it was conceived and conducted by the highly-regarded National Cancer Institute, published in a scientific journal of unquestioned repute, and fully endorsed by nutritional scientists who have a major responsibility for the official dietary recommendations that are exacerbating the epidemics of the modern nutritional diseases.

PSEUDOSCIENCE STILL PREVAILS: A more egregious example of the substandard quality of research used by the nutrition establishment to set official nutrition policy occurred more recently with the publication claiming that consumption of red meat is associated with an increased risk of premature mortality from all causes (22).

This paper was not only published in a highly reputable journal but among its authors were members of the Harvard nutrition establishment who have a singular interest in protecting their professional validation of a proscription against saturated fat and cholesterol. The study violates a number of principles of competent epidemiology, the most important of which is that it implies cause/effect without proving it; it did not "remove the pump handle" (see the lessons of Dr. Snow, Chapter Eleven). The abstract carefully states that consumption of red meat is only associated with the risk of a number of chronic diseases. However, it implies cause/effect by offering extensive data showing that substitution with other so-called healthy protein sources would present a lesser risk.

Further evidence that the authors had no explanation (no proof) for why red meat consumption would be associated with an increased risk of mortality is demonstrated by speculations offered in comments at the end of the paper. Among the few possible explanations suggested for the effect were the old saws of saturated fat and cholesterol from red meat. If the study had actually proved cause/effect there would have been no need for guesses, and if the authors had a good foundation in nutritional biochemistry there would have been no need for the study.

The Reality

The heart-healthy diet has not only failed its mission of preventing heart disease but has also brought with it serious, unintended consequences in the form of overweight, obesity, type-2 diabetes, and cancer. Attack rates of these aliments and have grown tremendously in the past several decades. In more recent years, mental disorders with which the public is less familiar, such as depression, aggression, and dementias, are also on the rise. These diseases, too, have been shown to have nutritional links.

The dietary changes that have occurred over the past century have had a marked effect on the nutrition of the American public. What is the relationship between diet and nutrition, and why does a change in one influence the other? Diet refers to the foods that comprise the daily fare, and nutrition refers to the substances (nutrients) that the body requires for growth, maintenance, and repair, which are provided by foods.

Although the number of foods available for consumption is great and varied, all are composed of only the same few basic nutrients (proteins, carbohydrates, fats and other lipids, vitamins and minerals). Excluding physical and esthetic qualities, the only difference among foods is that their basic nutrients are present in different quantities and different ratios. The nutritional quality of a diet is completely dependent on what foods are selected to be in it. Thus, if diet contributes to or causes a chronic debilitating disease, the fault must lie in the kinds and quantities of the foods that are selected for the diet.

The nutritional road map drawn decades ago by national dietary policy to direct a whole nation down an unhealthful dietary path seems to have been created using the simplistic but faulty logic that the fat and cholesterol that clog arteries must have come from fat and cholesterol in the diet. That this logic is not founded on facts is explained by innumerable studies conducted over the past 25 years that have shown that it is sugar, starches, and polyunsaturated vegetable seed oils, not saturated fat and cholesterol, that are underlying causes of heart disease, stroke, type-2 diabetes, mental illnesses, and probably many cancers. The verity of the conclusion that sugar, starches, and polyunsaturated vegetable seed oils are the culprits is confirmed by biochemistry in Part Two.

It is important to note that the wholesale adoption of bogus epidemiology by the nutrition community is the lynch pin of the current so-called heart-healthy diet. If sound nutritional science is not able to dislodge the lynch pin, the massive human feeding experiment foisted on the American public decades ago will continue to take its toll. Thus, the reality appears to be that the four horsemen of the apocalypse may have once again come to visit us. This time, however, they ride as false prophets preaching of low-fat and high-carbohydrate diets. Instead of bringing pestilence, famine, war, and death, they bring malnutrition, drug-induced nutrient depletions, chronic diseases, and death.

Revisiting the Lessons of History

The concept that diet could be responsible for disease was unheard of a century ago when outbreaks of beriberi and pellagra occurred. The experts believed that only bacteria could cause epidemics. Hence, when health officials were confronted with epidemics of these diseases, it was reasonable for them to assume that the etiologic agent for each was a pathogen. The search for the infectious agents was fruitless, and investigators remained baffled for many years because the underlying causes were not infectious organisms.

CLASSIC NUTRITIONAL DISEASES

BERIBERI: The symptoms of beriberi included fatigue, mental confusion, nerve damage, weight loss, diarrhea, swelling of the limbs, high blood pressure, weakened cardiac muscle, and heart failure. Beriberi was born of the fact that the germ in whole raw grains became rancid during storage. To solve this problem, machines were invented that removed the oily, vitamin-containing germ from grains such as rice.

The absence of important vitamins, particularly the B-vitamin thiamin, in polished rice, caused the debilitating and often fatal disease in very large population groups. When it was discovered that beriberi was associated with polished rice, even though the causative agent was unknown, this information was used to prevent this disease. Today, beriberi is prevented by fortifying polished rice with thiamin.

PELLAGRA: Pellagra is a malady characterized by an itchy rash, no appetite, sore tongue, depression, dementia, diarrhea, headaches, dizziness, weight loss, and eventual death. The underlying cause of pellagra was the high consumption of maize (corn). Because of its low cost, good taste, and availability, corn became the staple food in poor countries and displaced traditional diets that included sufficient amounts of meat, eggs, and dairy products. Eventually, corn was found to be devoid of the vitamin niacin (B_3).

THE LIST EXPANDS: In the early 1900s, researchers began to accept that not only beriberi and pellagra but also scurvy and rickets might be caused by specific dietary deficiencies.

This opened an era of active research aimed at discovery of the chemical identity of nutrients that prevented specific diseases.

The number of classic nutritional diseases for which the etiological agents were unknown gradually decreased as new vitamins were discovered. By the mid-20th Century, all of the major vitamins were known, important dietary minerals were recognized, and epidemics of the classic nutritional diseases became afflictions of the past.

Scurvy: Scurvy, which is caused by a deficiency of vitamin C, is probably the most famous of the classic nutritional diseases because of its early history as a curse of sailors who spent long periods of time at sea. They suffered from spongy, bleeding gums, large bruises, swollen joints, heart failure, and ultimately death.

In 1794, James Lind, a Scottish naval surgeon demonstrated that addition of oranges or limes to the daily ration could cure scurvy. His experiment, however, did not lead him to consider scurvy a nutritional deficiency disease. Instead he believed that scurvy was associated with warm air (23, p. 295). By the end of the Eighteenth Century, provision of lemon juice or limes brought an end to outbreaks of scurvy in the British fleet.

Rickets: Vitamin D deficiency may cause calcium and phosphorus deficiency in bone and result in the metabolic bone disease known as rickets in children and osteomalacia in adults. The disease results in softening of bones and is characterized by muscular weakness, listlessness, aching and bowing of long, weight-bearing bones. The bowing is especially prominent in adults whose vitamin D deficiencies occurred in early childhood and remained uncorrected during the growth period. Vitamin D is created in the body by sunlight, but in northern climates, sunlight is often not sufficient. The discovery of the exact chemical structure of vitamin D made it widely available for the fortification of milk and for sale as a dietary supplement.

Goiter: The element iodine is of critical importance for production by the thyroid gland of thyroxin and triiodothryonine. These thyroid hormones are essential for proper function of cellular oxidative reactions throughout the body. Because the main source of iodine is seafood, iodine deficiencies tend to be endemic in areas inland from the seacoasts. Iodine deficiency prior to adulthood may cause cretinism, a disease characterized by dwarfism, mental retardation, potbelly, dry skin, and coarse, brittle hair. In adults, deficiency causes varying degrees of hyperplasia of the thyroid gland with consequent tumorous swelling of the neck. Today, table salt is fortified with iodine and pills that contain iodine are available as dietary supplements.

The Lessons for Today

The dietary changes and disease patterns we are witnessing today resemble those that led to the great epidemics of pellagra and beriberi, which occurred more than a century ago. These long-forgotten nutritional diseases, along with others such as goiter, rickets, and scurvy, were once scourges of mankind. These diseases serve to show how fragile people really are when it comes to the impact of diet on their lives and well being. Beriberi and pellagra are especially important models for today's modern nutritional diseases because they demonstrated that large scale, man-made dietary changes are capable of causing great epidemics of non-infectious debilitating diseases.

The classic nutritional diseases resulted from dietary deficiencies of a single micronutrient – a vitamin or mineral. A diet lacking in a vital nutrient can result in severe illness and increased susceptibility to infectious and life shortening diseases. How quickly the illness occurs and how severe the symptoms might be depends on the degree of the deficiency and its duration. The greater the deficiency and the longer its duration, the more severe are the symptoms and the damage. Small deficiencies, on the other hand, tend to cause only minimal or subclinical effects. In the ill or the elderly patients, they usually go undetected.

Unlike the classic nutritional diseases, the modern nutritional diseases are primarily the result of excesses or imbalances among dietary macronutrients – proteins, carbohydrates, and/or lipids – rather than deficiency of a single micronutrient. Because of the great interdependence and complexity of interactions among the macronutrients, determination of which and how much of each contributes to a disease process has been difficult; however, current biochemistry is helping to solve this problem. It is because of the need to evaluate a multiplicity of variables that makes the epidemiology of modern nutritional diseases so complicated. When a disease is caused by a single agent, an association of the agent with the disease is easier to detect because it not confounded by the presence or absence of other variables.

Actually, epidemiological studies of the association of diet with chronic diseases done over the past several decades have been inconclusive, despite a tremendous investment of time and money (13). These studies have failed to include vital dietary variables such as sugar and starch consumption. Despite this failing, great advances in the sciences of biochemistry and physiology have overcome this problem by elucidating the biological impacts of macronutrient excesses and imbalances on human health.

Today's great epidemics of inflammatory diseases, while different in details, parallel the great pellagra and beriberi epidemics of long ago. As then, large-scale, man-made dietary changes were brought about by innovations in food production. However, a century ago, when reliable scientific studies uncovered the true causes of pellagra and beriberi, reasonably prompt actions were taken to control these nutritional diseases. Today, underlying causes of the modern nutritional diseases are known and available in the scientific literature. Yet no credible preventive or remedial action has been taken by the nutrition community or anyone else. Instead, the focus has been on medical treatment, primarily in the form of early detection, treatment with prescription drugs and surgery, and advice to reduce intake of animal fats and increase exercise.

Revisiting these classic nutritional diseases is also valuable in understanding the cause of some of the maladies of the elderly, a major fraction of whom suffers from some degree of malnutrition. For example, it is shocking to learn that scurvy, a disease that was conquered more than a century ago, not only exists in all ages in the United States (24) but also in developed countries throughout the world (25). In studying the classic nutritional diseases, one may speculate on how many of them exist unrecognized among seniors and other populations at risk.

To illustrate this point, note that symptoms of almost all of the classic deficiency diseases include some form of mental dysfunction such as lassitude, anxiety, dementia, fatigue, depression, mental confusion, nervousness, or vague pains. Balch writes that the early symptoms of pellagra may be misinterpreted as mental illness (26, p. 422). Pauling devotes a whole chapter of his book to the relationship between poor mental function and nutritional deficiencies (27, p. 181ff). Suffice to say that a number of cases of the mental deterioration that are occurring among the aged may well be related to some form of borderline deficiency of one or more nutrients. Those caring for seniors with vague memory or attention difficulties should ensure that diets are nutritionally adequate before concluding that their mental problems are a natural part of old age and, therefore, not preventable or reversible.

Aside from the fact that the classic nutritional diseases may still be occurring among us, recalling their histories hopefully will rekindle an appreciation of the fundamental importance of vitamins, minerals, and other essential nutrients to good health. Diseases such as scurvy, pellagra, and beriberi destroyed the health and the shortened lives of millions of people. They demonstrate how very dependent humans are on certain minor but essential components of our diets.

Adverse Drug Reactions

Adverse drug reactions are mentioned in this chapter because one type of adverse reaction, specifically depletion of a vital nutrient by use of a drug, can create a nutritional deficiency with its associated health problems. Adverse reactions to drugs constitute one of the most serious and least talked about health problems faced by Americans. A study done in 1994 estimated that among patients in hospitals alone properly and legally administered drugs caused about 106,000 fatalities and more than two million serious adverse drug reactions per year. If adverse drug reactions among nonhospitalized patients had been counted in this study, the total number of adverse drug reactions would have been far higher (28). These data reinforce the advice that, for a long healthy life, one should avoid prescription drugs whenever possible (29).

Adverse drug reactions are not included in government health statistics and, therefore, are not officially counted or acknowledged as being a cause of death. If the estimated 106,000 deaths caused annually by legally administered drugs in hospitals alone were included in the national statistics, adverse drug reactions would rank as the fifth leading cause of death in this country. Only the number of fatalities caused by heart disease (599,413), cancer (567,628), chronic lower respiratory diseases (137,353), and possibly stroke (128,842) as reported for the year 2010 (30), would be more numerous.

Parenthetically, it is worth noting that if all of the 225,000 deaths caused annually by medical care (iatrogenic deaths) in hospitals were included, this category would be the third leading cause of death in America. Of 225,000 annual iatrogenic deaths, 12,000 are caused by unnecessary surgery, 7,000 by medication errors, 20,000 from other errors in hospitals, 80,000 from hospital-caused infections, and 106,000, as mentioned above, caused by adverse effects of properly and legally administered drugs in hospitals (31).

WHY ADVERSE DRUG REACTIONS OCCUR

To accomplish their pharmacological objectives, all drugs, including prescription drugs, must be administered in doses that are large enough to overcome the body's natural defense mechanisms. For most drugs, small doses cannot be effective because they are promptly metabolized (detoxified) and excreted from the body. For this reason, a drug dose is designed to be large enough so that the drug will remain in the bloodstream for a number of hours before the body's defense mechanisms can eliminate it.

Drugs, like all chemicals, have threshold doses below which no effects occur – beneficial or harmful. Drug doses are therefore carefully calculated to ensure that they are high enough to have the desired therapeutic (beneficial) effects, but not so high as to cause adverse (harmful) effects. Some drugs have large differences between the therapeutic dose and the harmful dose, and some drugs have small differences. The greater the difference between the two points, the safer the drug.

In understanding why adverse drug reactions occur in some people but not in others, it is important to recognize that individuals display a range of reactions to equal doses of the same drug. The reason for the range of adverse drug reactions is that no two people utilize their biochemical pathways to exactly the same degree. Even people of the same age, sex, and health status can vary slightly in this respect. Thus, a slightly different reaction to any given drug can produce a range of health effects.

Another important reason for differences in susceptibility to adverse drug reactions is age. Older adults have higher risks. According to an article in *Geriatrics*, individuals who are 60 years or older suffer 51 percent of the total deaths due to adverse drug reactions, yet they make up only 17 percent of the total population. And about 14 percent of hospitalizations of older patients are related to an adverse drug reaction (32).

DRUG-INDUCED NUTRIENT DEPLETION

There are three basic mechanisms by which a drug can cause harm: Interference with a metabolic pathway in the body; alteration of the action of another drug taken concomitantly; or by depletion of one or more nutrients. The latter effect, drug-induced nutrient depletion, is essentially unrecognized by the medical community.

The mechanism whereby drug-induced nutrient depletion occurs depends on the drug and the nutrient or nutrients involved. For example: the drug may interfere with the absorption of an important nutrient; prevent a nutrient from being metabolized or synthesized; or deplete a nutrient by reacting with and destroying it. Drug companies are not required to warn doctors about possible nutrient depletion or to include this hazard on drug labels. And drug reference books usually do not mention drug-induced nutrient depletion.

There are perhaps 150 commonly used prescription and nonprescription drugs that have been found to deplete essential nutrients. These are described in the thoroughly-referenced *Drug-Induced Nutrient Depletion Handbook* (28), which lists the commonly used prescription and nonprescription drugs according to the specific nutrients affected. Pharmacists are also excellent sources of information on nutrient depletion by drugs.

EXAMPLES OF DRUG-INDUCED NUTRIENT DEPLETION: The information presented in the following two examples does not constitute a complete review of contraindications, dietary considerations, or drug interactions associated with these drugs. The intent of these examples is to alert the reader to the fact that many commonly used drugs, both prescription and over-the-counter, can significantly alter nutrient status.

The first example, statin drugs, are a family of cholesterol-lowering agents that are regularly used by many middle-aged and older adults to lower blood cholesterol levels and ostensibly reduce the risk of heart attack and stroke. The second example, acetaminophen, is the most commonly ordered in-hospital and over-the-counter nonprescription pain reliever used in this country.

Cholesterol-Lowering Drugs: The statin drugs are commonly termed cholesterol pills. Their use is prescribed and promoted by official guidelines to lower blood cholesterol to levels deemed healthful by the National Heart, Lung, and Blood Institute (33). The number of Americans currently using statin drugs is approximately 13 million. However, because their use is prescribed by the NHLBI, it is estimated that the number regularly using statin drugs will rise in the next few years to an estimated 36 million, or approximately 18 percent of the U.S. population (34).

Depletion of Coenzyme Q$_{10}$: The statin drugs reduce cholesterol levels by inhibiting the enzyme HMG-CoA reductase (hydroxymethylglutaryl-coenzyme A). Inhibition of this enzyme slows the biochemical conversion of acetyl CoA to cholesterol (see Figure

6-4) and reduces the amount of cholesterol in the blood. It is worth stressing here that, in normal good health, the body makes only the amount of both HDL and LDL cholesterol that it requires for its cellular and tissue functions. Biochemical textbooks clearly indicate that, except in rare cases of familial hypercholesterolemia, excess cholesterol in the blood is the result of excess dietary sugar and starch (Chapters Six and Eight).

By inhibiting the synthesis of cholesterol, statin drugs also inhibit all of the intermediate steps in the metabolic pathway between HMG CoA and cholesterol. The first step in this pathway is the synthesis of mevalonic acid. Mevalonic acid (or mevalonate) is the precursor of an extremely important coenzyme called coenzyme Q_{10} (Co Q). Thus, inhibition of cholesterol also inhibits the biosynthesis of Co Q. All brands of statin drugs cause approximately the same adverse reactions and carry approximately the same precautions (28), none of which warn of the inhibition of CoQ.

CoQ is required to provide energy for cellular function. Because of the heart's great and constant demand for energy, its need for CoQ is greater than for any other cells of the body. Over time, the deficiency of CoQ resulting from inhibition by statin drugs leads to a range of cardiovascular problems. These include congestive heart failure, high blood pressure, stroke, heart valve damage, and cardiac arrhythmia.

Other potential adverse effects of CoQ deficiency include lack of energy, gum disease, and weakening of the immune system. Taken as a dietary supplement, CoQ can offset the depletion of CoQ caused by the statin drugs (28). Long-term use of statin drugs can cause serious disease by depleting a vital biochemical normally synthesized by the body.

Acetaminophen: This drug is sold over-the-counter for pains, headaches, and other minor ailments. It is essentially the only analgesic prescribed in hospital settings. Among the group of drugs that contain acetaminophen, the most common and best known brand name is Tylenol™. Acetaminophen is only a painkiller, whereas the NSAIDs and aspirin are not only painkillers but they are also anti-inflammatory.

Depletion of Glutathione: Acetaminophen is a somewhat unusual over-the-counter drug because of the narrow range between its pharmacologically effective dose and the dose that causes serious toxic effects. In other words, the toxic dose is not very much greater than the recommended safe dose. Thus, even when used as directed, this particular drug provides a relatively small margin of safety. In the United States, poison control centers report that acetaminophen is the leading cause of death as a result of overdose (35).

With long-term or excessive short-term use, acetaminophen can adversely affect liver function and damage kidneys. The symptoms are principally the result of destruction of glutathione, which is required as a metabolite and/or an antioxidant by a host of vital biochemical reactions in the body. Glutathione is a tripeptide, consisting of the amino acids glycine, cysteine, and glutamic acid. Glutathione is normally produced by the body from dietary protein. In the liver, one function of glutathione is as a detoxifying agent. Acting in this capacity, glutathione reacts with acetaminophen and converts it to a chemical that is excreted in the urine. This process of detoxification of acetaminophen depletes the body's stores of glutathione (36).

As with all chemicals, people vary in their susceptibility to the adverse effects of acetaminophen. The majority of people who use acetaminophen do so without apparent harm. This drug, like all other drugs, carries extensive warning labels that provide instructions about adverse drug reactions, interactions, and limitations on dosage and use, but they do not warn of glutathione depletion. Suffice to say here that Consumer Union's *Complete Drug Reference* indicates that before using acetaminophen, patients should inform their doctors about allergies, alcohol abuse, or other medical problems (37).

One illustration of the importance of glutathione to long-term health is a study of a large population group in which the effect of pain-relieving drugs on chronic diseases was examined (38). The study looked at acetaminophen, which is known to deplete glutathione, and NSAIDs, which are analgesic drugs that do not deplete glutathione. This study showed that the risk of developing Alzheimer's disease was reduced by 74 percent by aspirin, reduced 40 percent by NSAIDs, and increased 35 percent by acetaminophen.

These results suggest that important underlying causes of Alzheimer's disease may be a combination of uncontrolled inflammation and depleted glutathione. This study showing protection against Alzheimer's disease plus other studies showing that aspirin or NSAIDs reduce the risk of cardiovascular disease suggest that the choice of something as simple as a pain reliever may be important to long-term health.

References

1.)   http://www.framinghamheartstudy.org/about/history.html/ Accessed Sept. 26, 2012.

2.)   Sullivan MG. Now is the time to prepare for the onslaught of Alzheimer's disease. Caring for the Ages. 2007; 8(8): 12. http://www.caringfortheages.com/ Accessed Sept. 26, 2012.

3.)   Taubes G. Good Calories, Bad Calories. New York, NY: Alfred A. Knopf, 2007.

4.)   Keys, A. Atherosclerosis. Journal of Mount Sinai Hospital. 1953; 20: 118-139.

5.)   Enig MG, Fallon S. The Oiling of America. Nexus Magazine. Dec./Jan.1999, Feb/Mar 1999. (Available at http://www.westonaprice.org/know-your-fats/the-oiling-of-america). Accessed Sept. 26, 2012.

6.)   Kannel, W.B. et al. The Framingham Study: An epidemiological investigation of cardiovascular disease. Bethesda, MD: National Institutes of Health, 1969.

7.)   Krehl, W.A. The nutritional epidemiology of cardiovascular disease. Annals of the New York Academy of Sciences. 1977; 300: 335-359.

8.) Yudkin, J. Sucrose and cardiovascular disease. Proceeding of the Nutrition Society. 1972; 31: 331-337. Cited in reference 7, above.

9.) Mann GV. The Way It Seems. New York, NY: Vantage Press, 1988.

10.) Mann GV, Editor. Coronary Heart Disease: The Dietary Sense and Nonsense. An evaluation by scientists. London, England: Janus Publishing Company, 1993.

11.) Ravnskov U. The Cholesterol Myth: Exposing the Fallacy that Saturated Fat and Cholesterol Cause Heart Disease. Washington, DC: NewTrends Publishing Inc., 2000.

12.) Yerushalmy J, Hilleboe HE. Fat in the diet and mortality from heart disease: a methodologic note. New York State Journal of Medicine. 1957; 57(14): 2343-2354.

13.) Ottoboni A, Ottoboni F. Low-fat diet and chronic disease prevention: The Women's Health Initiative and its reception. Journal of American Physicians and Surgeons. 2007; 12(1): 10-13.

14.) Kantrowiitz, B, Kalb C. Food news blues. Newsweek, March 13, 2006, pp 44-50.

15.) Willett WC. Eat, Drink, and Be Healthy: the Harvard Medical School Guide to Healthy Eating. New York, NY: Free Press, 2001.

16.) Shellenbarger S. Canceling a vacation could cost you dearly in the long run. Wall Street Journal. April 11, 2001; B1.

17.) Buchman AS, et al. Total physical activity and the risk of AD and cognitive decline in older adults. Neurology. 2012; 78(17): 1323-1329. http://www.neurology.org/content/78/17/1323.abstract/ Accessed Sept. 26, 2012.

18.) Stehbens, W.E. Coronary heart disease, hypercholesterolemia, and atherosclerosis: False premises I. Experimental and Molecular Pathology. 2001; 70: 103-119.

19.) Sinha, R., et al. Meat intake and Mortality: A prospective study of over a half million people. Archives of Internal Medicine. 2009; 169(6): 562-71.)

20.) http://edition.cnn.com/2009/HEALTH/03/23/healthmag.red.meat.lifespan/index.html/ Accessed Sept. 26, 2012.

21.) The Washington Post. March 23, 2009

22.) Pan A, et al. Red Meat Consumption and Mortality. Archives of Internal Medicine. 2012; 172(7): 555-563.

23.) Porter R. The Greatest Benefit to Mankind. New York, NY: W. W. Norton & Company, Inc., 1997.

24.) Hampl JS, et al. Vitamin C deficiency and depletion in the United States. American Journal of Public Health. 2004; 94(5): 870-675.

25.) Velandia, B., et al. Scurvy is still present in developed countries. Journal of General Internal Medicine. 2008; 23(8): 1281-4.

26.) Balch JF, Balch PA. Prescription for Nutritional Healing, Second Edition. Garden City Park, NY: Avery Publishing Group, 1997.

27.) Pauling L. How to Live Longer and Feel Better. New York, NY: W.H. Freeman & Co., 1989.

28.) Pelton R, et al. Drug-Induced Nutrient Depletion Handbook: 1999-2000. Hudson, OH: Lexi-Comp, Inc., 1999.

29.) Mindell E. The Mindell Report. 1999; 1(9): 4-5.

30.) http://www.cdc.gov/nchs/fastats/deaths.htm/ Accessed Sept. 26, 2012.

31.) Starfield B. Is US Health Really the Best in the World? Journal of the American Medical Association. 2000; 284(4): 483-485.

32.) Cohen J.S. Avoiding adverse reactions: Effective lower-dose drug therapies for older patients. Geriatrics. 2000; 55(2): 54-64.

33.) Press Release: 9:30 a.m., EST, Tuesday, May 15, 2001. NCEP Issues Major New Cholesterol Guidelines. National Institutes of Health, National Heart, Lung, and Blood Institute.

34.) Burton TM, Adams C. New U.S. Guidelines Would Triple Use of Cholesterol-Lowering Drugs. The Wall Street Journal. May 16, 2001: B1.

35.) Easton T, Herrera S. J&J's dirty little secret. Forbes Magazine. Jan.12, 1998: 42-44.

36.) http://emedicine.medscape.com/article/820200-overview/ Accessed Sept. 26, 2012.

37.) Consumer Reports. Complete Drug Reference, 2001 Edition. Englewood, CO: MICROMEDEX

38.) Thompson Healthcare. 2001.

39.) Greenwell I. Role of inflammation in chronic disease. Life Extension Magazine. February 2000: 44-7.

Part Two

The Science

Far more crucial than what we know or do not know is what we do not want to know. **Eric Hoffer. The Passionate State of Mind. 1954.**

It is difficult to get a man to understand something when his job depends on not understanding it. **Upton Sinclair**

The goal of Part Two is to present the scientific data that validate the nutrition facts and figures presented in this book. The six chapters that comprise this section briefly describe the chemistry, biochemistry, and physiology of the macronutrients and micronutrients; the biochemical pathways that nutrients travel in the body; how the nutrient composition of the diet governs which biochemical pathways are followed; and the impact of all on the eicosanoid control system that governs the biochemistry by which health or disease is determined.

The reluctance of the nutrition establishment to open its collective mind and explore beyond its dogma has resulted in a standoff between the establishment and scientists seeking to correct the wrongs in the official nutrition policy. This standoff, which has been very costly in terms of human suffering and medical care dollars, continues because clear, unassailable proof based on a hard biochemical and physiological sciences is largely ignored by the bureaucracies in charge of the nutrition policy.

Despite the fact that scientific writings do not make for enjoyable reading, except perhaps for other scientists, they are the *sine qua non* for establishing the soundness of the claim that the modern American diet is the cause of the epidemics of chronic diseases at issue in this book. With this in mind, an apology and a plea are offered to readers who consider the biochemical explanations tedious; an apology for the inconvenience and a plea for acceptance that they must be included.

To dispel a distaste of biochemistry, descriptions have been simplified to the extent possible and the suggestion is made to skip over parts that are too onerous and proceed with the rest of the passage. Despite a lack of public interest, biochemical science is too vital to ignore in view of America's devastating epidemics of chronic diseases.

Chapter Four

Diet Composition and Utilization

Nutrition is a personal matter, as personal as your diary or your income-tax report. The food you eat can make the difference between the day ending with freshness...or with exhaustion... **Adele Davis. Let's Eat Right to Keep Fit. (1, p. 15)**

When you are in balance you feel so good – mentally sharp, physically strong and well, emotionally stable – and when you vary from balance you feel so lousy that you will ask yourself..."Why did I eat that?" **Michael and Mary Dan Eades. Protein Power. (2, p. 137)**

The purpose of this and the following chapters on nutritional supplements, carbohydrates, proteins, lipids, essential fatty acids, and eicosanoids is to describe these components of the diet and what is known of the science that governs them in order to provide a background for an understanding of what happens to them in the body. It is necessary to know how nutrients, the substances that nourish the body, function normally in order to diagnose their malfunctions. A broken machine cannot be fixed without knowing how it works. So it is with the human body. Knowledge of the biochemical pathways that nutrients follow and how they influence each other is required for an understanding of which pathways foster health and which lead to illness. In order to plan a healthful diet that will prevent the modern nutritional diseases, one must know what makes for a healthful diet and why and how dietary imbalances promote disease.

Examination of the tremendous number and variety of cookbooks available in bookstores reveals that there are literally hundreds of different kinds of foods and many thousands of individual ways of preparing them for the table. Despite this great assortment of dishes from which daily meals can be assembled, all of the varied chemicals in them fall into two categories: nutrients, those that nourish; and nonnutrients, those that do not nourish.

Excluding water, a substantial fraction of the chemicals in foods are nonnutrients. The nonnutrient category includes all of the substances that the body does not use or need for energy or to make more of itself. The nonnutrients include nondigestible matter and a wide array of chemicals, primarily those that occur naturally in plants, which are absorbed into the body but serve no nutrient function. Nondigestible matter is labeled as fiber and all other nonnutrient chemicals are called xenobiotic, or foreign, chemicals.

Food Composition

There are six chemical elements that are considered to be the elements of life. All, living organisms are composed of biochemicals that are made from carbon, hydrogen and varying quantities of oxygen. In addition, some of these biochemicals contain small amounts of nitrogen, sulfur, and/or phosphorous. Foods consumed by nonphotosynthetic (heterotrophic) organisms, with the exception of a few essential inorganic elements, are carbon compounds made from these six elements. The fact that food compounds are based on carbon makes food chemistry one with organic chemistry, the chemistry of carbon, originally called the chemistry of life.

The unique properties of the carbon-to-carbon bond enable the formation of an almost infinite number of individual compounds (foods) from just their carbon, hydrogen, and oxygen moieties. The origins and complexities of organic chemistry and carbon-to-carbon bonding are reviewed in the chapter on lipids (Chapter Eight). The lipid group, with its very long chains of carbon atoms arranged in single file or in cross links best displays the unique capabilities and versatility of carbon bonding.

Nutrients

Nutrients are the food substances an organism uses for its life functions. Nutrients can be divided into two major groups. One group supplies building materials and fuel. The building materials are used for the framework and other structures of the organism; the fuel is used to provide the energy for construction, maintenance, and operation of the organism. The second group of nutrients includes all of the tools and supplies – pliers, hammers, nails, screws, glue, and so forth – needed to use with the building materials to provide form and function to the organism.

The body's building materials are obtained mainly from carbohydrates and proteins and the fuel is provided by carbohydrates and the fat and oil fraction of the lipid group. Because carbohydrates, proteins, and lipids, are needed in fairly large amounts, they are called macronutrients. The tools and supplies are primarily vitamins and minerals. They are needed in fairly small quantities and are called micronutrients.

ESSENTIAL-NONESSENTIAL NUTRIENTS

Nutrients are classed biochemically as either essential or nonessential. This is a very important but commonly misunderstood distinction. Essential nutrients are those that the body requires for life but is not able to make for itself. Essential nutrients must be supplied by the diet. An organism cannot survive if it is deprived of its essential nutrients. The essential nutrients for mammalian organisms are all of the vitamins, some minerals, a few amino acids, and a few fatty acids. There are no essential carbohydrates; if not supplied in the diet, the body can make any carbohydrate nutrient it requires from one of the nonessential amino acids.

Nonessential nutrients are nutrients a healthy body can make, independent of whether they are supplied in the diet. The body makes nonessential nutrients from the carbohydrates, proteins, and lipids in food. Examples of nonessential nutrients are: glucose, a sugar from carbohydrates; glutamic acid, an amino acid from proteins; and oleic acid, a fatty acid from the fat component of the lipid group.

The essential-nonessential classification of nutrients is misleading and, for many, difficult to understand. Are not all nutrients essential? Doesn't the body need all of them? The answers are, "No, not all nutrients are essential biochemically, but whether the body can make them or not, they are all necessary." and "Yes, the body does need and use all of them whether they are classed as essential or nonessential. Despite the seeming contradiction, nutritional and biochemical scientists must have a method for distinguishing between nutrients that an organism can make and those that it cannot make. The very practical reason is to identify those nutrients that are required for life and hence must absolutely be supplied by the diet.

MACRONUTRIENTS

The macronutrients are the well-known carbohydrates, proteins, and lipids (fats). Animal and vegetable products used as foods usually contain all three macronutrients in varying amounts. Because of the importance of these three dietary components to the modern nutritional diseases, each will be discussed more fully in following chapters. Each macronutrient has its own special metabolic functions in the body but, with few exceptions, all eventually find their way to the metabolic hub of energy production, the Krebs cycle, which is described later in this chapter.

MICRONUTRIENTS

Micronutrients are the nutrients that are present in relatively small amounts in foods. This category is a diverse one that includes all vitamins and minerals and an assortment of other trace biochemicals. The vitamins and minerals are all essential nutrients; they must be supplied in the diet because human biochemistry is not capable of making them. Various other biochemicals included in the micronutrient category are small organic compounds that, unlike vitamins and minerals, are not classed as essential because the body can synthesize them in the amounts normally sufficient for its needs.

Some nonessential micronutrients may become essential under certain conditions. The body may not be able to make them in sufficient quantities when there is increased demand or reduced absorption of them. For example, a large number of medications inhibit utilization or absorption of one or more micronutrients (3). In addition to drug-induced effects, a greatly increased demand for the same or other micronutrients often occurs during periods of illness or other stress. More importantly, the biochemical and physiological changes that accompany the aging process typically increase the need for a number of micronutrients, essential as well as nonessential.

Nonnutrients

From the beginning of time, all living organisms have had to deal with the nonnutrient chemicals that accompany all foods. In order to thrive, all living organisms, whether they are plant or animal, have to extract the nutrients from food and reject the accompanying foreign chemicals.

FIBER

Unlike micro- and macronutrients, fiber serves no nutrient function. It is, nevertheless, a valuable component of foods. Two types of fiber are recognized: soluble and insoluble. These designations are misleading, because both types are insoluble in the literal sense of the term. The distinction is that fibers classed as soluble are of sufficiently small size to remain suspended when mixed in water and, when present in large numbers, form gels. Fibers classed as insoluble, on the other hand, settle out of a liquid mixture because they are too large to remain suspended. The quantity of soluble fiber in plants is from a tenth to half that of insoluble fiber.

The actions of fiber in the gastrointestinal tract are numerous. Insoluble fiber can adsorb food components such as micronutrients. Micronutrients adsorbed on fiber are not available for transfer from the intestinal tract into the body. Thus, prolonged consumption of large amounts of fiber may result in a deficiency of one or more micronutrients by preventing them from being absorbed from the intestinal tract. Both soluble and insoluble fibers hold considerable quantities of water, which makes for more easy passage of food through the digestive tract. They also allow for more even and controlled absorption of macronutrients from the small intestine. The main benefit of fiber is as a hydrophilic filler to promote easy elimination and help the digestive system work more efficiently.

Plant foods are the only dietary source of fiber, which is composed primarily of cellulose, the structural carbohydrate of plants. Cellulose, a polymer of glucose, cannot be digested by the gastrointestinal system of nonruminant animals. Although dietary fiber is mostly carbohydrate, it is not counted as carbohydrate in diet planning because it is not digested and contributes no calories. Although no official recommendation has been forthcoming from government agencies on the amount of fiber that should be in the diet, it is generally agreed that the daily intake of fiber should be between 20 and 35 grams a day (14 grams fiber /1,000 kcal of diet). It is estimated that the average American diet contains about half the recommended amount.

XENOBIOTIC CHEMICALS

This category includes all the substances in foods that are absorbed from the intestinal tract but, like fiber, are not used as nutrients by the body. The category takes its name from the Greek word *xenos*, meaning *strange* or *foreign*. Foreign chemicals may be naturally occurring or they may be added to food products, deliberately or inadvertently, somewhere between the farm and the consumer.

The public is generally unaware of the fact that there are many chemicals in foods that are foreign to the body (4). Also not generally known is the fact that the quantities and kinds of foreign chemicals in foods that are naturally occurring are many times greater than the quantities and kinds that are synthetic. Most of the naturally occurring chemicals in foods that are foreign for humans are of plant origin. These natural plant chemicals include alkaloids, hydrazines, iso-thiocyanates, aromatic carboxylic acids, alkyl phenols, various glycosides, and catechols, just to name a few. The digestive and metabolic systems of animals selectively eliminate from their digestive tracts many of the foreign chemicals in their plant feed and retain only those that they can use. The result is that the flesh of animal used for human food is free of these nonnutrients.

All organisms must be able to distinguish between chemicals they can use and chemicals they cannot use. A foreign substance may be harmful or benign. If it is harmful, it must be eliminated before it exerts its toxic effect. If it is benign, it must be eliminated in order to prevent useless trash from collecting and interfering with bodily functions. The presence of small amounts of foreign chemicals in foods should not be of concern to anyone (4). Humans are the beneficiaries of the evolution over millions of years of a very effective system of enzymes designed specifically to handle xenobiotic chemicals.

Enzymes

Before discussing the digestion of the foods we eat or the changes nutrients undergo in the body, it is important to define enzymes and briefly explain their function. More detailed information about enzymes can be found in any college biochemistry book.

WHAT ARE ENZYMES?

Enzymes are biochemicals made by living organisms to accelerate the rate of the biochemical reactions that comprise its metabolism – the sum of all the biochemical reactions required by its life processes. Biochemical reactions are made up of three parts, the starting biochemical (substrate), an enzyme plus its cofactors, if any, to assist the reaction, and the biochemical (end product) that results from the reaction.

Enzymes may be likened to the chemical catalysts used in the chemical industry in that they enable chemical reactions to proceed and accelerate them without themselves being consumed or changed in the process. With few exceptions, all of the biochemical reactions that occur in living organisms are catalyzed by enzymes. Without enzymes, the biochemical reactions necessary for life functions could not proceed at the very rapid rate necessary to support life.

All enzymes are proteins, many of which require combination with a cofactor (coenzyme) to become active as catalysts. A coenzyme is a smaller, nonprotein chemical, such as a vitamin or mineral. A countless number and variety of enzymes exist in the plant and animal kingdoms. The rules that govern enzyme chemistry apply to all living beings.

NAMING OF ENZYMES: Many enzymes are named by adding the suffix –*ase* to the name of the substrate that they act on. For example, urease is the enzyme that acts on urea to convert it to carbon dioxide and ammonia. Other enzymes are named by adding –*ase* to the type of reaction they catalyze. For example, alanine racemase rearranges (isomerizes) the amino acid alanine from its L-form to its D-form (L- and D- refer to optical rotation). A few of the enzymes that were discovered decades ago, long before the system of naming enzymes was formulated, have retained their historic names, such as the digestive enzymes pepsin and trypsin.

EXTERNAL – INTERNAL ENZYMES

There are two major classes of enzymes, those that work outside the body in the gastro-intestinal system (although the digestive tract is generally thought of as being within the body, literally it is outside of the body) and those that work inside the body in cells and tissues. Enzymes that work in the digestive tract are relatively few in number and limited in function. They are produced by specialized cells in the mouth, stomach, and pancreas and are referred to as digestive enzymes because, as the name implies, their sole purpose is to catalyze reactions that break down food components. Some plant enzymes can perform the same digestive functions as do human digestive enzymes.

Unlike digestive enzymes, the enzymes that work in cells and tissues within the body are vast in number and varied in function. It is estimated that in every living cell there are tens of thousands of copies of a hundred or more different kinds of enzymes. Despite the fact that there are many different kinds of enzymes, only six basic types of enzymes, categorized according to general function, have been identified. They are oxidation-reduction reactions (electron exchange), transfer reactions (exchange), hydrolysis reactions (breakdown by H_2O), lysis reactions (breakdown), isomerization reactions (rearrangement), and ligation reactions (joining).

PROPERTIES OF ENZYMES

First, it must be remembered that enzymes are proteins and, as such, they are digested and metabolized by the same pathways that all other proteins are metabolized. Plant and animal enzymes in the foods we eat are modified and broken down in the gastrointestinal tract to yield their component amino acids. With a few exceptions, they do not function as enzymes in humans. These exceptions are several digestive enzymes of plant origin that can perform the same functions in the gastrointestinal tract that human digestive enzymes perform. These plant and human digestive enzymes, like all proteins, are eventually broken down to their component amino acids in the small intestines.

DENATURATION: All food proteins are denatured (changed in some way from their natural state) by heat or by chemicals such as acids and alkalis. If cooking or other pretreatment has not already done so, digestive processes will denature them. Denatured enzymes are deactivated, which means they cannot function as enzymes. The digestive tract does not recognize that enzymes are enzymes but only that they are proteins.

Some people with poor digestion often benefit by supplementation with a special group of plant enzymes known as digestive enzymes. However, to prevent denaturation of these supplements from the action of gastric juices, they are usually administered in coated tablets that deliver them to the small intestine in active form. Enzymes present in foods carry no such protective coating.

Effect of Temperature: The catalytic activity of enzymes is temperature dependent, with most enzymes having their greatest activity in the narrow range of the normal temperature of the human body (96.7-99.0 °F). The speed with which an enzyme works drops off rapidly on either side of its optimal temperature, and it is completely inactive outside of its range.

Effect of pH: As with temperature, the catalytic activity of enzymes is dependent on the pH of the medium in which they operate. The pH scale, which is a measure of the concentration of hydrogen ions (H^+), was designed by early biologists to describe the degree of acidity or alkalinity in biological fluids. These early scientists found that the concentrations of H^+ in biological fluids were infinitesimally smaller than the concentrations that occurred in the acid/base reactions of inorganic chemistry. Thus, calculations used in inorganic chemistry could not be applied to biological fluids. A special scale had to be designed that could be applied to solutions with very low concentrations of H^+ ions. This special scale became the now well known pH scale of biological sciences.

The pH of a biological fluid is calculated by the equation [$pH = -\log (H^+)$], where (H^+) represents the concentration of H^+. The pH scale runs from 0 to 14, with 7 representing neutrality, meaning that the number of H^+ and OH^- (hydroxyl) ions are equal. Solutions with a pH below 7 have an excess of H^+ and are acidic. Solutions with a pH above 7 have an excess of OH^- and are basic (alkaline). The concentration of H^+ is greatest at 0 and decreases by 10-fold with each number up to 14. Thus, H^+ is inversely related to pH; the smaller the pH number, the greater the acidity. The reverse holds for OH^-, the concentration of OH^- is smallest at 0 and greatest at 14.

Most biological fluids are just slightly more basic than neutral. The normal pH of human blood, for example, is 7.4, which is commonly accepted as the normal, physiologic pH value for most biological fluids. In certain disease states, the pH of the blood can vary by small amounts from normal. If the blood pH drops slightly below 7.4, the condition is termed acidosis; if it increases slightly above 7.4, it is called alkalosis. Fortunately, the human body has a great buffering capacity, which keeps deviations from 7.4 at an absolute minimum. The pH range compatible with life is estimated to be between 6.8 and 7.8. As would be expected from its great constancy, the physiologic pH of 7.4 is the pH at which most enzymes within the body display optimal activity. A few enzymes, notably a few digestive enzymes that must work in the acidic environment of the stomach, have greatest activity in pH ranges significantly lower (more acidic) than 7. These enzymes will be noted below in the section on digestion.

A note with regard to how organic acids are referred to in the scientific literature is appropriate here. Organic acids typically have names ending in -ic, such as acetic acid, oleic acid, or glutamic acid. Because of the physiological requirement that the pH of the internal milieu does not deviate significantly from pH 7.4, organic acids are not usually found in their free acid (-ic) state in biological systems, but rather as their salts (the -ate form). Consequently, in scientific literature organic acids are often referred by their salt names, such as acetate, oleate, or glutamate.

SPECIFICITY: Probably the most remarkable feature of enzymes is their high degree of specificity. They are specific for the species of biochemical they will act on or for the type of reaction they will perform. An enzyme links with the substrate for which it was designed, holds it while the reaction it catalyzes is carried out, and then releases the desired product or products to be used as needed by the organism. Because of this specificity, enzyme-catalyzed reactions almost always have yields of about 100 percent. There is little opportunity for side reactions to occur and unwanted products to accumulate.

This is in marked contrast to the notoriously low yields obtained in laboratories from organic chemical reactions similar to those undertaken by living organisms. Organic chemicals, like biochemicals, are complex and often have more than one reactive site within their molecules. Without a catalyst to control the reaction and direct it to the one site of interest, side reactions occur and a number of different end products would be formed. The yield of the desired end product is often less than 50 percent from synthesis of organic chemicals in a laboratory.

Substrate Specificity: One type of specificity is substrate specificity. Some enzymes act only on substrates with a certain chemical structure. Others act on any one of a small group of substrates that are closely related chemically. Alcohol dehydrogenase, for example, is associated most commonly with the alcohol (ethanol) in alcoholic beverages, but it will also accept as substrates any one of several other small organic alcohols closely related to ethanol.

Isomer Specificity: Some enzymes are not only substrate specific but also are stereoisomer specific; they further distinguish between stereoisomers of a single substrate. This is an extremely important property, because there are numerous organic chemicals of vital biochemical importance that are identical in molecular formula but differ in the arrangement of their atoms in space, resulting in pairs of chemicals that are mirror images. These pairs of stereoisomers rotate light in opposite directions. Those that rotate light to the left are designated as the L-form (levo-form), and those that rotate light to the right are designated as the D-form (dextro-form).

There are two major classes of biochemicals whose members form stereoisomeric pairs. These are amino acids and monosaccharides (sugars). There are a few naturally occurring d-amino acids; however, the only amino acids that serve as substrates in human metabolism are those in the l-form. Conversely, among the monosaccharides, the d-form predominates and is the form active in human biochemistry.

In laboratory synthesis of an amino acid or a sugar, in the absence of a catalyst to direct the production of one stereoisomer or the other, an approximately equal mixture of l-form and d-form is made. This mixture is called a racemic mixture.

Reaction Specificity: Some enzymes are specific for the kind of reaction they catalyze. Regardless of whether an enzyme serves only one substrate or several, it always performs the same reaction. Using alcohol dehydrogenase again as an example, the only reaction it catalyzes is conversion between an alcohol and an aldehyde. As the name dehydrogenase implies, it removes the H^+ from an alcohol group (-COH) and converts it to an aldehyde group (-C=O). The most common substrate for alcohol dehydrogenase in human biochemistry is ethanol (ethyl alcohol).

An interesting side note, methanol (methyl alcohol, or wood alcohol) is a highly toxic alcohol. It becomes toxic by action of alcohol dehydrogenase. Ethanol serves as an antidote for methanol poisoning by occupying the alcohol dehydrogenase enzyme, thereby giving time for the lungs and kidneys to excrete the methanol before it is acted upon by alcohol dehydrogenase and becomes toxic.

Like most enzymes, the alcohol dehydrogenase reaction is reversible. That is, the enzyme will catalyze the same reaction in either direction. If the substrate it is presented with is an alcohol, it will convert it to an aldehyde; if the substrate is an aldehyde, it will convert it to an alcohol. This quality of reversibility is of great importance in providing flexibility and control of metabolic reactions.

PRESENCE OF SUBSTRATE: All enzymes respond to the presence of their substrates. An increase or decrease in quantity of a substrate will be accompanied by a corresponding increase or decrease in the quantity of the appropriate enzyme(s). There are two types of enzymes; those that are always present in some amount and those that biosynthesized only when their substrates are present. The former are called constitutive enzymes and the latter are called adaptive or inducible enzymes.

Adaptive Enzymes: Adaptive enzymes are not normally present in cells and tissues but are synthesized when stimulated to do so by the presence of their substrates. They are induced by the presence of their substrates. The genetic codes for making adaptive enzymes exist but they are not called upon to make them unless the enzymes are needed.

The discovery of adaptive enzymes was made decades ago in the early research on the metabolism of sugars. Baker's yeast, the experimental organism commonly used at the time, starts to grow immediately when placed in a glucose solution, as evidenced by CO_2 production. The same yeast, when placed in a solution of galactose (milk sugar) shows no growth for a period of time. Then growth starts, slowly at first, and then increases until it reaches the same rate of growth as it had in the glucose solution. The presence of galactose induces the galactose-metabolizing enzymes. The final proof is that galactose-adapted yeast, when put in fresh galactose solution, begins growth immediately, as it did when put in glucose solution.

The recognition of the existence of adaptive enzymes led to speculation that perhaps all enzymes are adaptive and that the many constitutive enzymes involved in the metabolic processes of daily living are always present because their substrates are always present.

ENZYME REACTIONS, ACTIVITY

An exquisite and complex organization that directs and controls the innumerable enzyme reactions required to support life exists within all cells and tissues. Enzyme reactions are not random but highly regulated. A brief mention of how enzymes work together and how their activity is influenced by the presence of other biochemicals can help with an understanding of metabolic pathways described in later chapters.

Although some enzymes operate alone in a single reaction, the great majority of enzymes within cells and tissues work together in a series of sequential reactions. Enzymes that work alone link with the substrate, conduct the appropriate reaction, and then release the product (metabolite) into the surrounding medium. The metabolite is then directed to the next step in its metabolism, which may be another enzymatic reaction, absorption or translocation to another site, incorporation into a structure, or storage.

Enzymes that work in series, such as those in cell mitochondria, occur together in a chain on a membrane or in some sort of matrix that holds them in a fixed pattern. The substrate enters the chain at one end and, in assembly-line fashion, is acted on by the first enzyme, passed on directly to the next enzyme in line, and so on through the chain until the final reaction takes place and the final metabolite is released into the medium. Intermediary metabolites produced along the chain that are also required for some other function of the organism can be drawn off from the chain as needed. Enzymes that work in series are important in reactions that convert macronutrients to smaller, usable units and oxidation reactions that produce energy for metabolic reactions.

Stimulation and inhibition of enzymes are important tools to help assure that metabolic requirements of an organism are met in an orderly and timely fashion. Stimulation of an enzymatic reaction can increase production of a metabolite when an increased demand occurs, and inhibition can slow production of a metabolite when the quantity produced exceeds demand. Enzymatic activity can be stimulated or inhibited by internal factors, such as the presence of hormones or other biochemical regulators, temperature, and pH.

In addition, there are a number of external factors that can either stimulate or inhibit enzyme activity, such as viruses, drugs or other foreign chemicals, coenzymes, and metal ions. However, probably the most important factor in controlling enzyme activity is the concentration of a reaction's own substrate or one or more of its metabolites. An increase in the concentration of its substrate or a decrease in the concentration of a metabolite is stimulatory. Conversely, a decrease in the concentration of its substrate or an increase in the concentration of a metabolite is inhibitory.

Digestion

Digestion converts bites of food into units small enough to be capable of passing through the wall of the digestive tract into the body. This section will deal primarily with the macronutrients because the processes of digestion are much more complex for them than are those required for micronutrients. In general, micronutrients require little modification (digestion) to gain entry into the body. Size is not a problem for most micronutrients because their molecules are already sufficiently small.

THE GASTROINTESTINAL (DIGESTIVE) TRACT

Foods must first be broken down physically to smaller and smaller pieces and then chemically to simpler chemicals in the gastrointestinal tract before they can be absorbed into the body where they are converted to biochemicals that provide materials and energy for life functions. Digestion refers to changes that take place in foods between the time they enter the mouth and the time the nutrients they contain are absorbed from the intestinal tract into the body.

Mouth and Stomach: The primary task of both the mouth and the stomach is mechanical fragmentation of food. The teeth begin the job by cutting large pieces of food into smaller pieces, which are then passed down the esophagus to the stomach. The stomach may be likened to a food processor in that it holds, grinds, and mixes food bites delivered from the mouth to form a semi-solid/liquid gruel called chyme. The residence time of the chyme in the stomach depends on its liquid content. A very liquid meal may empty in as little as 45 minutes, whereas a solid meal may take more than two hours for complete emptying. On the other hand, a drink of water on an empty stomach can pass through to the small intestine within a minute or two. This difference in residence time between full and empty stomachs is of critical importance when taking oral medications.

In addition to mechanical modification of food, both the mouth and the stomach secrete substances that start the chemical breakdown of macronutrients and prepare the chyme for final processing by the small intestine. Salivary secretions in the mouth, in addition to water, are α-amylase (ptyalin), an enzyme that starts the digestion of polysaccharides (long-chain carbohydrates), and lingual lipase, an enzyme that starts the digestion of medium chain triglycerides (fats). In addition to its digestive enzymes, saliva also helps the digestive process physically by secreting the protein mucin, which gives saliva its viscosity and aids in chewing dry foods.

Gastric juices are highly acidic (pH 1.8 to 3.5) as a result of hydrochloric acid (HAc) secretion by specialized cells in the wall of the stomach. Ptyalin, which has a pH optimum of 7 (the pH of saliva), is soon inactivated by the acid pH of the stomach. Lipase, on the other hand, which works best at a pH of 4, continues working in the stomach, but at a slower pace. HAc secretion helps protect the intestinal tract from microbial invasion and aids in the emulsification of dietary fats. Other gastric secretions include two proteins, the enzyme pepsin, which begins the cleavage of proteins, and intrinsic factor, which immediately binds vitamin B_{12} liberated from animal proteins and protects it from destruction by HAc in the chyme.

SMALL INTESTINE, PANCREAS, AND BILE: The small intestine is a long tube-like structure that is made up of three parts, the duodenum, the jejunum, and the ileum, each with its own special absorption role in the process. However, the major overall task of the small intestine is to complete the digestive process and to absorb the products of digestion into the body.

When the chyme is sufficiently ground and mixed, it is gradually released from the stomach into the duodenum of the small intestine to begin the final stage of digestion. The chyme is immediately mixed with alkaline solutions to neutralize the highly acidic chyme and to thin the mixture. These solutions are secreted by the small intestine (2 to 4 liters) and by the pancreas (1 liter), a glandular structure located near and connected to the duodenum by a duct. The pancreas also releases a number of enzymes that break down proteins (proteases), carbohydrates (amylases), and lipids (lipases) into the duodenum. Enzymes in the small intestine work best at a neutral pH.

Bile, which is primarily a waste product from the metabolic activity of the liver, is also secreted into the duodenum. Biliary secretion into the small intestine not only furnishes an avenue of excretion from the liver but also provides soaps (bile salts) that greatly enhance absorption of fats and other lipids, such as the fat soluble vitamins.

Bile is constantly being secreted by the liver and stored in the gall bladder until emptying is triggered by the presence of food in the stomach. One of the most important triggers for emptying the gall bladder is the presence of dietary fat in the duodenum. Frequent and adequate emptying of the gall bladder is necessary for the prevention of gallstone formation. Dietary regimens that restrict fat intake pose a threat of gall bladder stasis (cessation of contractions), which is a condition that favors formation of gallstones.

Transit of intestinal contents, from entry into the duodenum to exit from the ileum, normally takes from 12 to 14 hours. During this time the contents are twisted, squeezed, and mixed thoroughly with digestive enzymes. As nutrients are released from the mix, they are absorbed and transported across the intestinal wall. Almost all of the substances absorbed into the body from the small intestine require active transport by special enzyme systems to cross through the intestinal wall. Once inside the body, water-soluble nutrients plus a few small lipids travel via the hepatic portal vein to the liver for further processing while lipids travel via the lymphatic system to the heart where they enter the circulating blood.

LARGE INTESTINE: As soon as the contents of the small intestine finish their passage through the ileum, they enter the large intestine. At this point, digestion and absorption are essentially complete. The main task of the large intestine is to recover the water from the mixture and prepare the residue for elimination from the body.

Metabolism

As with digestion, this section will deal primarily with macronutrients. Once absorbed, micronutrients need little change (metabolism) to perform their highly individualized tasks, which they undertake alone or in combination with other micronutrients. Metabolism refers to the chemical changes that take place in nutrients after they leave the digestive tract and enter the body. Metabolism is the sum of all of the biochemical reactions that take place within living organisms. Metabolism is divided into three parts, *catabolism*, *anabolism*, and a whole area of cellular work between catabolism and anabolism that is given the catchall term of *intermediary metabolism*.

Catabolism refers to the breakdown or degradation of molecules. These are the reactions that take place to release energy for life functions and to break large molecules down for excretion or to other molecules needed by the organism. Anabolism refers to build up or synthesis of biochemicals. These are the reactions that make molecules needed for maintenance, repair, and reproduction. Intermediary metabolism includes all the cellular reactions in between breakdown and build-up.

ENERGY AND THE KREBS CYCLE

The metabolic pathways followed by macronutrients are unique to each macronutrient and are described separately in later chapters. However, in all aerobic organisms, even in the most primitive cellular forms, the ultimate source of energy that drives all life is provided by a single catabolic pathway known as the Krebs cycle.

The Krebs cycle is a major metabolic pathway found in all aerobic organisms. The Krebs cycle was first discovered in yeast cells by Hans Krebs in 1937. The Krebs cycle, also known as the citric acid cycle or the tricarboxylic acid cycle, is the final set of biochemical reactions that convert fats and carbohydrates to carbon dioxide, water, and chemical energy, which is stored primarily as high-energy phosphate bonds in adenosine triphosphate (ATP). Metabolites from the Krebs cycle also can be drawn off to serve as starting points for the biosynthesis of many other biochemicals that the organism needs, including those that may be either deficient in amount or totally lacking in the diet. This use of the Krebs cycle is important in providing nonessential amino acids for protein synthesis.

The Krebs cycle is present in every cell of every living organism that uses oxygen to sustain life. Figure 4-1 is a simplified diagram showing how lipids, carbohydrates, and proteins funnel into the Krebs cycle. Fats and carbohydrates are ultimately converted to an important intermediary biochemical known as acetyl CoA. Acetyl CoA is formed from acetic acid (acetate) and coenzyme A (vitamin B_5, pantothenic acid).

The acetate fraction of acetyl CoA enters the Krebs cycle by combining with oxaloacetic acid, a 4-carbon biochemical. The combination of acetate and oxaloacetic acid forms citric acid, a 6-carbon biochemical. Citric acid goes around through the cycle, yielding chemical energy in the form of high energy phosphate bonds (36 adenosine triphosphate (ATP) molecules), two molecules of CO_2, and two of H_2O, and finally regenerating oxaloacetic acid in the process. Oxaloacetic acid is then ready to accept acetate from another acetyl CoA and start the cycle again.

The oxidation of proteins through the Krebs cycle is a bit more complicated than is the oxidation of fats and carbohydrates. Proteins, like fats and carbohydrates, must first be broken down to their component amino acid units. Amino acids provided by the diet are used first for synthesis of the body's own proteins. Certain amino acids that are in excess of the body's need have pathways into the Krebs cycle. These are the nonessential amino acids. Nonessential amino acids are first deaminated and then enter the Krebs cycle by a simple reversal of the pathway that makes them from the cycle.

Amino acids that the body cannot make, the essential amino acids, have no direct pathway of entry into the Krebs cycle. Their primary function is to serve as substrates for the synthesis of the body's own proteins. Any essential amino acid that is in excess of need is broken down and excreted by its own unique, complicated pathway of catabolism.

Most of the reactions that lead to the Krebs cycle can be reversed. When the need arises in some other metabolic pathway for any one of the biochemicals in the Krebs cycle, it can be provided by reversing the appropriate pathway of the cycle.

Calories

Although all of the macronutrient food components have distinct biochemical properties and serve different functions, they have one property in common, namely caloric value. No discussion of foods or food regimes would be complete without some mention of calories and an explanation of what they are. Despite the fact that the most important goal of diet planning is to ensure a proper balance among macronutrients and an adequate intake of micronutrients, calorie counting seems to be the main concern for most people. calories might be likened to little dictators. Even people who do not fear or are not slaves to calories know about them and consider them important. Why is this so? It is probably because calories are blamed as being responsible for weight gain and obesity.

FIGURE 4-1
METABOLIC PATHWAYS OF NUTRIENTS

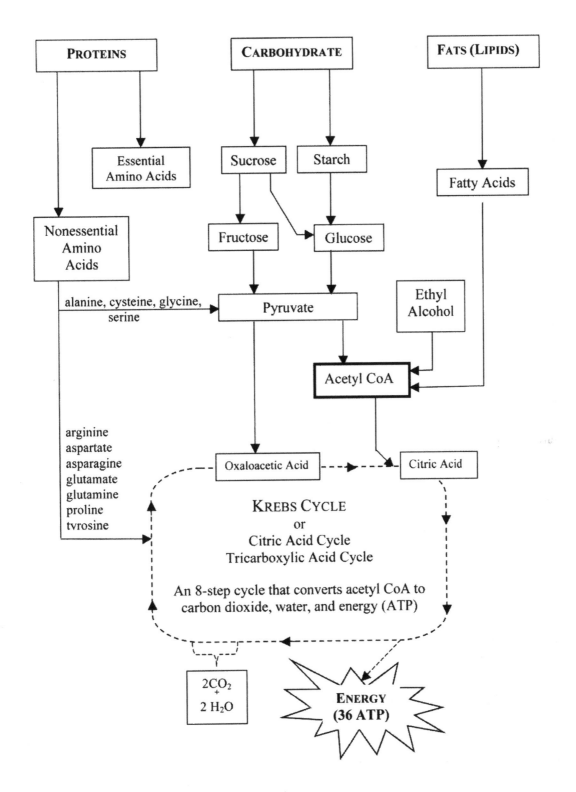

WHAT ARE CALORIES?

A feature common to all foods is that they are needed and used to supply energy for growth and life functions. A calorie is a unit of energy. The concept of the calorie came from the work of Lavoisier and other French chemists in the late eighteenth century. The calorie was defined as the amount of heat (energy) required to raise the temperature of one gram of water one-degree centigrade from $15°$ to $16°C$.

By the mid-nineteenth century, it was recognized that the heat produced by an animal body, called the physiological heat, was related to the animal's food intake. It was also found that similar kinds of foods, when combusted, consistently yielded the same number of calories per gram. Interestingly, the study of the caloric value of foods revealed that the calorie of physical chemistry was much too small to be used as the calorie for physiological measurements. It was not only much too small but also much too cumbersome – like using inches to measure the distance between two cities.

Creating a new calorie for food that contained 1,000 of the older, small calories solved the problem. The old calorie was still called the calorie, or small calorie. The new calorie was named the large calorie, also called the kilocalorie (kcal) or Calorie (calorie with a capital C). Today, the distinction between small and large calories seems to be lost in lay circles; a calorie with a small C is often used when referring to the large food calories.

The study of the Caloric value of food showed that the quantity of heat released by fat was constant at 9.3 Calories per gram, whether the combustion occurred outside in a calorimeter or inside an animal body. Carbohydrates behaved in the same manner except that the heat released was 4.1 Calories per gram. Proteins, on the other hand, were anomalous. They produced 5.3 Calories when burned in a calorimeter, but only 4.1 Calories when metabolized by an animal body. The reason for this is that when proteins are burned in a calorimeter, they are burned completely and all of the energy is released. However, when they are used to make energy in a living body, the amino groups are first removed. Amino groups are then excreted from the body as the waste product urea, which still contains some energy value, leaving only 4.1 Calories for use by the animal. Carbohydrates and fats, on the other hand, are completely oxidized and all the energy is extracted by both the animal body and the calorimeter.

The Caloric value for foods in carbohydrate, protein, and fat categories are not all 4.1, 4.1, and 9.3, respectively. These figures are just the averages of values determined for many hundreds of foods in each category. For example, starch yields 4.2 Calories per gram, and sucrose 3.9 Calories per gram. In order to make the calculation of Caloric value of a diet a reasonably achievable exercise, the values for Calories per gram in carbohydrates, proteins, and fats are rounded off and taken as 4, 4, and 9, respectively. Alcohol (ethyl alcohol), which is sort of a hybrid between the fat and carbohydrate categories, yields 7 Calories per gram.

In recent years, Calories have become a subject of controversy between the philosophies of traditional nutrition and what we will call alternative nutrition, as a parallel to alternative medicine. Traditional nutrition maintains that the amount of energy obtained from a food Calorie is independent of its source. Advocates of alternative nutrition propose that the amount of energy obtained from a food Calorie differs, depending on its source. This controversy alone is sufficient reason to explore the subject of Calories.

IS A CALORIE A CALORIE?

The obesity epidemic in America has been growing for years. Over these same years, official policy, based on the views of traditional nutritional experts, has been that Calories are independent of the type of food eaten. Very simply, if a person ingests more Calories than needed, the surplus Calories will be stored as body fat. On the other hand, intake of fewer Calories than required will result in weight loss. It does not matter if beefsteak, bread, or butter provides the Calories; too many Calories will cause weight gain and too few Calories will result in weight loss. Such diets have been tried and weight loss can be made to occur. However, the insurmountable problem is that the current high-carbohydrate, low-fat diet of the Food Guide Pyramid is a combination of food Calories that encourages hunger and obesity.

The alternative position, based on the views of a few interested scientists who have studied biochemistry and physiology, has been that not all Calories are equal because carbohydrates, proteins, and fat Calories are used differently by the body. Thus, all Calories are not the same. The macronutrient Calories are related largely to the composition of the diet. The traditional nutritional experts would be correct if they were studying the operation of furnaces. But the body is not a furnace that burns food; it is a finely tuned, biochemical system that utilizes food for many purposes in addition to energy. A very few examples are: carbohydrates influence insulin, a powerful hormone that controls body functions. Proteins provide the building blocks for muscle and bone. Fat provides energy and controls hunger.

Papers by Feinman and Fine (5, 6) explain the scientific basis for why this apparent contradiction does not violate thermodynamic principles, as claimed by traditional nutrition. An excellent and easy to understand discussion on the subject of thermodynamics and food Calories is available on the Protein Power web site (7).

More important than whether or not all Calories are equal is what the nutritional value of the food is that provides the Calories. Let anyone who believes that a Calorie is a Calorie try to survive on a diet in which all Calories are provided by table sugar. As a practical matter, the evidence that Calories are not metabolically equal is the basis for some very successful books and dietary strategies that have induced weight loss, controlled weight gain, and improved overall health (2; 8; 9; 10).

CALORIE RESTRICTION

The relatively new dietary practice of Calorie restriction has been seriously misunderstood by a number of people who reject it as a deprivation or starvation regimen. In actual practice, it is a diet that provides just the amount of food required each day rather than the greater amount that most people consume. Calorie restriction entails much more than simply reducing daily caloric intake. It requires that the diet contain the full complement of all essential nutrients, including vitamins, minerals, amino acids, a healthful ratio of essential fatty acids, a healthful balance of macronutrients, plus sufficient Calories to maintain a normal weight. When properly implemented, it is a satisfying diet.

The current interest in Calorie restriction had its beginnings decades ago in the early animal-feeding studies of pharmacological and toxicological effects of chemicals. Controlled feeding was a common and necessary practice because it was essential to know precisely how much feed experimental animals had ingested in order to calculate the dose they received of the chemical that had been added to their feed. Animals in control groups were often fed all they wanted (*ad libitum*) in order to save the time and labor of measuring their feed consumption. The determination of feed intake *per se* by control animals was not considered important.

These early studies gave rise to numerous reports that some groups of animals fed experimental diets were healthier and grew better than did the control animals (4, p. 73). Were the differences due to differences in quantity of feed consumed? Experiments were designed specifically to answer this question. They demonstrated that, all other conditions being equal, animals fed restricted but nutritionally adequate quantities of feed were healthier, had fewer tumors, and lived longer than animals that were permitted to eat all of the feed they wanted.

Such data were not only puzzling but also very disconcerting. For many years, no explanation was forthcoming on how diet restriction could possibly produce healthier animals with fewer benign and malignant tumors. Today, new knowledge and techniques in the fields of genetics and aging offer the promise of an explanation (11). There is every reason to believe that Calorie restriction would provide the same benefits to humans as it does to animals.

To avoid misunderstanding, it should be stressed here that Calorie restriction does *not* mean Calorie deprivation. It refers to the concept of balancing caloric intake in food with caloric expenditure required for life functions and activities. When a balance of Calories is achieved, there are no extra Calories that must be diverted to excess body fat or excess cholesterol. Calorie restriction is reported to be the only reliable method for extending maximum life span (11). Studies of the relationship between Calorie restriction and the genetic patterns of aging support the theory that this new nutritional approach to good health and longevity is a valid one (12). If Calorie restriction is the appropriate dietary model for humans, the current American diet should be labeled *Calorie extravagance.* Meanwhile, practicing Calorie restriction as intended certainly can do no harm.

A final suggestion for a person who wants to reduce food intake is to eat slowly. Because it takes about 20 minutes for the brain to realize there is food in the stomach, it is recommended that at least 30 minutes are spent in consuming a meal (13). When food is consumed rapidly, more than sufficient food is eaten before the sensation of hunger is appeased. Speed eating almost guarantees overeating.

MUCH ADO ABOUT NOTHING?

Despite the enormous importance attributed to Calories by the nutrition community, Calorie counting is little more than a pedantic exercise with little practical importance for the average person. In fact, a recent survey by the International Food Information Council Foundation found that only one out of every eight adults knows how many Calories he should eat in a day (14). Confusion abounds about Calories despite a sincere desire on the part of the public to eat a healthful diet.

The bureaucratic response is not to provide practical nutrition data, but rather to educate the public in the concept of Calories. The practical and much more user-friendly solution, as will be explained in Chapter Twelve, is to provide information on what foods are in the three macronutrient categories and what fraction of total intake should come from each category. Calorie restriction then becomes, very simply, a serving-size restriction.

References

1.)   Davis A. Let's Eat Right to Keep Fit. New York, NY: A Signet Book, 1970.

2.)   Eades MR, Eades MD. Protein Power, New York, NY: Bantam Books, 1999.

3.)   Pelton R, et al. Drug-Induced Nutrient Depletion Handbook. Hudson, OH: Lexi-Comp Inc., 2001.

4.)   Frank P, Ottoboni MA. The Dose Makes the Poison: A Plain-Language Guide to Toxicology, 3rd Edition. New York, NY: John Wiley & Sons, 2011.

5.)   Feinman RD, Fine EJ. "A calorie is a calorie" violates the second law thermo- dynamics. Nutrition Journal. 2004; 3: 9. http://nutritionj.com/content/3/1/9/ Accessed Sept. 26, 2012.

6.)   Feinman RD, Fine EJ. Thermodynamics and metabolic advantage of weight loss diets. Metabolic Syndrome and Related Disorders. 2003; 1(3): 209-219.

7.)   http://www.proteinpower.com/ Accessed Sept. 26, 2012.

8.)   Sears, Barry. Enter the Zone. New York, NY: Regan Books imprint of HarperCollins Publisher, 1995.

9.)   Simopoulos, Artemis P. The Omega Plan. New York, NY: HarperCollins Publishers, 1998.

10.)   Atkins, Robert C. Dr. Atkins' New Diet Revolution. New York, NY: Avon Books, Inc. 1999.

11.) Fahy, Gregory M. Aging Revealed. Life Extension Magazine. November 1999: 52-69.

12.) Greenwell I. Eat Less – But Do Eat Lots of Blueberries. Life Extension Magazine. Sept 1999: 26-34.

13.) Quillin P. Controlling Food Binges. Nature's Impact. Feb/Mar 1998:46-49.

14.) http://www.physiquespeak.com/2010/07/15/majority-of-americans-can't-count-calories/ Accessed Sept. 26, 2012.

Chapter Five

Nutritional Supplements

No vitamin, mineral, herb, food, drug or doctor ever "cures" any condition. The body cures itself when it receives the necessary raw materials.
Walter A. Heiby (1, p. 85).

Over the years, more and more Americans have discovered nutritional supplements. In spite of admonitions by government and nutrition organizations that nutritional supplements are unnecessary and perhaps even harmful, sales of supplements have grown steadily year by year. In 1982, supplement sales amounted to only two billion dollars. By 1999, sales were more than 15 billion dollars (2). From 2005 to 2009, the market grew by a total of 26 per cent (3). With increasing life expectancy and with the interest of people in health and nutrition, there is every reason to assume the trend will continue.

Several decades ago, the only micronutrients known to nutritional scientists were a few vitamins and minerals. These few micronutrients made up the sum of nutritional supplements available to the general public. Now the number of supplements known and available has increased exponentially. This is largely the result of the great strides that have taken place in the biochemical sciences in the past few decades.

So much more is known now about the biochemical reactions that occur within the human body and so much more about nutrients associated with optimum health. These nutrients include not only vitamins and minerals but also essential amino acids, essential fatty acids, antioxidants, hormones, enzymes, herbs, and assorted biochemicals that are used as intermediates in a variety of important functions in the body.

Are Supplements Necessary?

With the exception of vitamins and essential minerals, many of the hundreds of nutritional supplements now available in health food stores are biochemicals that can be synthesized by the human body. If the body can make them, why should anyone take them as supplements? And what about the many vitamins and minerals the body cannot make but are available in foods? Do people really need to supplement their diets with nutrients that are nonessential, or even those that are essential?

Depending on whom one asks, the answer is an emphatic "No" or an equally emphatic "Yes." The emphatic "No" comes from establishment nutrition. The consensus among the majority of nutritionists in academia and in government is that a proper diet that follows the USDA official dietary guidelines described in MyPyramid (4) provides all of the vitamin and mineral nutrients that a person requires. The emphatic "Yes" comes from what might be termed alternative nutrition, the nutritional counterpart of alternative medicine. Alternative nutrition maintains that the so-called proper diet that follows MyPyramid is nutritionally inadequate for many people.

THE "NO" ARGUMENT

The general argument against supplementation is that it is not necessary. This argument is based on information in two huge banks of records collected since the beginnings of nutritional science a little over a hundred years ago. One bank contains information on the human requirements for macronutrients and all or most vitamins and minerals. The other bank contains data on nutrient composition of practically every known or conceivable food. The findings contained in these two sources provided the basis for the ultimate achievement of nutritional science, the *Dietary Guidelines for Americans* (5), as detailed in MyPyramid. MyPyramid is calculated to contain all of the nutrients that are required; therefore, if MyPyramid is followed, supplementation is not necessary.

A less publicized argument against supplementation is nutritional science's professed concern for public health. It recognizes that the snake-oil phenomenon is still with us, even though the medicine show is a thing of the past. The medicine show has been supplanted by direct mail advertisements, infomercials, expert opinions, and "medical" reports in the popular press. Many useless nostrums are hyped as cures for everything from ingrown toenails to cancer. Exploiters of public ignorance are probably the principal reason why the American Dietetic Association (ADA), a voice of traditional nutrition, has adopted a rather inflexible position against individuals choosing their own supplements. One goal of the ADA is to protect a gullible nation against charlatans.

THE "YES" ARGUMENT

The argument for nutritional supplementation is based primarily on belief in the principle that a person has a right to make his own decisions about his own health. With regard to nutritional supplements, as mentioned above, this belief is contrary to official U.S. nutrition policy. Despite official disapproval, the nutritional supplement industry is thriving and expanding because increasing numbers of people are purchasing supplements. Why is this so? Why do Americans feel a need for nutritional supplementation? Most people will follow dietary recommendations they consider honest and accurate.

While official RDAs (recommended dietary allowances) and AIs (adequate intakes) provide some guidance for people, in most instances the recommendations are generally recognized as being too conservative, They are designed only to prevent overt deficiency disease. This leads to what is probably the most compelling argument for supplementation - to achieve optimum health as opposed to just enough for deficiency-disease prevention. Alternative nutrition generally follows the theory that even if a proper diet does provide all of the micronutrients necessary to prevent overt deficiency diseases, it may not contain amounts adequate for *optimum* health.

RDA INADEQUACY: There are many examples of nutrients that display increasing benefits with increasing doses above the minimum required for prevention of overt deficiency disease. Of these, ascorbic acid (vitamin C) is just one. The daily intake of vitamin C required to prevent scurvy is between 30 and 50 milligrams. Many years ago, the recommended daily intake for ascorbic acid was set at 60 milligrams, an amount just sufficient to prevent scurvy in the majority of people. Over a decade ago, the Food and Nutrition Board (FNB) of the Institute of Medicine recommended that the RDA for vitamin C be raised to 100 or 200 milligrams (6). This recommendation was a response to many clinical and other scientific studies showing that optimum health requires many times more than 60 milligrams of vitamin C. Despite a recommendation by FNB, essentially no change has been made in the RDA, and no change is expected in the near future.

Nutrition officialdom's reluctance to consider scientific data that challenge the minimal nature of its nutrient standards is counterproductive in assuring the public that those nutrient standards are sufficiently protective of their health. People are concerned about their health and are now much more knowledgeable about nutritional supplements than they have been in years past. The failure of the nutrition establishment to acknowledge that there is often a vast difference between the amount of a nutrient that will prevent overt disease and the amount that will foster optimum health contributes to public skepticism about the adequacy of official recommendations.

Further, rejection of scientific data that do not fit nutrition dogma casts doubt on the objectives of the bureaucracy that promulgates nutrient standards and the validity of their recommendations for all other nutrients. An excellent source of scientific information on all essential and nonessential micronutrients and macronutrients is the information center of the Linus Pauling Institute at Oregon State University (7).

THE REALITY

In the real world, there are many reasons why people do not receive sufficient amounts of some or many micronutrients from their food. One important reason is that nutritional needs change with age. It is common and accepted knowledge that the nutritional needs of infants and children are very different from those of adults. It is less commonly known that older people, even elders in apparent good health, also have special nutritional requirements. A complicating factor is the loss of appetite that the elderly frequently suffer. In addition to loss of appetite, other factors, such as dental problems, may make chewing difficult. Finally, for any number of reasons, the nutrients the elderly actually do consume are often poorly absorbed.

The needs of elders are often not recognized because changes in health and activity with age occur very slowly almost without notice. Prescription and over-the-counter drugs can alter nutritional needs, as can the illnesses for which the medications are taken. Lowered levels of physical activity can result in smaller appetite, which, in turn, reduces the normal intake of nutrients in food. Further, the loss of youthful vigor that is part of aging, if not recognized, can lead to irregular eating habits, overuse of fast foods, and loss of interest in preparing ample and balanced meals every day.

People have no inner alarm system that tells them their biochemistry is suffering from less than optimum supplies of vitamins or minerals. The human body is very forgiving. It struggles along, without complaint, on what is provided for as long as it can and as best it can. Fortunately, the body repairs quickly when given the nutrients it requires.

Another reality is that even healthy people often have different requirements for the essential nutrients. This fact is based on the concept of biochemical individuality, pioneered by the late nutritional biochemist Roger J. Williams. Dr. Williams demonstrated that it is a biological reality that there is no such thing as an average person. Most people require greater amounts of one or more specific nutrients than the amounts recommended by the Food and Drug Administration (FDA). They cannot achieve optimum health if those nutrients are not added as supplements to their diets. In written testimony to the FDA, Dr. Williams argued for nutritional supplementation as insurance against deficiency (8, p. 119).

Dr. Williams' appeal for nutritional insurance prompts one to ask, "If I am deficient in one or more nutrients, why am I not ill?" The answer lies in the fact that, for most essential nutrients, there is a minimum amount that will prevent overt deficiency disease and a greater amount that is used to serve other important functions. While minimum amounts of essential nutrients are present in most diets, larger amounts are often required for optimum health. Thus, because obvious cases of nutritional deficiency are uncommon, it is easy to assume that none exist. Moreover, nutritional deficiencies cause cognitive decline with the result that the victim tends not to recognize the problem.

FOOD FORTIFICATION: Despite their conviction that nutritional supplementation is not necessary, the ADA and federal bureaucracies concerned with the nutritional status of the American people acknowledge that, in certain circumstances, there is justification for nutritional supplementation. To this end, the Food and Drug Administration (FDA) was charged several decades ago with administration of food fortification regulations (9). Examples of food fortification requirements set by the FDA include: vitamin B12 for strict vegetarians (vegetables do not contain B_{12}); folic acid for women of childbearing age (prevention of spina bifida); vitamin D for people with limited sources of vitamin D (exposure to sunlight); calcium for people who have lactose intolerance (lactose is the disaccharide in milk); and the B-vitamins niacin and thiamin for the general public (to prevent pellagra and beriberi).

The subject of food fortification brings up an interesting philosophical point. It is nutrition officialdom's position that a proper diet provides all of the nutrients that are necessary, yet it supports a policy of food fortification to provide the public with certain micronutrients that may be wanting in the food supply. The question is if the food supply is lacking in certain nutrients, how can a proper diet be planned without including supplementation? The practice of fortification is tacit proof that supplementation is necessary for some nutrients and for some people; it has been of inestimable health benefit for a great many people.

The fact is that food fortification by government regulation is a formally approved form of nutritional supplementation. Thus, it appears to be official FDA policy that nutritional supplementation is acceptable if done under the direction and control of the government, but not acceptable if done by individuals to meet their own personal needs.

Nutrient Standards

A brief explanation of the history and definition of the several acronyms commonly used in the nutrition literature and on food labels may be helpful in the study of micronutrients. These acronyms refer to nutrient standards set by the FDA. The first standard was the MDR (minimum daily requirement). Prior to World War II, MDRs were set for the few vitamins that had been identified up to that time. By the late 1930s, as a result of the tremendous expansion of the nutrition database, it was recognized that the few MDRs that were in existence had become outdated. Thus, the RDA (recommended dietary allowance) was created, which utilized more scientifically based nutrition data (10).

In 1990, the Nutrition Labeling and Education Act was passed to require that food labels list nutrient components and their daily requirements. After the act was passed, FDA realized that the number of RDAs in existence were insufficient to satisfy the food industry's labeling requirements. Because of the insufficiency of RDAs, FDA had to develop further standards to meet labeling needs. Thus began the development of an alphabet soup of nutrition acronyms that are quite confusing and very difficult to use by all but the most sophisticated of dietitians.

First, FDA created the DV (daily value) as the umbrella standard for all nutrients that must be listed on food labels (11). DVs include two sets of reference standards. One is the RDI (reference daily intake) for vitamins, minerals, and proteins. RDIs are based on RDAs or, in the case of nutrients for which no RDAs have been established, on the recommendations of the Food and Nutrition Board (FNB) of the National Academies' Institute of Medicine. The second reference standard is the DRV (daily reference value). DRVs are suggested daily intakes for food components for which no set of standards previously existed but which are important for health, such as fat and fiber.

In 1994, the FNB embarked on an ambitious initiative, with the support of the United States and Canadian governments, to develop a new and broader set of DRVs, which are collectively known as DRIs (dietary reference intakes). The DRIs were designed to expand upon and replace the RDAs issued in prior years. The DRIs were published as they were prepared between 1997 and 2005. They were issued collectively in 2006 in the DRI guide book (5).

DRIs include four nutrient-based reference values designed to assess and plan the diets of healthy people. The first DRI is the EAR (estimated average requirement), which is the average daily nutrient intake level estimated to meet the requirements of half of the healthy people in specific population groups. The second DRI is the well-known RDA, except that the new RDA varies with specific population groups whereas the former RDA was a one-size-fits-all value.

The new RDA is equal to the EAR minus two standard deviations. The third DRI, the AI (adequate intake), applies to nutrients or food components for which an RDA cannot be determined. It is based on fewer scientific data and is essentially a judgment call on the part of the FNB. The fourth DRI is the UL (tolerable upper intake level), which refers to the highest level of daily intake that is likely to pose no risk of adverse effects. For each DRI reference value, 24 specific population groups have been identified (twelve life-stage groups for each gender).

Any recommended intakes or supporting data mentioned in the balance of this chapter are for adults. Recommended intakes for other life stages, plus further information about dosages, requirements, deficiency signs and symptoms, and beneficial effects on which the intakes were based, can be found in the DRI guide (5). Readers who recall RDAs from prior years will find that many of these have been replaced with AIs because of more stringent criteria established by FNB for setting of new RDAs.

Vitamins

The late 19th and early 20th centuries are appropriately referred to as the period of the discovery of vitamins. It was through the recognition that some diseases, now referred to as the classic nutritional diseases, could be cured by certain foods that the existence of vitamins was made known. Cause-effect relationships could be established relatively easily because the symptoms of a disease resulting from a deficiency of a vitamin are specific to that vitamin. In 1906, Frederick Gowland Hopkins labeled the "astonishingly small amounts" of certain substances in food that were curative as "accessory food factors." In 1912, Casimir Funk named these unknown substances "vitamines," meaning "vital amines," because he thought they were amine (NH_2) compounds. When it was found that not all vitamins were amines, the final "e" was dropped (12, p. 554).

There are thirteen officially recognized vitamins. These are vitamin A, vitamin C, vitamin D, vitamin E, vitamin K, and eight B vitamins. The eight B vitamins are B1 (thiamin), B2 (riboflavin), B3 (niacin), B5 (pantothenic acid), B6 (pyridoxine), B12 (cobalamin), biotin, and folic acid. The first vitamin to be discovered was thiamin in 1897. This was followed by vitamin A in 1909, vitamin C in 1912, and vitamin D in 1918. The last vitamin to be discovered was folic acid in 1941. All of the known vitamins were isolated in pure form by 1948 and synthesized by 1972 (13, p. 3).

A great deal has been learned about the functions and interactions of vitamins since the discovery of thiamin over 100 years ago. The minimum amount required to prevent overt disease is well known for each vitamin, but the *optimum* amount, the amount that affords and sustains maximum good health, is not known for any vitamin. As a result there has been a great deal of controversy about what amounts of which vitamin supplements, if any, people should take. More complete information about individual vitamins, minerals, or other nutritional supplements can be found in the DRI guide (5), the Oregon State University website (7), or any popular nutrition textbook or handbook.

MULTIVITAMIN PREPARATIONS

Interesting findings on the benefits of multivitamin supplementation are coming from continuing evaluation and follow-up of the subjects in the famous Harvard Nurses' Study (14). In the Nurses' Study, roughly 90,000 women who were free of cancer in 1980 provided updated assessments of their diets and multivitamin use from 1980 to 1994. The objective of the investigation reported here was to evaluate the relation between folate (folic acid, a B vitamin) intake and the incidence of colon cancer.

Statistical evaluation of the data indicated that folate intake from dietary sources alone was associated with a modest reduction in risk for colon cancer. It also showed that long-term multivitamin intake appeared to be beneficial. The study concluded that long-term use of multivitamins may substantially reduce the risk for colon cancer and that this effect may be due to the folate present in multivitamin preparations (15). Hence, a good brand of multivitamin pill taken daily provides insurance that minimum needs are met.

Reputable manufacturers of multivitamin pills follow FDA guidelines on which and how much of each vitamin to include and what the appropriate daily dose should be. Each vitamin has its own special functions; thus, depending on personal health needs, some people may want to increase the daily intake of one or more of the vitamins. However, anyone considering increasing the intake of any one or several vitamins in addition to a multivitamin pill should not do so without some study and without some idea of what the supplementation is expected to achieve. With the exception of vitamins A and D, vitamins are essentially nontoxic, but imbalances in intake can create health problems.

WATER-SOLUBLE VITAMINS

Water-soluble vitamins (vitamin C and the B vitamins) are present in the aqueous medium of the body. They do not have storage sites in the body, thus must be supplied in the diet on a regular basis. Amounts greater than what the body uses each day are excreted primarily in the urine.

Claims that excretion of water-soluble vitamins only occurs after all the needs for them have been satisfied and that any excretion indicates excessive intake are not biochemically valid. Because of the great complexity of metabolic interactions, some fraction of whatever the daily intake of a water-soluble vitamin will be excreted. The most basic and easily satisfied function of a vitamin will be taken care of first, with a certain fraction of the intake being excreted. As intake increases, more of the vitamin's different functions are served, with a certain fraction still being excreted. It is only when an optimum amount is ingested (which is not known for any vitamin at any given time for any individual) that a further increase in intake produces no further benefit. It is only at this point that the amount excreted is truly an excess of the vitamin and that the label of "expensive urine" would be appropriate.

A helpful example of what might be termed the multilevel requirement for nutrients is a water bucket with a series of holes in it running from top to bottom on one side. As water is poured into the bucket, the water level rises until water begins to flow out of the lowest hole. As water continues to be poured into the bucket, the level rises further and water starts flowing out of the second hole, then the third hole, and so on until water reaches the top and spills over. Each hole in the bucket can be thought of as representing a different function of the vitamin, with the top of the bucket representing optimum requirement.

The Institute of Medicine apparently accepts the concept of multilevel requirements for nutrients. In setting DRI values for vitamin C, the Institute of Medicine used vitamin C's nutrient adequacy for immune system protection, rather than the lesser requirement for prevention of scurvy, as the criterion (5, p. 9).

VITAMIN C (ASCORBIC ACID): If the public were permitted to have only one vitamin supplement, a strong case could be made that vitamin C should be that vitamin. The tremendous amount of scientific interest in the role of vitamin C in human health is evidenced by international conferences on the subject, such as those convened by the New York Academy of Sciences in 1960, 1974, and in 1986 (16). It is well known that vitamin C is both a potent antioxidant for normal cells and a lethal oxidant for cancer cells. Further, the evidence is compelling that it is a vitamin that is virtually impossible to obtain in amounts adequate for optimum health from diet alone. In addition, dietary intakes of many thousands of times larger than the RDA have not been shown to be harmful; on the contrary, they have been shown to have strong anticancer properties (17).

Beneficial Effects: The benefits of vitamin C are many and varied because it participates in so many different biochemical mechanisms. In addition to promoting the nonspecific benefits of general good health, vitamin C fosters good dental health, furthers wound healing, and aids in prevention and cure of colds and other infectious diseases through its role in immune function (18). Probably the most publicized benefit of vitamin C relates to its antioxidant properties and protection of essential fatty acid double bonds. Vitamin C works together with other antioxidants such as vitamin E to help prevent and reverse damage done by oxidation of critical biochemicals. Thus, as an antioxidant, vitamin C is credited with possessing not only anti-aging properties but also anticancer properties.

The effect of high doses of vitamin C on the development and course of various heart-related illnesses has been the subject of numerous scientific studies since that time. Excellent reviews of the findings of these and other studies confirm that large doses of vitamin C do have beneficial effects in the treatment of heart-related illnesses (19; 20).

Deficiency Symptoms: Deficiencies of vitamin C that are severe enough to result in frank scurvy are rare in developed countries, but mild deficiencies may be fairly common, particularly among the elderly and people suffering debilitating diseases. Smokers also have a much greater need for vitamin C than do nonsmokers. Among the symptoms of mild deficiency (borderline scurvy) are tender or bleeding gums, frequent upper respiratory infections, prolonged healing of cuts and scrapes, and tendency to develop black and blue marks.

Because full-blown scurvy is no longer common, its clinical features are no longer well appreciated. As a result, patients with mild scurvy are often misdiagnosed (21). This is particularly true among the elderly. Vitamin C supplementation is of special importance for the elderly; they are the people at greatest risk of developing subclinical scurvy.

A review of the literature suggests that some hospital deaths attributed to multiple organ failure may be the result of subclinical scurvy in patients whose illnesses have depleted their systems of the last of their vitamin C reserves, which give rise to fatal scurvy (22).

Human Requirements for Vitamin C: The optimum daily intake of vitamin C for guinea pigs, a species that, like humans, requires vitamin C, is 5 milligrams per 100 grams of body weight (23). Accordingly, the amount required by a guinea pig would be the equivalent of approximately 3,500 milligrams for an adult human. In an effort to estimate the probable need of vitamin C for humans, numerous studies have investigated the quantities of vitamin C synthesized by species that can make their own vitamin C.

Burns (16, p. 535) found that laboratory rats synthesize daily an amount of vitamin C that would be equivalent to approximately 2,000 milligrams for a 154-pound human. Most animals, including cows, sheep, cats, and dogs, synthesize vitamin C in amounts that would be equivalent to about 10,000 milligrams a day for an adult human (24, p. 77).

The foregoing data provide a strong argument for the theory that the human requirement for vitamin C is in gram quantities, with a minimum of one-gram (1,000 milligrams) rather than the milligram quantities of the RDA. There is no reason to assume that, for optimum health, humans need less vitamin C than do other animals. Animals would not synthesize so much vitamin C a day if it were not necessary. As a general rule, living organisms are very frugal. They do not waste energy in making biochemicals they do not need or in amounts greater than they need.

THE B VITAMINS: B vitamins are water-soluble organic chemicals that are present in all animal, yeast, and plant cells. It was first thought that there was only one B vitamin. It was designated as "the water soluble growth vitamin" and later named vitamin B (vitamin A had already been discovered). It was soon realized that vitamin B was actually two distinct substances rather than one. Accordingly, thiamin, the first to be isolated, became B1, and riboflavin, the second to be isolated, became B2. As other B vitamins were discovered, the group became referred to as the vitamin-B complex.

The question of why B vitamins appear not to be numbered in sequence is explained by the fact that in the early days of discovery, more and more compounds were being isolated from liver or yeast brews. As new ones were found, they were given numbers in series, until finally there were about seventeen B vitamins. Scientists then decided that there had to be more specific criteria for classifying a substance as a B vitamin, other than merely finding it in water extracts of B-vitamin-rich sources such as liver or yeast.

It was decided that for a vitamin to be classed as a B vitamin, it must be water-soluble, must be essential for all living cells, and, perhaps most important, it must function as a coenzyme. As a result, many already-numbered B vitamins were dropped from the category, along with the numbers assigned to them, because they did not function as coenzymes, even though they might be essential nutrients in other respects. Later, when additional vitamins that fit the B-vitamin definition were discovered, they were given names rather than numbers. Examples are biotin and folic acid.

B vitamins do not have long-term storage sites in the body. Therefore, they should be supplied each day in food. Any B-vitamin molecules that are not used soon after absorption are excreted, even if they may be needed somewhere else in the body. As a result, as mentioned above, the presence of a water-soluble vitamin in the urine does not necessarily signify that an excess of the vitamin has been ingested. Some amount of the vitamin will always appear in the urine, even with intakes that are less than optimal.

Coenzyme Functions: As pointed out earlier, in order for a nutrient to be classed as a B vitamin, it must function as a coenzyme. The B-vitamins, the coenzymes they form, and the enzymatic functions they serve are listed in Table 5-1.

TABLE 5-1
B-VITAMIN COENZYMES

Vitamin	Vitamin Name - Coenzyme	Metabolic Function
Vitamin B1	Thiamin Pyrophosphate	Transfer of two-carbon units
Vitamin B2	Riboflavin - FAD (flavin adenine dinucleotide)	Oxidation-reduction reactions (2 electrons)
Vitamin B3	Niacin - NAD (nicotinamide adenine dinucleotide)	Oxidation-reduction reactions (1, 2 electrons)
Vitamin B5	Pantothenic Acid - Coenzyme A	Transfer of acyl groups
Vitamin B6	Pyridoxine - Pyridoxal Phosphate	Transfers to and from amino acids
Vitamin B12	Cobalamin - Adenosylcobalamin	Relocations, methyl group transfer
Biotin	Biotin - Biotin	Carboxyl group transfers
Folic Acid	Folic Acid - Tetrahydrofolate	Transfer of one-carbon units

Cautions and Toxicity: When taking supplements of individual B vitamins, it is extremely important to understand that most vitamins of the B complex work together and that great excesses of any one can result in deficiencies of one or more of the others. It is recommended, for example, that vitamins B1, B2, and B6 (thiamin, riboflavin, and pyridoxine, respectively) should be taken in equal quantities. Although, the B vitamins are of a low order of toxicity, an imbalance of them in the diet can cause serious problems. For this reason, anyone designing his or her own dietary regime should not include megadoses of any supplement without first studying and learning about it.

Homocysteine Regulators: The relationship between elevated blood levels of homocysteine and heart disease was first proposed by Kilmer McCully in1969 (25). It is now known that proper regulation of homocysteine metabolism (26), which is crucial for cardiac health, requires participation of three B vitamins. These are B_6, B_{12}, and folic acid.

These three B vitamins are often referred to, along with trimethylglycine, as homocysteine regulators. Homocysteine and its important biochemical role in the methyl transfer cycle are discussed in Chapter Seven (see Figure 7-1).

McCully recommends supplementation with a minimum of 3 milligrams of vitamin B6, 100 micrograms of vitamin B12, and 400 micrograms of folic acid to prevent homocystein-emia (25). Interestingly, the Institute of Medicine's DRI publication (5) mentions only that vitamin B$_{12}$ is a coenzyme in the conversion of homocysteine to methionine and that the evidence that folic acid is of benefit in vascular, cancer, or mental diseases is insufficient to use in setting folic acid requirements.

LIPID-SOLUBLE VITAMINS

The lipid-soluble vitamins, A, D, E, and K, are themselves lipids and are present in the lipid fraction of the diet. All have structures that contain both carbon rings and straight chains, and all are strongly hydrophobic. Low-fat diets tend to be deficient in lipid vita-mins, and their absorption from the intestinal tract is diminished in the absence of dietary fats. Despite their similarity to each other in their physical properties, they differ widely from each other in function.

VITAMIN A (RETINOL): The RDAs for retinol are given in micrograms, which is very confusing to most people because they are accustomed to seeing supplements of vitamin A expressed as IU (international units). One IU equals 0.3 micrograms of retinol (preformed vitamin A). The adult RDAs for vitamin A are 900 micrograms for males and 700 for females, which translate to 3,000 IU and 2,334 IU, respectively. The Tolerable Upper Intake Level (UL) for adults is 3,000 micrograms (10,000 IU). Several carotenoids found in plant foods, known as provitamin A carotenoids (α-carotene, β-carotene, and β-cryptoxanthin), are converted to retinol in the body. Retinol occurs only in animal-based foods; therefore, vegetarians must depend on provitamin-A carotenoids to meet their vitamin A requirement.

Retinol, which can produce toxic effects when in excess, is stored in the liver. Single doses of 150,000 micrograms (500,000 IU) can produce transient symptoms of hypervitaminosis A. Chronic toxicity can occur with daily doses of 30,000 micrograms (100,000 IU) for a period of months or years. The developing fetus is especially subject to teratogenic effects from exposure to high levels of retinol.

High intakes of β-carotene, up to the equivalent in 4 to 8 pounds of raw carrots, do not cause retinol toxicity. They are apparently without adverse effect other than a harmless, but unsightly yellowing of the skin known as carotenodermia (27). In general, conversion of provitamin-A carotenoids to retinol is inversely related to serum retinol levels; thus, they may serve as a storage form of retinol.

VITAMIN D: Like vitamin A, RDAs for vitamin D are given in micrograms but vita-min D supplements list them by IU. One IU equals 0.025 micrograms of vitamin D. The RDA for vitamin D has long been accepted as 400 IU. However, when the FNB set out to design and implement a new method for determining nutrient intakes, it was decided that sufficient information was not available to set an Estimated Average

Requirement (EAR) for vitamin D; therefore, an RDA could not be calculated. Instead, Adequate Intakes (AI) of 5, 10, and 15 micrograms for ages to 50 years, 51 to 70 years, and over 71years, respectively, were set, which translate to 200 IU, 400 IU, and 600 IU, respectively. A tolerable Upper Intake Level (UL) for adults was set at 50 micrograms (2,000 IU).

The body has two major sources of vitamin D. One is the action of sunlight on a metabolite of cholesterol (7-dihydroxycholesterol) in the skin to form 25, hydroxycholecalciferol, also known as cholecalciferol or D_3, which is ultimately metabolized in the kidneys to the most active form of vitamin D (1,25-dihydroxycholecaciferol). The other source is the diet, which contains two forms, vitamin D_2 (ergocalciferol) from plant foods and vitamin D_3 (cholecalciferol) from animal foods. Sunlight is the much more efficient source of vitamin D than is diet because, except for the flesh and oils of fatty fish, few foods are naturally rich in vitamin D. Studies published more than a decade ago suggested that, in the absence of sun exposure, 1,000 IU of cholecalciferol is needed by both children and adults to maintain a healthy serum level of vitamin D (28).

Because of the difficulty of obtaining sufficient vitamin D from foods, especially during winter months and in far-northern latitudes, a few foods such as milk products are required by United States and Canadian governments to be fortified with vitamin D. Vitamin D_2 is the form most commonly used as a food additive and supplement, but vitamin D_3 is now more widely available as a dietary supplement.

Vitamin D and the Flu: It has long been recognized that influenza epidemics are seasonal (29). They occur primarily during winter months and in latitudes with the least solar radiation. These temporal and geographic associations with the incidence of influenza strongly point to a beneficial effect of sunlight on the course of the illness. Analysis of morbidity and mortality data from the 1918-1919 influenza pandemic revealed that the incidence of fatal complications from secondary bacterial infection, such as pneumonia, was lowest in geographic areas with highest sunlight exposure and, as a result, vitamin D synthesis (30). This suggestion is in accord with the known role of vitamin D in protection against bacterial endotoxins and in production of the antibacterial peptide cathelicidin.

Vitamin D and Statin Drugs: As mentioned above, cholesterol is a precursor of 7-dihydroxycholesterol, which is converted by the action of sunlight to vitamin D_3. In general, cholesterol-lowering drugs known as statins interfere with the synthesis of cholesterol by inhibiting the enzyme (HMG CoA reductase) that synthesizes mevalonate, a precursor of cholesterol (see Figure 6-4). If a substance, such as a drug, inhibits a metabolic pathway at some point in a sequence of reactions, it will also inhibit synthesis of all of the other biochemicals that are synthesized between the point of inhibition and the last product of the metabolic pathway.

It is known that statin drugs inhibit the synthesis not only of cholesterol but also of coenzyme Q_{10}, a critically important metabolite that is produced in the metabolic pathway between mevalonate and cholesterol. Therefore, it is logical to assume that statins would also inhibit metabolites that are further down the chain from cholesterol, such as 7-dihydroxycholesterol. A reduction in the supply of cholesterol would be expected to result in depletion of vitamin D stores.

Despite the therapeutic relevance of the relationship, a review of the scientific literature reveals that no more than three or four studies have been undertaken to study the effect of statin administration on vitamin D synthesis (31). Although the few studies that have investigated this relationship reported negative results, a report by Ahmed et al. found that myositis-myalgia (muscle inflammation), a serious symptom of coenzyme Q10 depletion, could be reversed by vitamin D administration.

Vitamin D status was determined in a group of 621 statin-treated patients, 20 percent of whom had myalgia. Vitamin D deficiency was found in 43 percent of the asymptomatic patients versus 64 percent in patients with myalgia. Resolution of myalgia occurred in 92 percent of the myalgia patients given vitamin D administration along with continued statin therapy (32). In his review, Kaufmann notes that it is possible that some side effects of statins are not due directly to low cholesterol levels but with concomitant low vitamin D levels (33).

VITAMIN E: Vitamin E is Nature's antioxidant; plants protect the double bonds of their polyunsaturated fatty acids against oxidation by synthesizing them in combination with vitamin E. It is believed that the primary function of vitamin E is as an antioxidant in protecting unsaturated lipids and lipid structures, such as cell membranes, from destruction by free radicals formed during normal metabolism. It is therefore logical that the dietary requirement for vitamin E would increase with increasing intakes of essential fatty acids. Vitamin E does not appear to have a specific role in any metabolic pathway.

Vitamin E is a member of a family of complex organic chemicals known as tocopherols and tocotrienols. There are four naturally occurring tocopherols (alpha, beta, gamma, and delta) and four corresponding naturally occurring tocotrienols. Although all members of the tocopherol/tocotrienol family have antioxidant activity, the only one considered to be of nutritional significance is alpha-tocopherol (vitamin E).

The remaining members are not considered to have vitamin E activity because they are not converted to alpha-tocopherol in the body (5, p. 237). To further confound the vitamin E picture, it has eight possible stereoisomers, only four of which (2R forms) occur naturally in foods. Only the vitamin E activity of the 2R forms is used in establishing vitamin E requirements (5, p. 236).

VITAMIN K: There are three forms of vitamin K: vitamin K_1 (phylloquinone) found in plants; vitamin K_2 (menaquinone) produced by bacteria in the intestinal tract; and synthetic vitamin K_3 (menadone), which has been associated with liver damage. There are no known toxic effects from high intakes of vitamins K_1 or K_2. As with other fat-soluble vitamins, absorption of vitamin K is enhanced by dietary fat.

Vitamin K is known primarily for its role in production of clotting factors; thus, it counteracts the anticoagulant action of drugs such as warfarin. Long-term use of anticoagulants can result in a cellular vitamin K deficiency. Vitamin K has also been shown to modulate calcium levels and play an important role in bone metabolism. Although clinically significant vitamin K deficiency is considered to be extremely rare, it may be a factor in osteoporosis and arterial calcification.

Vitamin K's role in prevention of cardiovascular disease may be more important than previously recognized. A recent Dutch study found that high levels of vitamin K_2 were associated with protection against aortic calcification and a 50 percent reduction in risk of death from cardiovascular disease (34). Deficiency of vitamin K can mimic symptoms of diabetes and may also be associated with chronic inflammatory conditions due to high levels of C-reactive protein (35, p. 469).'

Minerals

Minerals are the inorganic chemicals that form the rocks and soil and sand that give structure to the inanimate world. Minerals are made from one or more chemical elements, ninety-two of which occur naturally. Of these ninety-two elements, twenty-one are known to be essential for the life processes of plants and animals. That these inorganic chemicals are essential for humans is illustrated by the fact that approximately 4 to 5 percent of the human body is composed of minerals. But why minerals, the chemicals that form the structures of the inanimate world, are essential for living creatures is not readily apparent. The answer may be found in a study of biological evolution.

The very first living organisms arose in ancient seas that were dilute soups of dissolved inorganic chemicals. These primitive creatures incorporated into themselves the minerals in which they were awash. Thus, they and the creatures that evolved from them came to require the minerals present in their environments. The evolutionary legacy of using inorganic chemicals as nutrients is the development of a dependence on them.

In the early 1900's, it was noted that the kinds and quantities of inorganic elements in human blood were very similar to those postulated for ancient seas. This led Macallum to advance a theory that human blood and body fluids had their ancestral origins in seawater (36). According to this theory, the earliest multicelled creatures had canal systems open to their watery environments through which oxygen and nutrients could flow in to the innermost cells and waste products could be carried out.

As larger and more complex creatures evolved, the simple canal system became too inefficient. It also prevented movement of creatures out of the sea and onto land. Gradually, species with closed circulatory systems developed, and the fluids in the closed systems took the place of seawater. Macallum's theory states that the composition of the blood and body fluids of today's higher animals reflect what the composition of seawater was at the time the circulatory system was closed off from the seawater environment.

Although the concentration of salts in seawater today is between 3 and 4 percent, in geologic times, it was estimated to be about 0.9 percent, the same as that in blood plasma. Essential minerals are divided into two groups, those that are required in relatively large amounts and those that are needed only in trace quantities. The minerals required in relatively large amounts are referred to as macrominerals or major minerals. Those required in small amounts are called microminerals or trace minerals. The major mineral nutrients required by humans are calcium, chlorine (as chloride), magnesium, phosphorous, potassium, sodium, and sulfur.

Probably the most familiar names among the trace minerals are copper, iodine, iron, manganese, selenium, and zinc. Other essential trace minerals that often are not recognized as being required by humans include boron, chromium, cobalt, fluorine (as fluoride), germanium, molybdenum, silicon, and vanadium.

With the great advances in the fields of biochemistry and molecular biology, increasing numbers of inorganic elements are being identified as having a role in some living organism. Many of these ultra trace minerals have little practical significance for human nutrition because, if they are essential, they are required in such infinitely small quantities that deficiencies are all but impossible to occur or detect.

MAJOR MINERALS

The essential minerals are not independent of each other, although they are usually treated in textbooks as if they were. They can interact with each and with other nutrients. Like vitamins, they can serve as coenzymes. The interactions among minerals may be accretive or antagonistic. Thus, any plan of supplementation with single minerals should not be undertaken without consideration for potential imbalances. As with other nutrients, healthful mineral nutrition planning requires study.

CALCIUM/MAGNESIUM: A prime example of a nutritional interdependence between two minerals is that of calcium and magnesium. Calcium and magnesium share equal importance in our bodies. They have different biological functions yet they function as a team (37, p.14). Neither can act without eliciting a reaction from the other in what Dr. Dean aptly refers to as "The dance of calcium and magnesium" (38).

Calcium is one of the main elements in the human body, accounting for about 2 percent of the total body weight. Magnesium is a relative lightweight; it contributes about 0.1 percent to the body weight. Skeletal structures, bone and teeth contain 99 percent of the body's calcium and about 65 percent of its magnesium. Both calcium and magnesium serve functions that may be divided into two categories. One category relates to their roles in providing for the structural parts of the body, the bones and teeth. Magnesium is often mentioned as an antagonist of calcium, but the relationship between the two is much more complex than mere antagonism (37; 38). The structural function of calcium is given more attention because of its well publicized association with osteoporosis.

The other category of calcium/magnesium function could be called a management or operational category. It includes their participation in numerous biochemical and physiological reactions. Calcium has essential roles in nerve transmission, muscle contraction, blood clotting, vasodilation and vasocontraction. Magnesium is an excellent tissue calcium channel blocker; it helps prevent deposition of calcium in arterial walls and soft tissues (37). It also serves as a coenzyme in more major enzyme systems than any other mineral (37; 38). In addition to being essential for general well being, a good balance of calcium and magnesium may also promote cardiovascular health, provide protection against colon cancer, and increase resistance to the chronic diseases attributed to the aging process.

Current research indicates that the most beneficial ratio of calcium to magnesium appears to be about 3:2 with average optimal amounts being 1,000 milligrams of calcium and 600 milligrams of magnesium (38, p.231). Thus, it is obvious that an RDA of 300 or 400 milligrams for magnesium is inadequate for a calcium AI of 1,000 milligrams (5).

Interestingly, many people depend on dairy products for calcium and magnesium intake, but the magnesium content of milk is only about 10 percent that of calcium and of cheese only about 6 percent. For example, a quart of 4 percent milk will supply approximately 1,200 milligrams of calcium, 400 IU of vitamin D, but only about 130 milligrams of magnesium – clearly a need for supplementation.

SULFUR: Although sulfur is an important and relatively abundant mineral in the human body, it seems to be an orphan as far as medical and nutritional sciences are concerned.

An extensive literature search for information on the biochemical and physiologic roles of sulfur in the human body and on the sulfur content of foods yields little or no data. There is a great deal of information on sulfur metabolism in microorganisms, but virtually nothing concerning sulfur metabolism in higher organisms. Jacob confirms the fact that the reason a literature search for sulfur in human nutrition yields no information is because there is no information (39, p. 34).

This lack of information on nutritional needs for sulfur is surprising in view of the fact that almost one percent of the human body is sulfur. It is present in every tissue, structure, and cell of the body, primarily in the form of two sulfur-containing amino acids, cysteine and methionine. These amino acids are components of a wide variety of proteins that serve the needs of hair, nails, skin, organ tissues and linings, hormones, enzymes, carriers of essential nutrients, messengers, and helpers of all sorts. Sulfur is also a component of numerous other important biochemicals, including glucosamine sulfate, glutathione, alpha-lipoic acid, coenzyme A, and the vitamins biotin and thiamin.

One example of the nutritional importance of sulfur is that it makes possible the formation of skin, hair, and nails. The cysteine molecules in long strands of protein link with cysteine molecules in other strands by chemically connecting their sulfhydryl groups (-SH) together to form disulfide bonds (-SS-). The amino acid formed from two cysteine molecules linked together by a disulfide bond is known as cystine. The cystine bridges that tie long strands of proteins together are vital structural elements of the body.

Every person who has had her (or his) hair permanently waved – or straightened – is the benefactor of chemistry involving disulfide bonds. In the process of waving or straightening hair, a chemical solution that breaks some of the disulfide bonds is applied to the hair. This breaking separates individual hair protein fibers from each other. The hair is then secured firmly in a curled or straight configuration that realigns the individual protein strands. Then another solution that reforms disulfide bonds is applied to the secured hair. The new disulfide bonds are permanent.

The body's inorganic sulfate requirement is provided for almost entirely by sulfates from catabolism of the cysteine and methionine content of food proteins. Other organic sulfur compounds, such as those found in onions, garlic, cabbage, broccoli, and cauliflower, make a minor contribution to the body's need for sulfur. MSM (methyl sulfonylmethane) is a valuable organic sulfur supplement. The body apparently cannot use elemental sulfur efficiently or at all, and inorganic sulfur (sulfates) from foods seems to be of little biological value. The body does not appear to require inorganic sulfates for synthesis of proteins or other organic metabolites.

TRACE (MINOR) MINERALS

In addition to the minerals that are required in relatively large amounts, there are at least fourteen more that are needed in very small amounts, perhaps as little as a few micrograms or milligrams a day. As mentioned earlier, the known trace minerals are boron, chromium, cobalt, copper, fluoride, germanium, iodine, iron, manganese, molybdenum, selenium, silicon, vanadium, and zinc.

The finding that some trace minerals are required in very small amounts gives evidence to the conclusion that they do not serve as structural elements in the human body. Instead, they function as helpers, messengers, or activators of various sorts. Some trace minerals, similar to vitamins, work as coenzymes (zinc, like magnesium, serves 100 or more enzyme systems). Others combine with organic chemicals and become essential components of vitamins, enzymes, or hormones. Precise biochemical roles have been established for some of the trace elements. However, numerous others are known to be essential only because organisms are found to suffer adverse effects when those particular trace elements are absent from the diet.

CHROMIUM PICOLINATE: Chromium is a trace mineral worthy of special mention because of the problem of sugar craving that many people have. Sugar craving makes it very difficult for some people to control their appetite for sweets. It has been known for years that long-term sugar intake depletes chromium and that, in turn, chromium depletion causes a powerful sugar craving. Thus, a vicious cycle is created: the greater the sugar intake; the greater the chromium depletion; and the greater the sugar craving. This problem may be solved by supplementing the diet with a chromium compound (40).

Chromium supplements that are available are chromium picolinate or chromium polynicotinate. In these forms, chromium is non-toxic and can be used to end sugar craving. An initial dose of 200 micrograms per day will prove helpful for some. If sugar craving persists, another 200 micrograms per day may be added. After the sugar craving stops, the chromium dose should be reduced to 100 to 200 micrograms per day.

ULTRA TRACE MINERALS

Essential ultra trace minerals are minerals required in extremely small quantities – less than a fraction of a microgram a day. A few, such as vanadium, nickel, tin, and germanium, are known to have some function in mammalian systems. Others, such as arsenic, bromine, cesium, and rubidium, are suspected of having minor roles but there is no clear-cut evidence that they do. It cannot be assumed that a chemical is essential because traces of it are found in animal tissues. It may only be an inert contaminant.

Nutrients that are required in minuscule amounts are very difficult and costly to study. They are usually already present in food or environment in amounts greater than are amounts that may be required. Essential ultra trace minerals are of little practical importance for nutritionists concerned with unintended deficiency states in humans or animals, because foods and the general environment have normal background levels of ultra trace minerals that are well above any possible nutritional requirement.

Biochemical Intermediates

In addition to vitamins and minerals there are many other supplements available to the general public that do not fit in either of these categories. Most of them are not essential in the strict sense of the term, because they are biochemicals the body normally makes. Nevertheless, they can be valuable as supplements, particularly in the elderly or the debilitated, when they are needed in quantities greater than the body can supply for optimum health. Two biochemical intermediates that are of particular value as supplements are alpha lipoic acid and coenzyme Q_{10}.

ALPHA-LIPOIC ACID

Alpha-lipoic acid, also known in past years as thioctic acid because of its sulfur content, was recognized as an essential nutrient for microorganisms in the early 1930's. For a number of years, it was classified as a B vitamin, a nutrient essential for all living cells. When it was found that animal cells can synthesize alpha-lipoic acid, it was removed from the vitamin category. Even though it is not a vitamin, it is a very important coenzyme for the production of energy from nutrients.

In addition to its role as a coenzyme, alpha-lipoic acid also serves as a free-radical scavenger, an antioxidant, and a chelating agent. It has a complex relationship with other antioxidants, such as vitamins C and E, and with glutathione and coenzyme Q_{10} (CoQ). It has an interesting structure that enables it to exist in an oxidized form and in a reduced form. Both forms are biologically active, which makes it a very versatile biochemical that can regenerate antioxidants that have served their purpose as well as regenerate itself. Although the body is able to synthesize alpha-lipoic acid, its production declines while its requirement apparently increases with age. For this reason it is worth considering as a dietary supplement (41).

COENZYME Q10 (COQ, Q10)

CoQ is a made by all plant and animal organisms, including humans. CoQ, known chemically as ubiquinone, has a complex structure that can accept or donate electrons in biochemical reactions. This ability to accept or donate electrons makes it a valuable coenzyme partner for a number of enzymes that store or release energy in biochemical reactions. All cells require ubiquinone to provide energy for metabolic processes. Heart tissues have a much greater energy demand and, hence, a much greater need for CoQ than most other tissues in the body.

The ability to synthesize CoQ declines with age. General symptoms of deficiency are a lack of energy, gum disease, and susceptibility to age-related diseases (42). However, because of its greater demand for energy, the decline in CoQ synthesis occurs more rapidly in heart tissue than in other bodily tissues (42; 43). Thus, symptoms of CoQ deficiency are related primarily to the heart. A deficiency state manifests itself primarily as congestive heart failure (44).

The statin drugs, widely prescribed for hypercholesterolemia, not only inhibit the body's synthesis of cholesterol but also its synthesis of CoQ (see Figure 6-4). Over a decade ago, Langsjoen and fellow scientists predicted problems from this drug-induced depletion (42). In 2004, a study showed that heart muscle weakness, which was reversible with supplemental CoQ, occurred in 70% of previously normal patients treated with statin drugs for six months (45; 46). Therefore, it is important for people who take statin drugs on a long-term basis to consider CoQ supplementation.

BUY WITH CARE

As a general rule, biochemical supplements are more expensive than are vitamin, mineral, or herbal supplements. This is because most are fairly complex organic chemicals and, as a result, are costly to isolate from natural sources or synthesize in the laboratory. Some of these supplements have very well documented histories of use and benefit, whereas others are of more theoretical value. Finally, some of these supplements have no demonstrable merit, but are mere fads that, like hula-hoops, enjoy great popularity for a time and then quietly disappear from the scene.

Beyond the obvious questions of what does the substance claim to do and what is the documentation that it does do what it claims, one should ask for evidence that the substance actually survives digestion and is able to reach the site of its intended action. Another question to pursue is whether some dietary deficiency is responsible for the need for the supplement. As mentioned above, supplementation should not be a substitute for good nutrition and healthful lifestyles.

Herbs

The use of plant materials for medicinal purposes is a comparatively new concept for most people (47), but plant components were the foundation of the healing arts in ancient cultures, not only for curing illnesses but also for preventing them. Many modern drugs had their origins in herbal medicines. The salicylates (see aspirin below) came from the willow tree. The foxglove plant provided the heart medicine digitalis. Quinine from cinchona bark, the medicine used successfully against malaria, was a gift from the ancient Peruvian Indians (48, p. 418). A wide variety of plant or animal remedies have been used for thousands of years in China and India. Prehistoric cultures must have known from experience that certain plants had healing powers. Even today, there are still many parts of the world in which age-old remedies are the preferred therapies.

Before embarking on any program of herbal use, readers are strongly urged to remember that herbal preparations have pharmacological actions - they are drugs. Herbs can be of benefit when used cautiously and with knowledge, but even when used with care they can present a variety of unanticipated and untoward problems. For example, the use of herbal medications can adversely affect the course of emergency medical care or routine surgical procedures (49), especially if the attending physician is unaware of their use. To avoid any such problem, people who routinely take herbs should inform their physicians of the fact. Further, anyone who has a chronic illness or other medical problem or who is taking prescription medications for any reason should not take any herbal preparation without first discussing the matter with his or her health care provider.

Aspirin – an Exceptional Supplement

Aspirin (acetylsalicylic acid) is included here for several important reasons. It is a very old and familiar pain remedy that most people, particularly the elderly, would find difficult to do without; it has become a daily requirement for every adult, much like a vitamin pill, by virtue of being prescribed in baby aspirin dosage to prevent cardiovascular disease; and perhaps most important, it has been shown within the past decade to be of great importance in supporting the body's natural healing processes as a result of its unique and vital in role eicosanoid metabolism.

The story of aspirin starts with the methyl ester of salicylic acid, the principle ingredient of oil of wintergreen obtained from natural sources such as willow bark. Oil of wintergreen is a centuries-old liniment for the aches and pains of rheumatism. However, because of its considerable toxicity, it could not be taken internally. Throughout the decades, many derivatives of salicylic acid were synthesized in an effort to find a less toxic form that would be acceptable for internal use. Some, including salicylic acid itself, were used internally and found to be very effective in relieving pain, but they were difficult to tolerate because of unpleasant side effects.

In the mid-nineteenth century, the acetic acid derivative of salicylic acid was synthesized by a chemist at the German chemical company now known as Bayer. Bayer patented the process for making acetylsalicylic acid and the name they gave it (Aspirin) in 1899. In the 100-plus years since aspirin was introduced to the public, it became the most widely used medication in the world with a yearly production of 50,000 tons and a daily consumption by Americans of about 80 million tablets per day.

In 1982, the Nobel Prize in Medicine was granted to Sune Bergstrom, Bengt Samuelsson, and Sir John Vane (50) for their discovery that the analgesic effect of aspirin was due to its ability to prevent conversion of the EFA arachidonic acid to inflammatory prostaglandins by cyclooxygenase, the enzyme now known to the general public as COX enzyme. It was assumed that this meant that aspirin inhibited the COX enzyme.

Thus began a massive program by the pharmaceutical industry to develop COX inhibitors as competitors for aspirin. Importantly, aspirin was no longer under patent protection or patentable. Thus, aspirin became the model for the class of new patentable pharmaceuticals known as NSAIDs (nonsteroidal anti-inflammatory drugs).

During NSAID development, it was discovered that the COX enzyme has two forms: COX-1 and COX-2. It was also discovered that COX-1 is the constitutive (always present) form that, among other things, contributes to protection against stomach bleeding. COX-2 was found to be an inducible (made when needed) form that was a cause of the pain associated with illness or injury. The ultimate goal of the pharmaceutical effort was to find drugs that would inhibit only COX-2 without interfering with the ability of COX-1 to protect against stomach bleeding.

In the last few decades many different versions of the NSAIDs have been synthesized, most of which are available only by prescription. A small number of them that had relatively few side effects, such as ibuprofen and naproxen, are available as over-the-counter painkillers. However, to date, none have been found to be more effective or safer than aspirin; a few have been recalled because of unacceptable adverse effects.

The difference between aspirin and the NSAIDS was not known until a few years ago when Serhan and co-investigators discovered that aspirin does not do what the pharmaceutical industry assumed it did; aspirin does *not* inhibit the COX-2 enzyme (51). This profound revelation apparently has not yet been recognized by main stream medicine.

What is the significance of COX-2 inhibition? As explained in Chapter Nine, COX-2 is more robust than COX-1. When acetylated by aspirin, COX-1 is completely inhibited. However, only one of the two catalytic sites in COX-2 is inhibited and this remaining site produces an intermediate metabolite that is instantly converted in the body to anti-inflammatory eicosanoids (52; 53). The pharmaceutical industry assumed that aspirin worked by inhibiting the COX-2 enzyme; this was an error.

Another disadvantage of NSAIDs is that when they inhibit the COX-2 enzyme, the arachidonic acid that is not metabolized by the now-inhibited COX-2 enzyme is diverted to the lipoxygenase-5 enzyme where it is converted to highly inflammatory leukotrienes. Instead, aspirin converts the AA to anti-inflammatory, pro-healing lipid mediators.

As important as aspirin is in its fundamental role in modifying inflammatory eicosanoid pathways, perhaps of even greater consequence for the health and well being of present and future generations are the more recent discoveries of the hitherto unsuspected role of aspirin in resolution (the healing process) and the unanticipated existence of whole new classes of aspirin-triggered anti-inflammatory eicosanoids that have been uncovered by the research into aspirin's mechanism of action (see Chapter Nine).

Water

Water is not considered a nutritional supplement, but it is mentioned here because of its great importance for optimum health. The water content of the body is approximately 70 percent by weight, with blood consisting of about 90 percent water. Body fluids, which are largely water, have many vital functions:

- Transport of oxygen and carbon dioxide across lung surfaces.
- Transport of nutrients (sugars, amino acids, vitamins, minerals) throughout body.
- Removal of waste product from cells and tissues to ultimate excretion in the urine.
- Maintenance of the water content of cells and tissues.
- Regulation and maintenance of a constant body temperature.
- Regulation of the normal functioning of the body by delivering biochemical substances such as hormones or antibodies to appropriate target organs or sites.

Our bodies are constantly losing water through the skin, from the lungs, from the urinary bladder, and from the gastrointestinal tract. The eyes, nose, and any moist parts of the body are minor avenues of water loss. If losses are not made up, the body goes into a semi-dehydration mode. The most critical functions for preserving life are attended to first. Functions that may not be immediately essential, but may be extremely important for long-term health and well being, are neglected. Repeated periods of water deprivation do not contribute to longevity.

Thirst is the body's warning system that there is a water deficit. Drinking sufficient water each day so that the sensation of thirst is never felt is the best way to provide adequately for the body's water needs. People who make water drinking a habit are doing one of the kindest things they can do for themselves.

References

1.)   Heiby WA. The Reverse Effect: How vitamins and Minerals Promote Health and CAUSE Disease. Deerfield, IL: MediScience Publishers, 1988.

2.)   Faloon W. Americans are getting healthier… But the FDA remains a major impediment. Life Extension Magazine. May 2000: 7-8.

3.)   http://www.marketresearch.com/Packaged-Facts-v768/Nutritional-Supplements-Edition-2642045/ Accessed Sept. 26, 2012.

4.)   http://www.mypyramid.gov/ Accessed Sept. 26, 2012.

5.)   Dietary Reference Intakes: The Essential Guide to Nutrient Requirements. Washington, DC: The National Academies Press, 2006. Levine M, et al. Criteria and recommendations for vitamin C intake. Journal of the American Medical

6.)   Association. 1999; 281(15): 1415-1423.

7.)   http://lpi.oregonstate.edu/infocenter/ Accessed Sept. 26, 2012.

8.)   Williams R J. You Are Extraordinary. New York, NY: Random House, 1967.

9.)   McNamara SH. Food fortification in the United States. Nutrition Reviews. 1995; 53(5): 140-144.

10.)   http://en.wikipedia.org/wiki/Reference_Daily_Intake/ Accessed Sept. 26, 2012.

11.)   http:/www.fda.gov/fdac/special/foodlabel/drv.html/ Accessed Sept. 26, 2012.

12.)   Porter R. The Greatest Benefit to Mankind. New York, NY: W. W. Norton & Company, Inc., 1997.

13.)   Sauberlich HE, Machlin LJ, editors. Beyond deficiency – new views on the function and health effects of vitamins. Annals of the New York Academy of Sciences 1992; 669: 1-6.

14.)   Willett WC, et al. Intake of trans fatty acids and risk of coronary heart disease among women. Lancet.1993; 341(8845): 581-585.

15.)   Giovannucci, E., et al. Multivitamin use, folate, and colon cancer in women in the Nurses' Health Study. Annals of Internal Medicine. 1998; 129(7): 517-524.

16.)   Burns JJ, Rivers JM, Machlin LJ, editors. Third Conference on Vitamin C. Annals of the New York Academy of Sciences: 1987; 498.

17.)   Hickey S. Roberts H. Ascorbate: The Science of Vitamin C. Lulu Press, 2004.

18.)   Ottoboni F, Ottoboni A. Ascorbic acid and the immune system. Journal of Orthomolecular Medicine. 2005; 29(3): 179-183.

19.)   Wand P. The vitamin C controversy. Life Extension Magazine. June 2000: 18-25.

20.)   Faloon W. How vitamin C prevents heart attacks. Life Extension Magazine. February Suppl. 1999: 23.

21.)   Reuler JB, et al. Adult scurvy. Journal of the American Medical Assoc. 1985; 253: 805-807.

22.) Kieffer P, et al. Multiple organ dysfunctions dramatically improving with the infusion of vitamin C:More support for persistence of scurvy in our "welfare" society. Intensive Care Medicine. 2001; 27(2): 448.

23.) Yew MS. "Recommended Daily Allowances" for Vitamin C. Proceedings of the National Academy1973; 70: 969-972.

24.) Pauling L. How to Live Longer and Feel Better. New York, NY; W. H. Freeman and Company, 1986.

25.) McCully K, McCully M. The Heart Revolution. New York, NY: Harper Collins, 1999.

26.) Horton HR, et al. Principles of Biochemistry, 2nd Ed. Upper Saddle River, NJ: Prentice Hall, 1996.

27.) Murray MT. Encyclopedia of Nutritional Supplements. Rocklin, CA: Prima Publishing, 1996.

28.) Holick MF. The vitamin D epidemic and its health consequences. Journal of Nutrition. 2005; 135: 2739S.

29.) http://www.vitamindcouncil.org/health-conditions/infections-and-autoimmunity/influenza/ Accessed Sept. 26, 2012.

30.) Grant WB, Giovannucci E. The possible roles of solar ultraviolet-B radiation and vitamin D in Reducing fatality rates from the 1918 influenza pandemic in the United States. Dermatology and Endocrinology. 2009; 1: 1-5.

31.) http://www.westonaprice.org/fat-soluble-activators/seafood-to-sunshine/ Accessed Sept. 26, 2012.

32.) Ahmed W, et al. Low serum 25 (OH) vitamin D levels (<32 ng/mL) are associated with reversiblemyositis-myalgia in statin-treated patients. Transl.Res. 2009; 153(1): 11-6. Epub 2008 DEC 6.

33.) Kaufmann JM. Benefits of vitamin D supplementation. Journal of American Physicians and Surgeons. 2009; 14(2): 38-45.

34.) Vitamin K: New functions and mechanisms of action. The Linus Pauling Institute Research letter. 2009: fall/winter, p. 3.

35.) Disease Prevention and Treatment, 4th Edition. Hollywood, FL: Life Extension Media, 2003.

36.) McCallum I. Ecological Intelligence: Rediscovering Ourselves in Nature. Fulcrum Publishers, 2009,

37.) Seelig MS, Rosanoff A. The Magnesium Factor. New York, NY: Avery: Penguin Group, 2003

38.) Dean C. The Miracle of Magnesium. New Your, NY: Ballentine Books, 2003.

39.) Jacob SW, Lawrence RL, Zucker M. The Miracle of MSM. New York, NY: G.P. Putnam's Sons, 1999.

40.) Docherty JP, et al. A double-blind, placebo-controlled, exploratory trial if chromium picolinate in atypical depression: effect on carbohydrate craving. Journal of Psychiatric Practice. 2005; 11(5): 302-314.

41.) Berkson B. The Alpha Lipoic Acid Breakthrough. Rocklin, CA 95677: Prima Health, 1998.

42.) How CoQ10 Protects Your Cardiovascular System. Life Extension Magazine. April 2000: 19-28.

43.) Martin R. Report: Co Q10's new benefits. Life Extension Magazine. August 2006.

44.) Langsjoen PH, Langsjoen A. Coenzyme Q10 in cardiovascular disease with an emphasis on heart failure and myocardial ischemia. Asia Pacific Heart Journal. 1998; 7(3): 160-168.

45.) Langsjoen PH et al. Treatment of statins adverse effects with treatment with supplemental coenzyme Q10 and statin drug discontinuance. Biofactors. 2005; 25: 147-152.

46.) Langsjoen PH. Alleviating congestive heart failure with coenzyme Q10. Life Extension Magazine. February 2008: 45-53.

47.) Runestad T. Reading between the lines of supplement labels. Delicious Living. 2001; 17(3): 34-38.

48.) Price WA. Nutrition and Physical Degeneration, 6th ed. Los Angeles, CA: Keats Publishing, 1998.

49.) Ang-Lee, MK, et al. Herbal medicines and perioperative care. Journal of the American Medical Association. 2001; 286(2): 208-216.

50.) Serhan CN. The Allergy Archives: The discovery and characterization of the leucotrienes. Journal of Allergy and Clinical Immunology. October 2006: 972-976.

51.) Claria J, Serhan CN. Aspirin triggers previously undescribed bioactive eicosanoids by human endothelial cell-leukocyte interactions. Proceedings, National Academy of Sciences. 1995; 92(21): 9475-9.

52.) Serhan CN et al. Resolution of inflammation: State of the art, definitions and terms. The FASEB Journal. 2007; 21 (2): 325-332.

53.) Serhan CN, et al. Maresins: Novel macrophage mediators with potent anti-inflammatory and Proresolving actions. The Journal of Experimental Medicine. 2009; 206(1): 15-23.

Chapter Six

Carbohydrates

Have you heard of the Sugar-Plum Tree? ...The fruit that it bears is so wonderfully sweet (As those who have tasted it say) That good little children have only to eat Of that fruit to be happy all day. **Eugene Field (1850-1895) The Sugar-Plum Tree. Poems of Childhood.,**

Some carbohydrate foods are the delights of the diet. They are the candies and cookies, soft drinks, sweet rolls, and sticky buns – all treats that taste so good. But carbohydrate foods are also broccoli, carrots, spinach, and kale – all the foods that are nutritious but not very exciting. Between these two extremes are many hundreds of carbohydrate foods that are considered staples of the diet: breads of all sorts, cereals, potatoes, pastas, beans, and rice. In addition to their function as food sources, carbohydrates serve as vital structural components of plants, as energy sources for animals, and as constituents of many important biochemicals in both plants and animals.

Carbohydrate Units

When the simplest formula for carbohydrates was discovered to be CH_2O, early French chemists labeled this class of compounds *hydrate de carbone*. Thus, carbohydrates received their name from their chemical composition – carbon (carbo) plus water (hydrate). As the science of carbohydrate chemistry developed, it became clear that carbohydrates did not behave chemically as hydrates, but the name persists to this day. Carbohydrates are also known as saccharides because of the sweet taste of the simplest members of the group. Saccharide comes from *saccharum,* the Latin word for sugar. With few exceptions, carbohydrate units are named using the suffix *-ose.*

MONOSACCHARIDES

Carbohydrates are composed of simple units called monosaccharides. Monosaccharides contain from three to six carbons. The six-carbon monosaccharides, glucose, fructose, galactose, and mannose, are the monosaccharides of most importance in human nutrition; however, they make only a small contribution to the diet as free monosaccharides. Most carbohydrates are present in the diet as disaccharides or as the polymers of the monosaccharide glucose (starch and cellulose).

Chemically, glucose, galactose, and mannose are identical to each other. They are stereoisomeric aldoses with the chemical formula $C_6H_{12}O_6$. Aldose is the chemical term for a carbohydrate aldehyde. An aldehyde is an organic chemical whose first carbon is linked to an oxygen atom by a double bond. Fructose has the same chemical formula as the aldoses but differs chemically from them in that it is a ketose. Ketose is the term for a carbohydrate ketone. A ketone has the oxygen atom linked by a double bond to an interior carbon rather than a terminal carbon. In fructose, the bond to oxygen is on carbon 2.

All monosaccharides exist in nature in ring form. In the case of glucose, galactose, and mannose carbon 5 of the carbon chain links through the aldose oxygen on carbon 1 to form a six-member ring. With fructose, carbon 5 links through the ketose oxygen on carbon 2 to form a five-member ring. This difference is seemingly very small, but it is very important biochemically, as will be illustrated later in this chapter.

Glucose is the most abundant carbohydrate in the human diet and the most important of the monosaccharides for humans and all higher animals. It not only provides energy throughout the body but also, as a vital component of blood, helps maintain homeostasis – the stability and constancy of the internal milieu. The normal range of glucose in blood is from 80 to 120 milligrams per 100 milliliters. Significant excursions outside of this normal range can be life threatening. The contribution of other monosaccharides to this homeostatic function of glucose is only to extent that they are metabolized to glucose.

The quantities of monosaccharides in the diet depend on the macronutrient composition of the diet: glucose (as maltose or sucrose) is the major constituent of all breads, cereals, pastas, grains, and sugars; fructose (free or as sucrose) is a component of fruits and products, primarily soft drinks, containing high fructose corn syrup; and galactose (as lactose) is present in milk and dairy products. Mannose, most commonly found in cranberries, is the least abundant monosaccharide in the human diet and of least importance in carbohydrate metabolism. However, in combination with certain proteins, it serves a variety of metabolic functions. It has also been shown to be of therapeutic value in the treatment of urinary tract infections (1; 2).

DISACCHARIDES

Disaccharides are combinations of two monosaccharides. The only disaccharides of human nutritional importance are maltose, sucrose, and lactose. Maltose, made from two glucose units, is a product of the digestion of starch. Sucrose (table sugar), formed from glucose and fructose, is the most abundant disaccharide in nature and is synthesized only by plants. Lactose (milk sugar), a combination of glucose and galactose, is synthesized only by lactating mammary glands of animals.

POLYSACCHARIDES

Polysaccharides are polymers containing from a few to hundreds of monomers, the most common of which is glucose. Polysaccharides important in human nutrition are glycogen, starch, and cellulose, all of which are polymers of glucose. Glycogen is an animal polysaccharide that is made and used as a storage form of glucose. Starch and cellulose are polysaccharides made by plants. Plants use cellulose as a structural material, and starch, like glycogen in animals, as a storage form of glucose.

Digestion of Carbohydrates

The digestion of carbohydrates begins in the mouth with the action of the enzyme ptyalin that is secreted with saliva. Ptyalin starts the degradation of starches to the disaccharide maltose, which is continued in the small intestine by amylase enzymes secreted by the pancreas and delivered to the intestines through the duodenum. Disaccharides and other small carbohydrates are further converted to monosaccharides in the small intestine, absorbed into the blood stream, and carried to the liver for further processing and/or distribution to other parts of the body.

The principal complex carbohydrates in the human diet are the polysaccharides cellulose and starch. The only difference chemically between cellulose and starch, both of which are polymers of glucose, is the way their glucose units are linked together. Their links are identical except that they are spatial opposites of each other. The glucose links in starch are α(alpha)-glycoside links and those in cellulose are β(beta)-glycoside links.

The α-glycoside linage is broken by α-amylase in the human digestive tract to yield glucose from starch. Human digestive enzymes, on the other hand, cannot break the links between glucose units in cellulose because they do not contain β-amylase. Thus, the value of cellulose in human nutrition is only as fiber. The major dietary source of fiber in the diet is cellulose from vegetables, fruits, and whole grains. Interestingly, cellulose can be used as a food by ruminant animals because the digestive systems of the microorganisms in their rumen possess enzymes that can break the β-glycoside links of cellulose to yield glucose. This glucose released from cellulose by the microorganisms in the rumen of animals is then used as a nutrient by ruminant animals in the same manner as glucose is used in humans.

Metabolism of Carbohydrates

Carbohydrate metabolism is, for all practical purposes, the metabolism of glucose. This is because almost all carbohydrate foods are composed of glucose units. The fate of the monosaccharides in the liver depends on the metabolic needs of the body. The liver uses some glucose to replenish stores of glycogen and sends the rest to the blood stream where it is carried to all cells of the body. Galactose and mannose that are not used to make other biochemicals are converted to glucose and metabolized as glucose. Fructose, discussed later, is not converted to glucose, but instead maintains its own identity separate from that of glucose.

GLYCOLYSIS

Glucose is used for energy by all cells of the body. Before its energy can be extracted, it must first be metabolized to pyruvate by a series of ten steps (enzymatic reactions) known as the glycolytic pathway or glycolysis (see Figure 6-1). The first three steps rearrange the glucose structure to a make a form of fructose (a diphosphate) that can be broken into two trioses (3-carbon units). The next seven steps rearrange the structures of the two trioses to yield two molecules of the triose pyruvate.

Glycolysis is a pathway from glucose to pyruvate employed by all anaerobic (oxygen independent) and aerobic (oxygen dependent) organisms to obtain metabolic energy from glucose without requiring oxygen. In anaerobes, pyruvate is converted to one of a number of different chemicals that serves as a metabolic endpoint (an electron receptor), which is necessary for glycolysis to continue. For example, in the anaerobic phase of yeast metabolism, pyruvate is converted to ethanol and carbon dioxide, thereby preventing the buildup of pyruvate. In some aerobic tissues, such as muscle tissue, during periods of strenuous exercise when oxygen supplies are limited, pyruvate permits continued glycolysis by donating its electrons to form lactic acid.

When conditions permit and sufficient oxygen is available, pyruvate conversion to lactic acid is no longer necessary. Pyruvate then switches to the aerobic Krebs cycle, which is its usual pathway. Meanwhile, the lactic acid produced in the muscles travels via the bloodstream to the liver where it is converted back to pyruvate. Pyruvate is then changed back to glucose by a pathway that is essentially the same as the glycolytic pathway. This cycle between muscle glucose/lactate and liver lactate/ glucose was named the Cori cycle for the scientists, Carl and Gerty Cori, who received the 1949 Nobel Prize in Medicine for its discovery.

There is no net energy gain from the reactions of the glycolytic pathway. The biochemical intermediates between glucose and pyruvate each contain the same quantity of energy as the glucose they came from. The energy from glucose is not obtained until pyruvate is converted to acetyl CoA and enters the aerobic Krebs cycle (Figure 4-1, Chapter Four).

The glycolytic pathway and the Krebs cycle together constitute a universal metabolic partnership that is present in all aerobic life forms, from simple one-celled organisms to complex humans. This system provides energy for all life functions including the formation and degradation of countless biochemicals. Many of the biochemicals in the Krebs cycle system also serve as substrates for other metabolic pathways, such as synthesis of the nonessential amino acids.

The interrelationship among carbohydrate, protein, and lipid biochemicals is made possible by the fact that all of the reactions in the glycolytic pathway are reversible. This reversibility, combined with the unique property of enzymatic reactions that enable them to be stimulated or inhibited by excesses or deficiencies of their metabolite, makes for very rapid responses to the needs of an organism.

FIGURE 6-1
GLYCOLYSIS

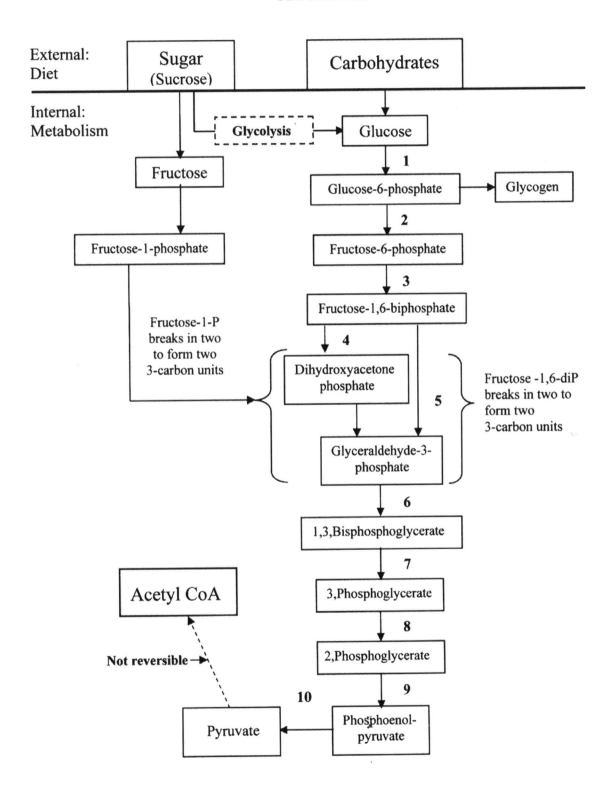

For example, if blood glucose levels fall to dangerously low levels, the body can convert nonessential amino acids to metabolites that enter the glycolytic pathway and, by reversal of glycolysis (gluconeogenesis), produce the glucose required for maintaining normal blood glucose levels. The only step shown in Figure 6-1 that is not reversible is the one from pyruvate to acetyl CoA.

Plants and microorganisms are able to make glucose from acetyl CoA by reversing the pyruvate to acetyl CoA reaction, but animal biochemistry does not include this capability. As a result, glucose cannot be made from fats because fats are broken down only to acetyl CoA (see Figure 4-1). Thus, with the exception of the glycerol moiety of triglycerides, the only sources for glucose synthesis in animals, other than carbohydrates, are the nonessential amino acids from proteins.

The fact that glucose can be synthesized from noncarbohydrate chemicals explains why, despite being a critically important carbohydrate in human biochemistry, glucose is not an essential nutrient (recall that an essential nutrient is defined as one the body cannot make but must be supplied in the diet). In fact, unlike a few members of the protein and lipid groups, there are *no* essential carbohydrates.

Figure 6-1 also shows that the fructose released from sucrose does not go directly to glucose or even to the fructose made from glucose in steps1-3 of the glycolytic pathway. This is because dietary fructose and fructose made from glucose are kept separate from each other in independent pools in the body by biochemical means (position of phosphate groups in the fructose molecule). In order for dietary fructose to be converted to glucose, it must first be metabolized to a triose and then, by reverse glycolysis, go back up the pathway to glucose.

GLYCEMIC INDEX: Before leaving the subject of carbohydrate metabolism, it is very important to explain the glycemic index (GI), which is a measure of the rate at which glucose from any given food enters the blood stream. The higher the GI, the more rapid is the entry of glucose into the blood stream.

The concept of the GI appears to have had its origins in the need for people with insulin-dependent (type-1) diabetes to avoid foods that caused rapid increases in blood glucose. Glucose itself is taken as the standard and assigned a GI of 100. Only the disaccharide maltose increases blood glucose levels more quickly than does glucose. Maltose has a GI of 110. The indirect pathway of fructose to glucose results in a GI of only about 20.

In general, foods that cause a fast rise in blood glucose levels have high GIs. Foods that cause a slow rise have low indices. However, inspection of GI tables, available on line from diabetes web sites (3), indicates that GI is influenced by cooking method, length of cooking, and perhaps by other factors. For example, parboiled rice has a GI of 47, yet instant rice has a GI of 91. Dried apricots have a GI of 30, while canned apricots (easy to chew) have a GI of 64. The lengthy and roundabout way of making glucose from fructose (Figure 6-1) helps explain why the GI for fructose is so very much smaller than the GI for glucose (20 versus 100).

The lists of specific numbers for glycemic indices can be obtained from the American Diabetes Association (3). However, note that an alternate method for rating the GI of foods has appeared in some nutrition books. In this rating system, the GI for white bread, rather than glucose, is taken as the standard and assigned a GI of 100. On this scale, glucose has a GI somewhere above 100. If readers are interested in using the glycemic indices in developing their own diets, it is suggested using information based on the glucose standard, because glucose is a pure chemical. Thus, unlike with white bread, the GI of glucose is less variable.

A detailed knowledge of GIs is probably more academic than practical for healthy individuals. It is more important for good health to follow a diet that excludes or strictly limits soft drinks, other sugary foods and starches and is moderate in carbohydrate calories. As a general rule, products high in sugars, refined flour products, and starchy vegetables have high GIs and should be avoided when possible. Green vegetables, nontropical fruits, nuts, beans, and dairy products have low indices. Proteins and fats have GIs of zero except when they occur in combination with carbohydrates.

Conventional wisdom says that high-glycemic diets tend not to satisfy hunger. People who have weight problems will be interested to know that recent nutritional research confirms this belief and provides a probable explanation. One study indicates that high-glycemic carbohydrates may promote overeating by increasing hunger (4). Another study postulates that the rapid absorption of glucose from high-glycemic foods induces a sequence of hormonal and metabolic changes that promote excessive food intake (5). Low-GI diets have shown promise in treating obesity in children (6). These data provide further reason to eliminate sugars and refined carbohydrates and to restrict carbohydrate calories to no more than 40 percent of the diet.

Glycemic Load: Criticism of the use of the GI in evaluating the nutritional quality of carbohydrates has pointed to the fact that many foods contain high-glycemic carbohydrates but in very small quantities. The concept of glycemic load (GL), which is considered to be more important than the GI, was proposed as an answer to this criticism. The glycemic load in a food is a number calculated from the GI of the carbohydrate, the grams of carbohydrate in the food, and the frequency of its intake. Another proposal for evaluating the glycemic potential of carbohydrates is the glycemic glucose equivalent (GGE), which refers to the grams of glucose that would induce a glycemic response equivalent to that induced by a specified amount of the carbohydrate food (7).

HEXOSE MONOPHOSPHATE SHUNT

The hexose monophosphate shunt is a metabolic pathway that makes a detour from glucose-6-P to fructose-6-P of the glycolytic pathway (see Figure 6-2). The HMP shunt is designed to support the heavy demands imposed on the immune system when dealing with threats from invading organisms or foreign cells. The shunt synthesizes 5-carbon sugars, known as riboses, which are used to make genetic material (DNA and RNA) for rapid proliferation of immune cells. The shunt is also active in producing niacin coenzyme NADPH used for synthesis of reactive oxygen species, the chemical weapon used by the immune system to kill invaders.

FIGURE 6-2
THE HEXOSE MONOPHOSPHATE SHUNT

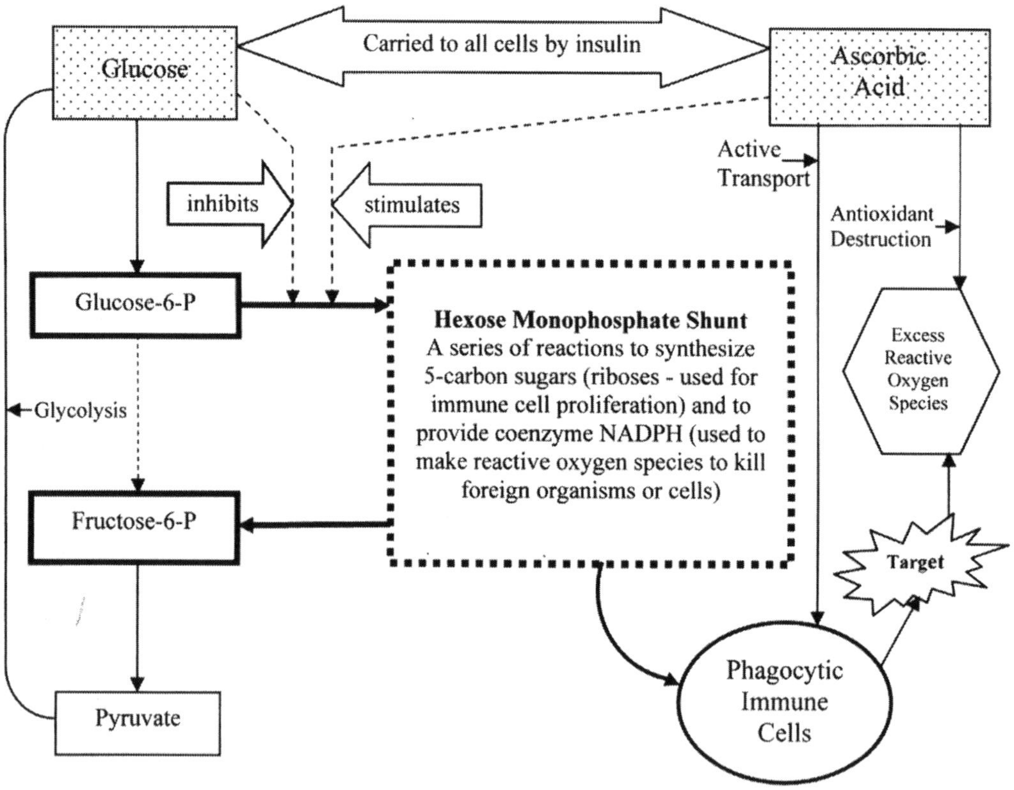

Ref, 8.) Ottoboni F, Ottoboni A. Ascorbic and the immune system. *The Journal of Orthomolecular Medicine.* 2005; **20**(3): 179-183.

As shown in Figure 6-2, the HMP shunt delivers riboses and NADPH to immune cells for attack on invaders. Reactive oxygen species in excess of the amount needed to eradicate invaders are, in turn, destroyed by the antioxidant action of ascorbic acid (8).

Activation of the HMP shunt is governed by the glucose/ascorbic acid concentrations in the blood. Glucose and ascorbic acid are both carried in the blood and delivered by insulin to all cells in the body. This common transport system combined with their structural similarity makes for a problematic relationship between them. As shown in Figure 6-2, glucose inhibits the shunt and ascorbic acid stimulates it. This competition stresses the importance of an appropriate balance between glucose and ascorbic acid for proper immune function. If glucose is present in great excess, it will effectively hinder the activation of the HMP shunt. Regular supplementation with ascorbic acid is essential to counter this glucose inhibition.

The tremendous importance of ascorbic acid for effective immune function is demonstrated by the fact that ascorbic acid is delivered to immune system cells by active transport. As a result, leukocytes, which are responsible for host defense, can have as much as 80 times the concentration of ascorbic acid as the surrounding plasma (9; 10). With passive transport, the intra- and intercellular concentrations would be the same.

Glucose, Insulin, and Glucagon

The monosaccharide glucose, the focal point of carbohydrate metabolism, has a singular role in nutrition. As an indispensable component of blood, it influences the metabolic fate of the other macronutrients. Thus, a review of how dietary macronutrients contribute to the blood glucose pool and how, in turn, blood glucose concentrations govern what metabolic pathways macronutrients take is basic to an understanding of the role of diet in the modern nutritional diseases.

Figure 6-3 outlines how the macronutrients affect blood glucose levels. With few exceptions, digestive and metabolic processes convert carbohydrates (sugars and starches) to glucose. Carbohydrates are the body's single most important source of blood glucose. Dietary proteins and fats do not have much effect on blood glucose levels. Nonessential amino acids are not used for glucose synthesis except when the amount of carbohydrate in the diet is insufficient to keep blood glucose levels in a normal range. Dietary fat, on the other hand, cannot be used by the animal body as a source of glucose (11, p. 375).

THE INSULIN/GLUCAGON RATIO

The singular role of glucose in nutrition is not related to its own metabolism but rather to its relationship with the hormones insulin and glucagon. Insulin and glucagon are complementary metabolic hormones secreted by special cells in the pancreas gland, the beta and alpha cells, respectively, of the Islets of Langerhans. In most instances, insulin and glucagon have opposite effects. The primary regulator of insulin secretion is blood glucose concentration. The dangers of high blood glucose and the importance of insulin in controlling it is demonstrated by the fact that the pancreas is continually prepared for a sudden marked increase in blood glucose by having a store of proinsulin available for rapid release of insulin (12). Insulin and glucagon are carried in the bloodstream to all cells throughout the body where they control cellular metabolism by regulating numerous biochemical processes.

FIGURE 6-3
IMPACT OF NUTRIENTS ON INSULIN AND GLUCAGON PRODUCTION*

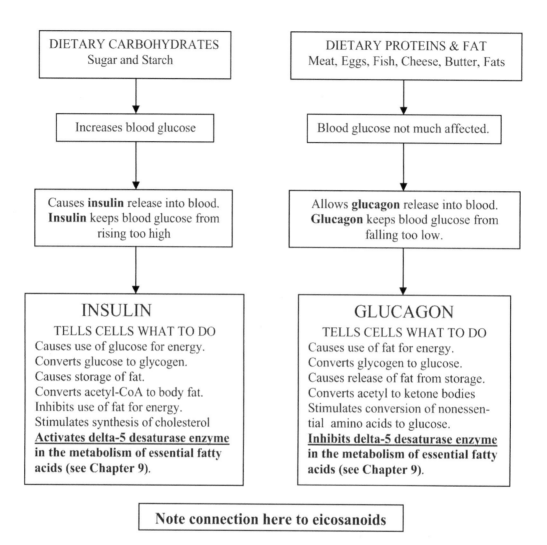

*Sources: Rhodes, RA,Tanner, GA. *Medical Physiology.* Boston, MA: Little Brown & Co. 1995.
Sears, Barry. *Enter the Zone.* New York, NY: ReganBooks, HarperCollins, 1995.

High blood glucose concentrations, such as occur after a high carbohydrate meal, stimulate the production of insulin. Several hours after eating, blood glucose concentrations drop and, as a result, blood insulin levels also drop. The resulting low glucose level stimulates glucagon secretion. The insulin/glucagon ratio can vary 100-fold or more during a 24-hour period. After a full meal, it is approximately 30; after an overnight fast, it can drop to 2; and after a prolonged fast it can drop to as low as 0.5 (12).

In proper balance, insulin and glucagon control and maintain blood glucose levels to within the normal range of 80 to 120 milligrams per 100 milliliters of blood that is essential for health. A brief excursion of insulin level related to food-intake history that is well above or well below the normal range is commonplace and is efficiently managed in healthy people by an appropriate insulin or glucagon response.

In its relationship with insulin and glucagon, glucose can be thought of as playing opposing roles of both master and servant. The concentration of glucose in the blood governs the release of insulin and glucagon; in turn, insulin and glucagon govern the concentration of glucose in the blood. Control of the balance between insulin and glucagon by blood glucose is one of the body's fundamental regulatory mechanisms for maintaining homeostasis, the stability of the internal environment of the body (12, p. 5). It is for this reason that the concentration of glucose in the blood must be kept within a relatively narrow range in order to maintain healthy life functions in all of the cells and tissues of the body.

Significance of Dietary Carbohydrate

Because of the obligatory relationship between blood glucose concentration and insulin/ glucagon status, the quantity of carbohydrate in the diet exerts a profound influence on how other dietary macronutrients are metabolized. This is best explained by reviewing the two dietary extremes, namely the high-carbohydrate diet shown in Figure 6-4 and the low-carbohydrate diet shown in Figure 6-5.

After eating carbohydrate foods, large amounts of glucose enter the bloodstream. As shown in Figure 6-4, the high glucose level stimulates release of insulin from the pancreas for the critical purpose of bringing the blood glucose level down into normal range. To do this, insulin initiates a number of actions that remove glucose from the blood. One, it withdraws glucose to make glycogen, a polymer of glucose used for storage in liver and muscle tissue; two, it stimulates glycolysis to yield acetyl CoA; and three, it furthers glycolysis by removing the acetyl CoA that is formed but not needed for energy and directing it to synthesis of body fat and cholesterol. In summary, if the diet provides more glucose than the body needs, the excess glucose is stored temporarily as glycogen, and when glycogen sites are filled, the energy from the excess glucose goes primarily to synthesis and storage of body fat and synthesis of cholesterol.

Excessive consumption of carbohydrates in the form of sugar and starch is a major factor in the development of high blood cholesterol (and atherosclerosis). However, if any specific carbohydrate foods could be singled out as important contributors to America's high blood cholesterol levels, such foods would have to be high fructose corn sweeteners and sucrose. Sucrose, common table sugar, is metabolized to yield equal amounts of glucose and fructose in the body.

FIGURE 6-4
HIGH-CARBOHYDRATE DIET
(LOW-PROTEIN, LOW-FAT DIET)

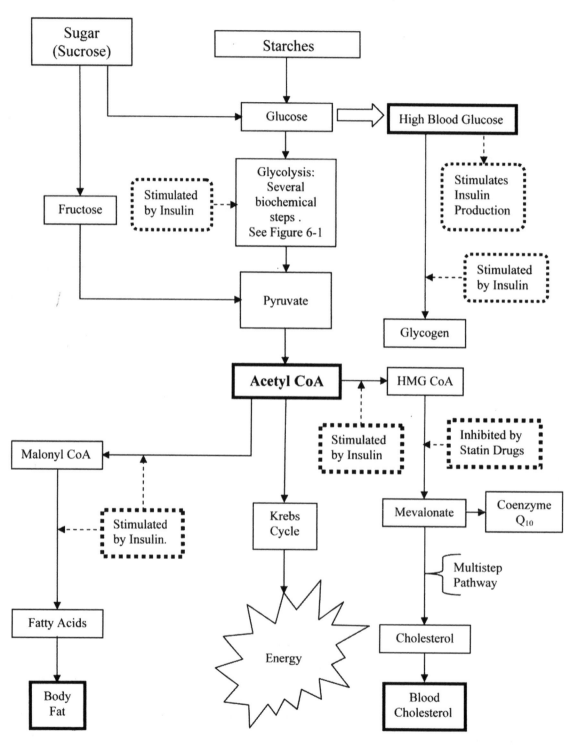

High fructose corn sweeteners are composed of roughly equal amounts of glucose and fructose. Once ingested, glucose enters the bloodstream and is metabolized by the glycolytic pathway. Fructose also enters the bloodstream, but takes a different path. It bypasses the constraints imposed by glycolysis and moves to acetyl CoA and the pathways that make cholesterol and body fat (see Figure 6-4). This difference in metabolism between dietary fructose and glucose makes dietary fructose a more direct precursor of cholesterol and body fat than glucose.

Figure 6-5 outlines the metabolic pathways followed when the blood glucose level falls below normal levels. This can occur after a high carbohydrate meal when the insulin has completed its job and excess glucose is utilized or when the carbohydrate content of the diet is very low. When blood glucose levels fall, insulin levels also fall, and the pancreas responds to the lowered levels with secretion of glucagon. The purpose of this response is to keep the blood glucose concentration from falling further to a dangerously low level. Glucagon helps maintain glucose in the normal range by first mobilizing stored glycogen and converting it to glucose, as needed, to help restore the normal blood glucose level.

As glycogen stores dwindle and blood glucose begins to fall again, glucagon prepares for the possibility that a new supply of dietary glucose will not be forthcoming soon. To this end, glucagon initiates release of body fat from adipose tissue and promotes β-oxidation of fatty acids to acetyl CoA and ketone bodies (see Figure 6-5). This provides an alternate energy source that spares glucose from being withdrawn from the blood for that purpose. This diversion of energy production from glucose to fatty acids represents a major shift in the body's metabolic energy control system, which is discussed in greater detail in Chapter Eight.

In addition to preparing for an alternate source of energy, glucagon also arranges for an alternate source of glucose, which can be made from nonessential amino acids, as mentioned earlier. Glucagon stimulates the body to make its own glucose; nonessential amino acids are deaminated, catabolized to pyruvate (see Figure 4-1) and, by reverse glycolysis, converted to glucose (see Figure 6-1). If these amino acids are available from dietary protein, they will be utilized first. After dietary proteins, the least critical of body proteins will be used. In severe starvation, the last proteins used are from muscle tissue.

A diet that contains sufficient carbohydrate to spare protein from having to be used to make glucose would be diagrammed by a composite of Figures 6-4 and 6-5. This composite would represent a normal, well-fed individual on a balanced diet. In such an individual, the insulin/glucagon cycle operates smoothly. The nutritional diseases that result from diets that disrupt the critical insulin/glucagon relationship (hypoglycemia, insulin resistance, obesity, and type-2 diabetes) will be discussed in Chapter Ten.

FIGURE 6-5
LOW-CARBOHYDRATE DIET
(HIGH-PROTEIN, HIGH-FAT DIET)

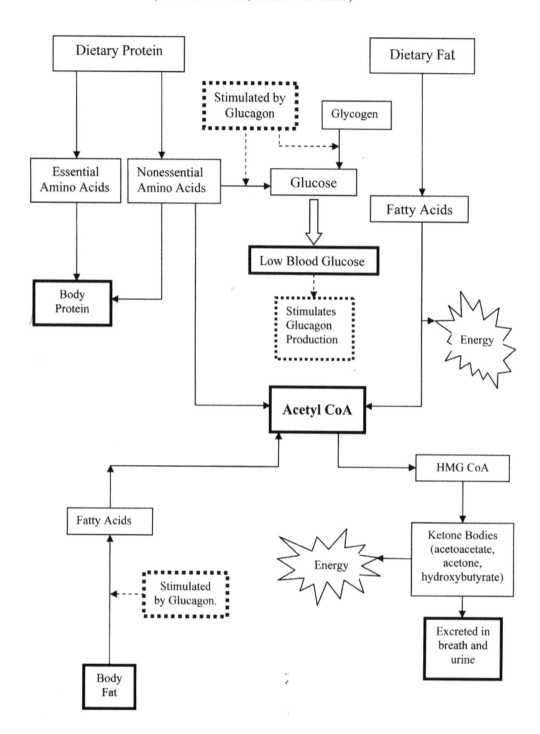

Nutritional Requirements for Carbohydrates

As mentioned above, there are no carbohydrates that are essential for humans. However, that must not imply that carbohydrate foods should not be included in a healthful diet. Although carbohydrates may not be essential in the strict biochemical sense, they are very important as vehicles for countless other essential micronutrients. Fruits and vegetables are a major source of fiber, minerals, and vitamins. They are especially important for their vitamins A, C, and E content. They are also the only sources of important phytochemicals such as carotenoids and flavinoids.

Perhaps one of the most valuable contributions that fruits and vegetables make to healthful nutrition is provision of antioxidants. It is only in recent years that the importance of anti-oxidants in food plants has been fully appreciated. The majority of these antioxidants are phytochemical pigments that confer on plant foods the great number and variety of colors. They seem not to have any specific functions in human biochemistry other than to serve in protecting its healthful internal reducing milieu. The redox environment of an organism is related to the antioxidant content of the diet.

The importance of an internal reducing environment is the result of the human body's need to constantly counter demanding oxidative pressures. The human organism has an oxidative biochemistry and lives in a sea of oxygen, both of which are circumstances that present numerous opportunities for injurious oxidations. The importance of a reducing environment within the body is underlined by the fact that just a moderate increase in the oxidative environment stimulates cell growth and division – an undesirable situation when defective cells are present.

Even though carbohydrates are not essential in the diet, the glucose that is derived from them serves as an important source of energy and more importantly as the blood component that helps the body maintain homeostasis – as described above. The amount of carbohydrate in the diet needed for energy depends largely on the age and activity level of the individual. Growing children and physically active adults have a much greater demand for energy than older or sedentary individuals. Empirically, the amount of carbohydrate that causes neither weight gain nor weight loss is the correct amount.

For adults of normal weight, the objective should be to eat just enough carbohydrate to prevent loss of muscle mass due to depletion of protein from muscle tissue and loss of normal weight due to depletion of fats from adipose tissue. The minimum amount of carbohydrate needed to prevent weight loss and spare protein from the need to replenish blood glucose has been estimated to be about 20 calories of carbohydrate (about 5 grams) for each 100 calories of diet (14, p. 126), which translates to 20 percent of diet calories. These data, combined with the fact that no carbohydrate is biochemically essential, makes one question why the official nutrition policy recommends a dietary intake of 55 to 60 percent or *more* of total calories from carbohydrates (15).

The carbohydrates that do not serve as vehicles for essential nutrients or fiber are the carbohydrates that should be used sparingly or not at all. This group includes foods that are largely sugar and/or refined grain products: candies, cookies, cakes, cereals, breads, rolls, pasta, and donuts. It also includes all varieties of soft drinks, which are labeled as *Liquid Candy* by the Center for Science in the Public Interest (16). Refined carbohydrate foods provide calories but little or no nutritive value. Table sugar (sucrose) is the perfect example of a food with blind or empty calories.

The label Liquid Candy is validated by a study of the relationship between soft drink consumption and obese children that found for each additional can or bottle consumed, the risk of becoming obese increased by 50 percent, independent of diet or exercise (17). The National Soft Drink Association issued a strong rebuttal disputing the findings and criticizing the study methods (18).

Dietary Recommendations for Carbohydrates

A review of the recommendations for carbohydrate intake that appeared in the 2010 revision (18) of the *Dietary Guidelines for Americans*, namely 45 to 65 percent, are essentially the same as those in the 2005 revision (15). Interestingly, the 2010 guidelines advise the higher percent, stressing that the 65 percent intake is preferable in order to obtain sufficient fiber.

The extensive data in the scientific literature that point to high-carbohydrate intake as a major factor in coronary heart disease (CHD) and type-2 diabetes (T2D) are still completely ignored in the 2010 report (19). With regard to the relationship of carbohydrates with CHD, T2D, behavior, and cognitive performance, it states "No detrimental effects of carbohydrates as a source of calories on these or other health outcomes were reported."

The American Heart Association, one of the sponsors of the official dietary recommendations, indirectly acknowledges the potential problems associated with high sucrose intake by suggesting that people use complex carbohydrate foods instead of sugar (sucrose). The fallacy in such a recommendation is that many complex carbohydrates have higher glycemic indices than sucrose. Examination of GI tables shows the following glycemic indices: sucrose, 59; baked potato, 98; carrots, 92; instant rice, 91; corn flake cereal, 80; wheat bread, 72; beets, 64; and bananas, 62 (3).

Sugar and Bread Substitutes

The subject of carbohydrates would not be complete without a mention of sugar substitutes (artificial sweeteners). The first of the sugar substitutes, saccharine, was developed many decades ago to provide people with insulin-dependent diabetes (type-1) a welcome relief from their otherwise sweet-free diet. As the years went by and other sugar substitutes came on the market, some clever entrepreneurs realized they could greatly increase the sales of these products to the general public by promoting them as diet aids. Thus, a whole new class of products was added to the grocery shelves.

Today, there are few sugar-containing foods that cannot be made in a sweet but sugar-free variety. Even table sugar has sugar-free counterparts in little single-serving packets. The use of sugar substitutes for weight control, rather than for their original purpose of providing diabetics with some sweetness in foods, has not prevented obesity. Although sugar substitutes contain no available carbohydrates, they do have the same insulin-stimulating and carbohydrate-craving properties as glucose (20, p. 55ff; 21, p. 59).

Stimulation of excess insulin promotes synthesis of body fat and cholesterol, regardless of whether the stimulation is caused by a noncaloric sweetener or by a carbohydrate. Apparently there has been no consideration by the nutrition community of the physiologic impact of stimulating insulin secretion in the absence of a glucose load. A substitute for bread is a different matter from that of a substitute for sugar.

The suggestion that there be a substitute for bread is probably alien to every culture, but the health benefits of eliminating bread from the diet, especially for sedentary individuals, would be immeasurable. Apples, a carbohydrate food that is tasty and satisfying, are excellent substitutes for bread. What is more, apples contain many vitamins, minerals, and beneficial phytochemicals. They are satisfying as substitutes for toast with a plate of bacon and eggs, for dinner rolls with a juicy steak, or for French bread with cheese and a glass of wine. The old adage "An apple a day keeps the doctor away" may contain more than just a grain of truth.

References

1.) http://www.healingtherapies.info/D-Mannose.htm/ Accessed Sept. 26, 2012.

2.) Healing Options: Nutritional alternatives for preventing and fighting urinary tract infections. Paraplegic News. 2002; 56(6): Part 1; 56(9): Part 2.

3.) http://diabetesnet.com/gi.html/ Accessed Sept. 26, 2012.

4.) Roberts SB. High-glycemic index foods, hunger, and obesity: is there a connection? Nutrition Reviews. 2000; 58(6): 163-9.

5.) Ludwig DS, et al. High glycemic index foods. Overeating and obesity. Pediatrics. 1999; 103(3): E26.

6.) Spieth, LE, et al. A low-glycemic index diet in the treatment of pediatric obesity. Archives of Pediatric and Adolescents Medicine. 2000; 154(9): 947-51.

7.) Monro JA, Shaw M. Glycemic impact, glycemic glucose equivalents, glycemic index, and glycemic load. American Journal of Clinical Nutrition. 2008; 87(1): 237S-243S.

8.) Ottoboni F, Ottoboni A. Ascorbic and the immune system. The Journal of Orthomolecular Medicine. 2005; 20(3): 179-183.

9.) Evans RM, Currie L, Campbell A. The distribution of ascorbic acid between various cellular components of blood in normal individuals, and to its relationship to plasma concentrations. British Journal of Nutrition. 1982; 47(3): 473-482.

10.) Moser U. Uptake of ascorbic acid by leukocytes. Annals New York Academy of Sciences. 1987; 498: 200-215.

11.) Horton, H, et al. Principles of Biochemistry, Second Ed. Upper Saddle River, NJ: Prentice Hall, 1996.

12.) Rhoades RA, Tanner GA. Medical Physiology. Boston, MA: Little, Brown and Company, 1995.

13.) Sears, Barry. *Enter the Zone*. New York, NY: ReganBooks, HarperCollins, 1995.

14.) Cantarow A, Trumper M. Clinical Biochemistry. Philadelphia, PA: W. B. Saunders Co, 1962.

15.) http://www.cnpp.usda.gov/ and/or http://www.mypyramid.gov/ Accessed Sept. 26, 2012.

16.) http://www.cspinet.org/liquidcandy/ Accessed Sept. 26, 2012.

17.) Ludwig DS, et al. Relation between sugar-sweetened soft drinks and childhood obesity. The Lancet. 2001; 357(9255): 505-508.

18.) http://www.spokesman.com/stories/2012/sep/22/soft-drink-industry-issues-rebuttal/ Accessed Sept. 26, 2012.

19.) http://www.cnpp.usda.gov/publications/dietaryguidelines/2010/dgac/report/d-5-carbohydrates.pdf/ Accessed Sept. 26, 2012.

20.) Gittleman AL. *Your Body Knows Best*. New York, NY: Simon & Schuster, 1997.

21.) Lipetz P. The Good Calorie Diet. New York, NY: Harper Paperbacks, 1996.

Chapter Seven

Proteins

Vegetables are interesting but lack a sense of purpose unless accompanied by a good cut of meat. **Fran Liebowitz (1).**

The importance of protein in the diet cannot be overstated. They are the most abundant of biochemicals. Proteins participate in virtually every biological process of living organisms. They provide essentially all the structural elements, the transport systems, and the control mechanisms of the marvelous machine known as the human body. There are probably few structures or functions in our bodies that do not require the use or participation of some protein. Because of their critical importance in all aspects of life function, the first task in planning a healthful nutritional regime is to determine one's protein requirement. The balance of the nutritional regime is filled in with appropriate additions of fats, carbohydrates, and essential micronutrients.

If necessary, proteins can be metabolized to provide the heat and energy required for life functions, but protein is not the best fuel for the purpose because it is inefficient. In fact, biological science has long known that humans cannot consume and digest sufficient quantities of protein to support their energy requirements on a long-term, continuing basis (2, p. 639). Ideally, energy production is the task of carbohydrates and fats.

Proteins are very large molecules composed primarily of carbon, hydrogen, oxygen, and nitrogen, with traces of sulfur. Protein molecules are polymers of smaller molecules, known as amino acids, linked together in long chains. There are two basic types of proteins; those that are like little globules that can move around easily and those that are like threads or fibers that stay in one place. Enzymes, hormones, antibodies, and oxygen-carrying molecules (hemoglobin and myoglobin) are examples of globular proteins that travel around in the aqueous media of the body; muscles, tendons, skin, hair, and nails are examples of fibrous proteins that are fixed in the body's structures.

Proteins do not have specific storage sites in the body like carbohydrates have in the form of glycogen in liver and muscle and fats have in the form of triglycerides in adipose tissue.

However, in times of ample protein intake, the blood plasma and all organs and tissues of the body accumulate variable amounts of extra protein (2, p. 633). The liver is capable of a considerable increase, perhaps as much as 20 percent, in its protein content. These accumulations are not considered storage, but rather reserves that help maintain an even amino acid supply in the face of uneven intake. This reserve supply is used to make up deficits when dietary proteins do not supply all the amino acids needed, either the appropriate quantity or the appropriate ratio.

Plants are the ultimate source of nitrogen for all animal life. Using carbon dioxide, water, inorganic nitrogen (N_2), plus the energy from sunlight, soil microorganisms (and some plants) convert (fix) nitrogen into a form that plants can use to make the amino acids they require for their proteins. Animals can make carbohydrates from proteins, and they can make fats from proteins, but they cannot make proteins or any other nitrogen-containing biochemicals without the nitrogen that plants fix in their amino acids. Plants make all of the same amino acids that animals do plus many more, but they make them in different proportions. Animal biochemistry obtains the ammonia (NH_3) it needs for other reactions by removing the amino groups from amino acids they cannot use.

Protein Units – Amino Acids

Amino acids are the building blocks of proteins. More than forty naturally occurring amino acids are known, but only twenty are commonly found in mammalian proteins. Of these twenty, ten are termed nonessential because the body can synthesize them from nutrients in the diet. The ten nonessential amino acids are alanine, aspartic acid, asparagine, cysteine, glycine, glutamic acid, glutamine, proline, serine, and tyrosine. Nine amino acids are labeled as essential because the body either cannot synthesize them or cannot synthesize them in sufficient quantities to supply the need for them. Thus, they must be provided in the diet. The essential amino acids are histidine, isoleucine, leucine, lysine, methionine, phenylalanine, threonine, tryptophan, and valine.

A twentieth amino acid, arginine, is listed as essential in some textbooks and nonessential in others. This is because growing animals cannot synthesize sufficient quantities of arginine for their needs; thus, arginine is essential for infants and children. It is not essential for adults because they can make all the arginine their bodies require. Despite the essential/nonessential distinction, all twenty of these amino acids are important and necessary for the proper functioning of the body.

Interestingly, the report on the recommendations for the 2010 revision of the *Dietary Guidelines for Americans* reassigns the above classic grouping of nonessential amino acids into nonessential and conditionally essential. The conditionally essential amino acids are listed as arginine, cysteine, glutamine, glycine, proline, and tyrosine. This new list indicates that although the body is capable of synthesizing these amino acids, there may be certain conditions in which the need for them is greater than the body's capability to make sufficient quantities of them (3). The essential group remains unchanged,

The amino acids in naturally occurring proteins are alpha-amino acids. They take their name from the fact that they share a common feature in their structures; they all have a carboxyl group (-COOH) as carbon one and an amine group (-NH$_2$) on carbon two, which is the carbon adjacent to the carboxyl group. They are called alpha-amino acids because the carbon adjacent to a carboxyl group is designated as the alpha (α) carbon.

With the exception of the simplest amino acid (2-carbon glycine), each α-amino acid has two forms. The two forms are identical to each other in composition, but differ in that they rotate light in opposite directions. Naturally occurring amino acids are called L-amino acids because they rotate light to the left (*levo*). Amino acids that rotate light to the right (*dextro*) are designated as D-amino acids. The *dextro* form can be made in the laboratory, but laboratory synthesis usually yields both D- and L-amino acids together in what is known as a racemic mixture.

Racemic mixtures of amino acids are optically inactive because laboratory synthesis produces equal amounts of the levo- and the dextro-form, which cancel each other's light rotation. As a general rule, only L-amino acids should be used as supplements. In some cases, the D-form is simply ignored by the body, but in others it can interfere with the utilization of the natural L-form.

Digestion of Proteins

Dietary proteins, whether animal or vegetable, cannot be used directly by the body but must first be broken down to their component amino acids by digestive processes. This begins in the stomach with denaturation of proteins by acidic gastric juices. Denaturation involves unfolding or unrolling of protein molecules so that the amino acid linkages are exposed and more accessible to action by digestive enzymes.

Heat as well as acid denatures proteins. A familiar example of denaturation is the conversion of egg white from a translucent gel to an opaque white solid by cooking. As with egg whites, proteins may already be denatured by cooking or other preparation before they reach the acidic medium of the stomach. Any protein that performs a specific function in its natural state, such as an enzyme, will be deactivated by denaturation, which means it can no longer perform that function.

Proteins are broken down in the small intestine to their respective amino acids or to peptides, which are combinations of two (dipeptides) or a few amino acids. Amino acids and peptides, primarily dipeptides, are transported by well-defined mechanisms across the lining of the small intestine into the hepatic portal vein and delivered to the liver for further processing and/or use. It is generally accepted that some tripeptides may be absorbed from the intestinal tract but, if they are, their quantities are not nutritionally significant. In normal individuals, no or negligible amounts of undigested or partially digested protein are absorbed from the digestive tract (4, p. 560).

A malfunction of absorption that permits entry of proteins or large peptides into the bloodstream can result in severe intestinal illnesses and/or life-threatening allergic reactions. The body is very sensitive to foreign proteins, which are proteins or protein fragments that it recognizes as not being made by itself. This ability to detect foreign proteins, although not specific for pathogens, is an important defense mechanism against infection or other unknown invaders.

Metabolism of Proteins

The metabolism of proteins and their component amino acids is somewhat different than that of the other macronutrients of the diet. Except for the singular role of glucose in homeostasis, by virtue of its concentration in the blood, a major function of carbohydrates and fats is to provide cellular energy. The main function of dietary proteins, on the other hand, is to provide the amino acid building blocks that the body uses to make its own particular proteins, which in turn become the structures and components of its operating system. Thus, the metabolism of proteins is primarily a process of degradation of proteins, new (dietary) or old (used), to yield their component amino acids followed by assembly of new proteins from the amino acids supplied by protein degradation.

PROTEIN TURNOVER

Amino acids are the building blocks the body uses to make its own unique proteins. In all organisms, proteins are constantly being broken down and resynthesized. The human body has a constant demand for a great number of proteins of varied sizes, shapes, and functions. In addition, many proteins within the body have half-lives (the time required for loss of half the number of molecules of a specific protein) from a few minutes to several weeks, depending on the kind of protein it is (5, p 515). The constant demand for new proteins, combined with the fact that, like most living things, proteins have limited lives results in a process called *turnover* in which there is almost continuous degradation and resynthesis. This creates a continual demand for amino acids. Thus, the need for a continuous supply of good quality protein cannot be overemphasized.

AMINO ACID METABOLISM

The body's shopping list for the amino acids is in continual flux. Its make-up at any moment depends on the kind of proteins needed and how many. Nonessential amino acids are obtained either by degradation (described above) or by *de novo* synthesis (anabolism), but essential amino acids are obtained only from degradation.

ANABOLISM: All of the nonessential amino acids are synthesized from a metabolite either in the glycolytic pathway or the Krebs cycle (see Figure 4-1); alanine, cysteine, glycine, and serine have their origins in metabolites of the glycolytic pathway and arginine (when it is nonessential), aspartate, asparagine, glutamate, glutamine, proline, and tyrosine in metabolites of the Krebs cycle. The detailed synthetic pathways for each can be found on the Internet on the Medical Biochemistry Page (6).

The final step in amino acid synthesis is the addition of an amino group in the alpha position (adjacent to the carboxyl group). A simple but highly efficient system for introducing ammonia (NH_3) into biochemical systems is used by animals as well as microorganisms and plants. It involves the addition of a molecule of NH_3 to α-keto- glutarate (from the Krebs cycle) to form the amino acid glutamic acid (glutamate). A second molecule of NH_3 is then added to glutamate to form the amino acid glutamine.

The second NH_3 (now called an amine group) is carried around in glutamine to sites of amino acid synthesis where it donates the amine group to the new amino acid. In the process, glutamine is converted back to glutamate, which in turn is free to go back and pick up another NH_3 molecule.

Glutamine serves not only as a transfer agent for amine groups in amino acid synthesis but also as a nitrogen donor in many other metabolic reactions. In mammals, glutamine acts as a carrier of nitrogen throughout the body, thereby avoiding the toxic effects of free ammonia in blood and tissues.

CATABOLISM: A pool of amino acids, which is kept supplied by the diet and/or by protein turnover, serves the demands of protein synthesis. Amino acids that cannot be used for protein synthesis or are in excess of the quantity needed are degraded (catabolized) and eliminated from the body.

The first step in the catabolism of amino acids is removal of the α-amino group by a process called deamination. Deamination yields ammonia (NH_3), a chemical that is toxic to tissues of the body. Thus, under normal circumstances, ammonia is attached to a carrier biochemical (usually glutamine) immediately upon release. If the NH_3 unit is not required for the synthesis of another nitrogen-containing biochemical, it is rapidly converted in a series of reactions called the urea cycle to form the less toxic urea (NH_2CONH_2) Urea is eliminated from the body chiefly in the urine with small amounts eliminated in perspiration. Urea is the principal form for elimination of nitrogen

After deamination, the carbon residues of the nonessential amino acids are eliminated fairly directly by conversion to pyruvate or one of the intermediates of the Krebs cycle and then on to CO_2 and H_2O via the Krebs cycle (see Figure 4-1). These are the amino acids that are used to supply glucose when blood glucose levels fall to low or below normal levels. They do this by reversal of the pathway through the Krebs cycle and then reversal of the glycolytic pathway ultimately to form glucose. The carbon residues of the essential amino acids each follow their own metabolic pathways. Their primary role is for use in protein synthesis. When their role is completed, they find their way to CO_2 through acetyl CoA or some component of the Krebs cycle.

A word of caution is appropriate here for anyone taking amino acid supplements. Keep in mind that amino acids in excess of the body's requirements must be broken down in the liver and excreted by the kidneys. Deamination and urea formation are reactions with a significant metabolic cost that could stress compromised liver or kidneys. For this reason, people with liver or kidney disease should keep protein intake, including amino acid supplements, to a level prescribed by a healthcare provider.

SPECIAL ROLES FOR AMINO ACIDS

In addition to serving as monomers in protein chains, several essential and nonessential amino acids participate in important intermediary metabolic functions.

GLUTAMATE-GLUTAMINE: As mentioned above, the nonessential amino acid glutamine provides the pathway for entry of nitrogen into mammalian biochemistry; it serves as a carrier of nitrogen, in the form of ammonia, throughout the body; and it participates in the biosynthesis of amino acids with its transaminase function.

CYSTEINE: Cysteine, a small nonessential amino acid containing a sulfhydryl (or thiol group -SH), is of vital importance in stabilizing protein structures by virtue of its ability to cross link with another cysteine molecule to form a disulfide bond (SS). The dimer formed by linking two cysteine molecules through a disulfide bond is named cystine. Cystine is of little biochemical significance as a free molecule, but its importance as an internal or external member in a protein structure is inestimable.

The formation of disulfide bonds makes for stability of the folded structures of globular proteins and the sheet or rope-like structures of fibrous proteins. Disulfide bonding occurs when two cysteine molecules within the same protein chain (internal), in the case of globular proteins, or in adjacent protein chains (external), in the case of fibrous proteins, come into apposition. Disulfide cross-linking makes possible such diverse protein forms as the globular protein hemoglobin and the fibrous protein collagen.

METHIONINE: The essential amino acid methionine is the entry point of what might be labeled the methyl transfer cycle (see Figure 7-1). Methionine is a major source of methyl groups ($-CH_3$) for a number of important synthetic reactions in intermediary metabolism. It is the immediate precursor of S-adenosyl methionine (SAMe), which is the activated methyl-donor form of methionine. When SAMe loses its methyl group in a transmethylation reaction, it becomes S-adenosyl homocysteine. Loss of the adenosyl group yields homocysteine. Homocysteine can complete the methyl transfer cycle by adding a methyl group to become methionine or it can leave the cycle via a pathway that ultimately can yield the amino acid cysteine.

In this cycle, the essential amino acid methionine, provided by dietary proteins, is converted to S-adenosyl methionine (commonly referred to as SAM or Sammy). SAM is the donor of virtually all methyl groups used in biosynthetic reactions. After donating a methyl group, SAM becomes S-adenosyl homocysteine, which, in turn, sheds the adenosyl group and becomes homocysteine. As shown in Figure 7-1, homocysteine has two pathways open to it. It can be catabolized by a pathway that requires vitamin B_6 as a coenzyme or it can be remethylated to methionine by a pathway that requires vitamins B_{12} and folic acid. The catabolic pathway involves a series of steps, one of which produces the nonessential amino acid cysteine.

Although homocysteine can be remethylated by a nonenzymatic pathway that uses methyl groups from trimethylglycine (betaine), a substantial deficiency of B_6, B_{12}, or folic acid can result in an increase in homocysteine levels in the blood. The relationship amid homocysteinemia, cardiovascular and Alzheimer's disease is discussed in Chapter Ten.

FIGURE 7-1
THE METHYL TRANSFER CYCLE

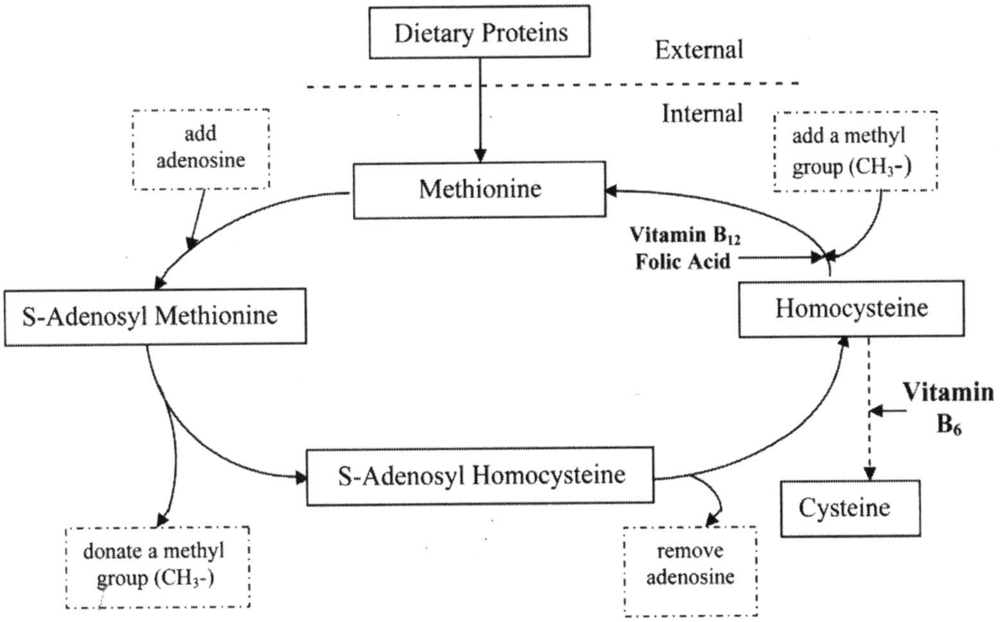

As important as the methyl transfer cycle is in intermediary metabolism, its normal functioning is of even more critical significance for the prevention of chronic nutritional diseases. Deficiencies of vitamins B_6, B_{12}, and folic acid can interfere with the metabolism of homocysteine and result in its build up to damaging levels in blood, as discovered by Kilmer McCully more than forty years ago (7).

GLUTATHIONE: Glutathione is an amino acid trimer (tripeptide) consisting of three nonessential amino acids, glutamic acid, cysteine, and glycine. Glutathione is synthesized by the body primarily from animal proteins, which are the major source of sulfur-containing amino acids. Glutathione is of major importance as an antioxidant, with particular value in preserving the efficacy of vitamin C.

It is generally accepted that the largest peptides capable of being absorbed from the small intestines are dipeptides with a question about the absorbability of tripeptides (4). Supplements of glutathione are available in health food stores; however, clinical trials show that oral administration is of no value because ingested glutathione is largely broken down to its component amino acids in the digestive tract (8).

If any glutathione is absorbed intact, the amount is too small to be detected. Presumably, adequate dietary protein will ensure ample glutathione synthesis within the body. Acetylcysteine (8) and alpha-lipoic acid (9) are recommended as valuable dietary supplements for biosynthesis of glutathione.

Protein Quality

The quality of a food protein is a measure of its nutritive value – how well it serves the amino acid requirements of its animal host. Many decades ago, investigations by pioneer nutritionists working with laboratory animals found that the best quality protein was in beef liver and kidney. They also found that dietary proteins with lesser nutritive value had to be fed at higher levels to maintain optimum health in the test animals. These scientists listed the foods they tested in descending order of value as follows: beef liver and kidney, whole egg, beef muscle, whole milk, soy beans, rolled oats, and whole wheat (2, p. 645). The highest protein quality is found in animal proteins.

Proteins from animal sources are similar to each other in the kinds and quantities of the various amino acids they contain. On the other hand, plant proteins differ considerably in amino acid composition not only among themselves but also from animal proteins. With few exceptions, plant proteins contain many unusable amino acids plus inadequate amounts of the amino acids that are essential for or usable by animals.

The difference in amino acid composition between plant and animal proteins is the reason why vegetarians must use a wide variety of plant proteins to obtain all of the essential amino acids they require. The reason for the higher protein quality of animal foods is because livestock break down plant proteins in feed to their component amino acids, select those they can use for synthesis of their own proteins, and discard those they cannot use. Thus, livestock animals save humans the metabolic energy of identifying and excreting unusable plant amino acids.

NUTRITIVE VALUE

The nutritive value of a food protein is dependent on its digestibility, biological value, and completeness. Any proper discussion of nutritive value must also include a consideration of protein quality. Today, the nutrition community apparently considers the matter of no consequence – it thinks of protein as protein, regardless of whether the source is plant or animal. Current governmental recommendations for daily protein intake put essentially no emphasis on protein quality (3). The concept that all proteins are of comparable nutritional value is flawed, and should be rejected by anyone interested in planning healthful diets.

DIGESTIBILITY: Digestibility in the sense used here refers to the percentage of a protein's amino acids that is absorbed and available for use by the body. Proteins of animal origin have the highest digestibility – 95 to 100 percent. The digestibility of proteins from wheat flours is slightly less than that of animal proteins. The digestibility of legumes and potatoes is about 75 to 80 percent.

BIOLOGICAL VALUE: More important than a protein's digestibility is its biological value, an attribute that is dependent on the amino acid composition of the protein. Biological value refers to the fraction of amino acids provided by the protein that can be used by the body to make its own proteins. A biological value of 70 percent, for example, means that 70 percent of the amino acids are usable; they are of the right kind and the right quantity. The greater the fraction of a protein's amino acids that can be used by the body to build its own proteins, the greater its biological value.

The biological value of proteins that supply a pool of amino acids for building the body's proteins might be likened to the value of a box of beads from which necklaces are made. If necklaces are made of alternating black and gold beads, a box of 1,000 beads containing half black and half gold beads has a much greater value than a box of 1,000 beads containing many different colors in addition to black and gold. The former will produce more necklaces than the latter and will have no wastage.

The great variety in form and function between animal and plant proteins makes for great differences between them in amino acid composition and, as a result, great differences in biological value. The biological value of animal proteins ranges from 70 to 95 percent; plant proteins from 35 to 65 percent.

Animal proteins have greater biological value than plant proteins because animals make proteins more similar to human proteins than plants do.

Table 7-1 shows the amounts of total protein and usable protein obtained from 100 grams of a few plant and animal foods for which information on protein digestibility and biological value are readily available. The amount of protein in 100 grams of food is multiplied by the percent digested to obtain the amount actually digested and absorbed into the body. The amount digested is multiplied, in turn, by the percent biological value to determine the amount of protein in the food that is actually usable by the body.

The data in Table 7-1 show that 21.3 grams of protein in 100 grams of beef flesh contain 14.1 grams of usable protein, whereas 22.5 grams of protein in 100 grams of cooked navy beans contain only 6.5 grams of usable protein. This is an example of the fact that, on a weight basis, the quantity of usable protein in plant foods is considerably less than that in animal foods. These data contradict the claim by proponents of vegetarian lifestyles that proteins found in plants are no different from the proteins found in animal products. The individual amino acids that are common to animal and plant proteins are identical to each other, but the animal and plant proteins made from these amino acids are very different both in quantity and kind of amino acids they contain.

TABLE 7-1
PROTEIN CONTENT, DIGESTABILITY, AND BIOLOGICAL VALUE
PER 100 GRAMS OF SELECTED FOODS

TYPE OF FOOD	Grams of Protein Per 100 Grams of Food	DIGESTIBILITY		BIOLOGICAL VALUE	
		% Digested (a)	Grams Digested per 100 Grams of Food	% Biological Value (a)	Usable Protein per 100 Grams of Food
Whole Eggs Cooked	13.2	100	13.2	94	12.4
Milk, Cow Whole	3.3	100	3.3	85	2.8
Beef Liver Cooked	20.4	90	18.4	77	14.2
Beef Flesh Cooked	21.3	96	20.4	69	14.1
Pork Flesh Cooked	25.0	100	25.0	74	18.5
Rolled Oats Cooked	16.7	90	15.0	65	9.8
White Flour Baked	10.8	100	10.8	52	5.6
Whole Corn Cooked	7.5	95	7.1	60	4.3
Potatoes Boiled	2.2	78	1.7	67	1.1
Navy Beans Cooked	22.5	76	17.1	38	6.5

(a) Source of data: Best CH, Taylor NB. *The Physiological Basis of Medical Practice, Fifth Edition.* Baltimore, MD: The William & Wilkins Company, 1950, page 644.

COMPLETENESS: Another argument against the vegetarian position that animal and plant proteins are of equal nutritional value relates to the completeness of their respective proteins. A complete protein contains all of the essential amino acids. An incomplete protein is one in which one or more of the essential amino acids are missing. The fact is that most animal proteins are complete and most plant proteins are incomplete. Notable exceptions are gelatin and soybeans. Gelatin is an incomplete animal protein. It is lacking in the essential amino acids tryptophan and tyrosine. Conversely, one of the numerous proteins in unprocessed soybeans is a complete plant protein that compares favorably with liver in amino acid composition (2, p. 646).

The adoption many decades ago of soybeans as a staple of the vegetarian diet was probably the result of reports of analyses, such as the above, showing that unprocessed soy beans contained a complete protein. Unfortunately, because raw soybeans contain so many unacceptable enzyme inhibitors and natural toxins, soy products must be subjected to a variety of treatments before they can be used as foods. Soy protein isolates are produced by high-temperature, high-pressure processing that destroys some of the essential amino acid content, thereby rendering all soybean proteins incomplete (10).

Incomplete proteins can be likened to the box of beads mentioned above. If the box contains no gold beads, no necklaces with gold beads could be made no matter how many extra beads the box contains. So it is with proteins. Incomplete proteins, no matter how ample the supply, cannot sustain animal life unless other proteins in the diet provide the missing essential amino acid or acids. This is the reason why it is very important for vegetarians to include a variety of vegetables in their diets. Vegetarians require much larger pools of amino acids in order to obtain a sufficient number and kind of suitable amino acids for synthesis of their own proteins.

Nutritional Requirements for Protein

The daily dietary protein requirement for humans has become a controversial subject among nutritionists, particularly since adoption of the so-called healthy-eating concept with its low-fat diets, weight-loss diets, detoxification diets, and the like. Over the past several decades, both private and government nutritional agencies have focused on reducing saturated fat and cholesterol in the American diet. In this effort they have advocated a reduction in the use of red meat, a very rich source of high quality protein, because of its cholesterol and saturated fat content. To justify the low protein levels in their low-fat (and hence low-meat) diets, these advocates have either ignored or downplayed both the importance of adequate dietary protein in the maintenance of optimum health and the significant differences between animal and plant foods in protein quality.

A reasonable estimate of daily protein requirement for adults is 1 to 1.1 grams per kilogram of body weight, which translates to about 1/2 gram of protein per pound of body weight per day. This estimate is based on studies by early nutritional scientists (2, p. 769; 11). These scientists concluded that a little over 1 gram of protein of high biological value per kilogram of body weight was an optimal daily intake, independent of total calories in the diet. Note the qualification "of high biological value.

The 2010 dietary guidelines revision of the adult RDA (recommended dietary allowance) for protein continues to be 0.8 grams per kilogram of body weight (3; 12). The RDA of 0.8 grams is the same as that set by the National Academy of Sciences (NAS) in 1989, but does not include the recommendation that daily protein intake should not exceed 1.6 grams per kilogram of body weight, or twice the RDA (13). Table 7-2 shows the protein requirements for various body weights based on the recommendations of 1 gram and 0.8 grams of protein per kilogram of body weight.

The 2010 dietary guidelines revision also does not include a UL (tolerable upper intake level) due to insufficient information about what an upper limit of intake should be, but it does add that 10 to 35 percent of calories should be derived from protein. The 10 percent recommendation is just slightly less than 0.8 grams of protein per kilogram of body weight for a 150 pound person on a 2,000 calorie diet. The 35 percent, which seems high for a DGA recommendation, is explained as being the percent necessary to provide the RDA for protein in low-calorie (low-fat) diets that are composed mainly of protein (3).

TABLE 7-2
PROTEIN REQUIREMENTS FOR VARIOUS BODY WEIGHTS

Body Weight in Pounds	120	140	150	160	170	180	190	210
Body Weight in Kilograms	54.5	63.6	68.6	72.7	77.3	81.8	86.4	95.5
Daily Protein Requirement in Grams – Based on 1 Gram per Kilogram	54.5	63.6	68.6	72.7	77.3	81.8	86.4	95.5
Daily Protein Requirement in Grams – Based on RDA of 0.8 Gram per Kilogram	43.6	50.9	54.9	58.2	61.8	65.4	69.1	76.4

A more scientific approach to estimating adult dietary protein requirements was pioneered by both Sears (14, p. 215ff) and the Eades (15, p. 312ff). This method is much more than a simple, one-diet-fits-all prescription; it is based on individual needs. The plan recognizes the fact that protein requirements vary depending on lean body mass and RDA for protein in low-calorie (low-fat) diets that are composed mainly of protein (3). The lean part of the body is, for all practical purposes, the only metabolically active part; thus, it is the part that needs most of the protein nourishment.

The greater the level of physical activity, the greater the wear and tear inflicted on tissue proteins and the greater the need for dietary protein to repair and rebuild them. Sears and the Eades have published tables that enable a person to calculate personal protein requirements using activity level and body measurements such as waist circumferences, weight, and height (14; 15). This method probably is the most accurate available today to a lay person for determining optimum personal protein requirements. Based on these data, Table 7-3 gives the daily protein requirements for selected lean body weights of adult females and for selected lean body weights of adult men.

Dietary Recommendations for Protein

A discussion of the adequacy of protein in many of today's popular diet plans is confused by the fact that protein and other macronutrient recommendations usually are given as percent of total daily calories. For example, a recommendation of 10 percent calories from protein equals 200 calories (50 grams) of protein on a 2,000-calorie diet but only 120 calories (30 grams) of protein on a 1,200-calorie diet. Thus, on a percent-of-daily-calories scale, an individual's daily protein intake is determined by the total number of calories consumed.

Using this system, the fewer calories a person eats, the less protein he or she takes in despite the fact that, on a body weight and activity basis, he or she may require more. The result is that diets that restrict total calories can be deficient in protein, often seriously. Table 7-4 gives the protein intake in calories per day and grams per day for diets with varying total calories and percent protein calories.

LOW-PROTEIN DIETS

Low-fat diets such as those espoused by Nathan Pritikin (16) and Dean Ornish (17) limit protein calories to about 10 percent of the total dietary calories. These diets are similar in quantity of protein to that of the Unified Dietary Guidelines, which are based on the U. S. Department of Agriculture's MyPyramid and recommended by such groups as the American Heart Association, the American Dietetic Association, and the American Cancer Society (3; 12). With the exception of Ornish, proponents of low-protein diets usually recommend avoiding or excluding only protein from red meat. Ornish's diet excludes meat of all kinds, including chicken and fish (18).

TABLE 7-3
HUMAN PROTEIN REQUIREMENTS FOR ADULT FEMALES AND MALES [a] ACCORDING TO BODY WEIGHT AND LEVEL OF ACTIVITY

FEMALES

Body Weight (lbs)	120			140			160		
Ave. % Fat (a)	32			32			32		
Lean Body Wt (lbs)	82			95			109		
Activity Level	Sed.	Lt.	Mod	Sed.	Lt.	Mod	Sed.	Lt.	Mod.
Required Grams of Protein/Lb (a)	0.5	0.6	0.7	0.5	0.6	0.7	0.5	0.5	0.7
Required Total Gm of Protein	41	49	57	48	57	67	55	65	76

MALES

Body Weight (lbs)	150			170			190		
Ave. % Fat (a)	23			23			23		
Lean Body Wt. (lbs)	116			131			146		
Activity Level	Sed.	Lt.	Mod	Sed.	Lt.	Mod	Sed.	Lt.	Mod.
Required Grams of Protein/Lb (a)	0.5	0.6	0.7	0.5	0.6	0.7	0.5	0.6	0.7
Required Total Gm of Protein	58	70	81	66	77	92	73	88	102

(a) Adapted from: Sears B. *Enter the Zone*. ReaganBooks, HarperCollins Publishers, New York, NY 1995 (pages 215, 261) and Eades MR, Eades MD. *The Protein Power Lifeplan*. New York, NY: Hachette Book Group, 2000 (pages 312, 313).

A comparison of Table 7-4 with Tables 7-2 and 7-3 shows that a 1,000-calorie diet containing 10-percent protein (25 grams) is inadequate for all body weights, and a 2,000-calorie diet (50 grams) is inadequate for all but a small or sedentary person. Further, if Table 7-4 were applied to vegetarian diets, adjustment would have to be made for the differences in nutritional value between plant and animal proteins in order to prevent protein deficit. The reason, as indicated in Table 7-1, is that the fraction of vegetable protein that is actually useable by the body is only about half that of its total protein content. In low-fat diets, the real target of the recommendation against meat is not the protein in meat but rather the accompanying fat or, more precisely, saturated fat and cholesterol.

In order to reduce the fat component of the diet to what is considered an acceptable level, meat and especially red meat, the major sources of saturated fat and cholesterol, must be restricted. When the fat and protein components of the diet are reduced, the deficit in protein calorie requirement can only be replaced by carbohydrate foods. The usual result is a diet that is not only inadequate in protein but excessive in carbohydrates.

TABLE 7-4
COMPARISON OF PROTEIN INTAKE IN CALORIES PER DAY;
GRAMS PER DAY FOR DIETS OF 1000, 2000, AND 3000 CALORIES

TOTAL DAILY DIET	10% of total daily Calories	20 % of total daily Calories	30 % of total daily Calories
FOR A 1000 CALORIE/DAY DIET			
Protein intake in calories/day	100	200	300
Protein intake in grams/day	25	50	75
FOR A 2000 CALORIE/DAY DIET			
Protein intake in calories/day	200	400	600
Protein intake in grams/day	50	100	150
FOR A 3000 CALORIE/DAY DIET			
Protein intake in calories/day	300	600	900
Protein intake in grams/day	75	150	225

Note: Daily protein requirement for a 160 pound person based on the standard of one gram per kilogram of body weight equals 72.7 grams per day.

IMPACT OF LOW-PROTEIN DIETS: When protein intake is inadequate to supply the demands for replacing or repairing tissue proteins, the body will cannibalize its own muscle tissue to obtain the essential amino acids and nitrogen it requires for its life functions. The elderly are at special risk of protein depravation due to poor appetite and poor absorption. The inevitable result is loss of muscle mass, the degree of which depends on the degree of protein malnutrition. A pot belly in an otherwise normal-weight person suggests weak stomach muscles due to protein deficiency.

In addition to loss of muscle, protein malnutrition causes a generalized impairment of all systems responsible for the body's defenses against disease and debility. There is a large volume of evidence from studies of primitive people that support the thesis that physical fitness and resistance to disease are associated in populations with higher protein intakes (2, p. 768; 19, p. 402ff; 20).

Insufficient protein in the diet can be a cause of peptic ulcer. The diet of evolutionary man contained almost no carbohydrates. It consisted mostly of protein and fat from animals and fish. Then as now, human gastric juices contained hydrochloric acid to help digest proteins and fats. Protein and fat buffer and quickly weaken the strength of the corrosive gastric juices and, as a result, they did not penetrate and damage the mucosa that lines the inside of the stomach and duodenum.

The modern American diet tends to be low in fats and proteins, and snacks usually consist of soft drinks and sweet carbohydrates with no proteins or fats. With little or no protein and fat, gastric juices are more liable to attack the mucosa and the tissues that underlie it, which, over time, can predispose to ulceration. Dr. Hoffer advised that the cure is to add fiber and remove the carbohydrates (21, p. 25).

The answer to why very low-fat diets appear to have some benefit for cardiac patients may very well relate to a beneficial effect of calorie restriction, as described in Chapter Four, rather than to low fat intake. However, in the long term, calorie restriction in the absence of an adequate balance and supply of essential nutrients can be detrimental. For a period of a few months or even a few years of deprivation, the human body is very forgiving. It will take whatever is provided, adapt to privation, and struggle along for years as best it can to maintain a semblance of health and well being. Holocaust survivors are extreme examples of what the human body is capable of tolerating.

A person accustomed to less than perfect health and energy level, as most people are in today's stressful world, would hardly notice mild protein malnutrition. But that does not mean that there is no insidious damage or that longevity is unaffected.

MODERATE-PROTEIN DIETS

Food plans that balance carbohydrate, protein, and fat calories in a 40:30:30 ratio fall in the moderate protein category. The 40:30:30-diet concept of calorie balance was introduced to the general public by Sears with publication of *Enter the Zone* in 1995 (14).

A highly successful weight loss diet plan that basically follows the moderate protein concept is that of the Drs. Eades, which they first described more than a decade ago in their earlier *Protein Power* book (15). The Eades' plan has been erroneously labeled by some nutritionists as a high-protein diet. The Eades have made effective application of the low-carbohydrate, moderate protein-concept in their medical practice specializing in weight control.

The fact that "high-protein" is a gross misreading of the Eades' diet is demonstrated by their recommendations of from 0.5 to 0.9 grams of protein per pound of lean body mass, depending on physical activity. Table 7-3 shows these recommendations are the same as those for a moderate-protein diet. Table 7-4 shows [that] diets containing 30-percent protein are adequate in protein for all body weights and levels of activity that are shown in Table 7-3 except for males on a 1,000 calorie diet who have moderate or greater activity levels than usual.

IMPACT OF MODERATE-PROTEIN DIETS: Moderate-protein diets based on a person's individual needs appear to offer a wise nutritional approach to good health. Moderate quantities of protein in the diet allow room for sufficient amounts of low-glycemic carbohydrates that contain essential vitamins and minerals and healthful amounts of fiber. Moderate-protein diets also provide sufficient opportunity for a good balance of saturated, monounsaturated, and essential polyunsaturated fatty acids.

HIGH-PROTEIN DIETS

The name "Atkins" immediately comes to mind whenever "high-protein diet" is mentioned. The late Dr. Atkins developed the so-called high-protein diet for use in treating patients who were excessively overweight or obese. Based on the success of his diet, he published the predecessor of *Dr. Atkins' New Diet Revolution* (20) in the 1970's. The earlier book introduced the Atkins' diet to a very receptive public and popularized a nutritional philosophy that today still raises the ire of nutrition academia.

In actual practice, the Atkins' diet is high in protein only in the initial induction phase during which there is close medical supervision. The purpose of the induction diet is to reverse weight gain and start the return of the patient to a more normal weight. When the patient has lost an appropriate amount of weight, the diet is gradually changed to a more moderate protein-intake plan called the maintenance diet (20).

Rather than high-protein diet, the Atkins' diet is more appropriately and more accurately called a controlled- or restricted-carbohydrate diet. It is based on sound nutritional biochemistry that shows that excess dietary carbohydrates, namely sugar and starch, through their stimulation of insulin release, are largely responsible not only for obesity but also are factors in many of the modern nutritional diseases. Thus, controlled-carbohydrate diets, which have been used successfully for many years in treating obesity, show great promise in the prevention and treatment of chronic nutritional diseases.

Diets that are truly high in protein, as opposed to that of Atkins, are composed solely of animal products, including meat, milk, and blood. Such diets are seldom encountered among people living in modern societies but were common in primitive cultures like those found among tribes in India, Africa, and New Guinea (2, p. 767ff).

IMPACT OF HIGH-PROTEIN DIETS: There is little or no evidence that high-protein diets cause adverse effects in healthy people. For example, renal and cardiovascular disease is uncommon among Greenland Eskimos, who eat enormous quantities of protein and fat (22). To the contrary, the data from primitive societies indicate that physical fitness and resistance to disease are associated with higher protein intakes (2. p. 768).

Books and articles that discuss the value of meat in the diet often cite the research and writings of Vilhjalmur Stefansson, an anthropologist and Arctic explorer, who was a credible proponent of high-protein diets. Convinced that the all-meat diet of the Eskimos he studied was a healthful one, Stefansson lived on the Eskimo diet for the more than 11 years he worked in the Arctic in the early 1900s (23).

Upon return from his years of study and exploration in the Arctic, Stefansson's excellent health after so long a period on an all-meat/fat diet prompted a yearlong, medically supervised study of his dietary regime at Bellevue Hospital in New York City (24). The controlled diet consisted of approximately 120 grams of protein, 230 grams of fat, and 5 to 10 grams of carbohydrate. Neither Stefansson nor Anderson, a fellow explorer who joined Stefansson in the experiment, showed any adverse effects on blood pressure, renal function, or general health at the end of the 12 months of the study.

Studies of populations suggest that diets high in protein promote good health (2, p. 769). On the other hand, proponents of low-fat, high-carbohydrate diets claim that diets high in protein, of necessity, contain large amounts of animal fats that promote high blood cholesterol and various cardiovascular diseases. They further argue that the heavy intake of protein puts an intolerable burden on the kidneys of having to dispose of excess nitrogen.

There is no question that dietary protein is detrimental to people with existing renal disease or that such people benefit from diets with minimal protein. However, normal kidneys in healthy people apparently can handle the burden of diets rich in protein without ill effect (25). In addition, they claim that the potential for ketosis is an unacceptable risk, which indicates a lack of understanding of the difference between dietary ketosis and diabetic ketosis (see Chapter Eight).

References

1.) Frank LR, ed. *Random House Webster's Quotionary* .New York, NY: Random House, 2000.

2.) Best CH, Taylor NB. *The Physiological Basis of Medical Practice, Fifth Edition.* Baltimore, MD: The William & Wilkins Company, 1950.

3.) http://www.cnpp.usda.gov/Publications/DietaryGuidelines/2010/DGAC/Report/D-4-Protein.pdf/ Accessed Sept. 26, 2012.

4.) Rhoades RA, Tanner GA. *Medical Physiology*. Boston, MA: Little, Brown and Company, 1995.

5.) Horton RH, et al. *Principles of Biochemistry*. Upper Saddle River, NJ: Prentice Hall, 1996.

6.) http://themedicalbiochemistrypage.org/ Accessed Sept. 26, 2012.

7.) McCully K, McCully M. *The Heart Revolution: The Vitamin Breakthrough that lowers Homocysteine, Cuts Your Risk of Heart Disease, and Protects your Health*. New York, NY: HarperCollins, 1999.

8.) Murray MA. *Encyclopedia of Nutritional Supplements*. Rocklin, CA: Prima Publishing, 1996.

9.) Berkson B. *The Alpha Lipoic Acid Breakthrough*. Rocklin, CA 95677: Prima Health, 1998.

10.) Fallon SA, Enig MG. Tragedy and Hype: The Third International Soy Symposium. *Nexus Magazine*. 2000; **7**(3). (from: http://www.westonaprice.org/soy-alert/tragedy-and-hype/) Accessed Sept. 26, 2012.

11.) Lewis HB. Proteins in Nutrition. *Journal of the American Medical Society.* 1948; **138**: 207.

12.) *Dietary Reference Intakes: The Essential Guide to Nutrient Requirements.* Washington, DC: The National Academies Press, 2006.

13.) National Academy of Sciences Report on Diet and Health, National Research Council, Washington, DC, March 1, 1989.

14.) Sears B. *Enter the Zone*. New York, NY: Regan Books imprint of HarperCollins Publishers, 1995.

15.) Eades MR, Eades MD. *The Protein Power Lifeplan*. New York, NY: Hachette Book G4roup, 2000.

16.) Pritikin N. *The Pritikin Program for Diet and Exercise*. New York, NY: Grosset and Dunlap, 1979.

17.) Ornish D. *Eat More, Weigh Less*. New York, NY: Harper Mass Market Paperbacks, 1997.

18.) http://www.fatfree.com/diets/ornish.html/ Accessed Sept. 26, 2012.

19.) Price WA. *Nutrition and Physical Degeneration, 6th Edition*. Los Angeles, CA: Keats Publish., 1998.

20.) Atkins RC. *Dr. Atkins' New Diet Revolution*. New York, NY: Avon Books, Inc. 1999.

21.) Hoffer A, Walker W. *Putting It All Together: The New Orthomolecular Nutrition*. New Canaan, CT; Keats Publishing, Inc, 1996.

22.) Thomas, W. A. *Journal of the American Medical Association*. 1927; **88**: 1559.

23.) Lieb CW. The effects of an exclusive long-continued meat diet. *Journal of the American Medical Association.* 1926; **87**:26.

24.) Lieb CW. The effects on human beings of a twelve-month exclusive meat diet. *Journal of the American Medical Association.* 1929; **93**:20.

25.) Bischoff F. The influence of diet on renal and blood vessel changes. *Journal of Nutrition.*1932; **5**: 431

Chapter Eight

Lipids

When accumulated data force a conclusion that runs counter to popular opinion and perceived wisdom, it is essential to stick to your guns. **The Trends Journal. August 2009, p.16.**

Lipids comprise a large and varied group of water-insoluble chemicals that are indispensable components of all living organisms. The lipid category of macronutrients includes all of the fatty substances in foods. With few exceptions, lipid chemicals contain only carbon, hydrogen, and oxygen. If macronutrients could be ranked in order of importance to human health, lipids would have to be listed second after proteins.

However, unlike proteins and carbohydrates, lipids vary widely in structure and function. Most people think of fatty substances as fuels that drive the human engine. But they are much more than fuels. Some are required in the diet for the absorption of fat-soluble vitamins. Some are packing materials that cushion the major organs and protect them against damage from jolts and sharp impacts. Some are thermal insulating materials that protect against cold and aid in temperature regulation. Some are structural materials that, in combination with proteins, form membranes in all cells of the body. Some are electrical insulation materials for nerve fibers and brain cells. Some serve as transport mechanisms for other nutrients and biochemicals. And some are hormone-like biochemical regulators, messengers, or mediators. Lipids serve many functions in the maintenance of life.

Lipid Categories

There are four major categories of lipids: fatty acids, fat-soluble vitamins, steroids, and terpenes. The first three categories, fatty acids, lipid vitamins, and steroids are important in human nutrition and biochemistry. The terpene lipids do not play any known role in human nutrition. They are plant lipids that are found primarily in the volatile oils of many trees, herbs, and flowers. Camphor, turpentine, and citronella are a few examples of the terpenes found in commercial products. The haze often seen over forests and mountain ranges is due in part to the action of sunlight on terpenes emitted by trees and plants. The Blue Ridge

Mountains and the Great Smoky Mountains owe their colorful names to the vast amounts of volatile oils produced by vegetation.

The fatty acids (the true fats) and steroids are the subject of this chapter. The lipid vitamins (A, D, E, and K) are discussed in Chapter Five. No further mention will be made of the terpenes because they have no known nutritive value and are not normal dietary components.

Steroids

Steroids are large complex lipids composed of carbon, hydrogen, and oxygen. All have the basic steroid structure, which is composed of four fused carbon rings, three with six carbons and one with five carbons. When diagrammed on paper, the steroid skeleton resembles a small section of chicken wire. There are literally thousands of steroid chemicals of plant or animal origin, but only one is of importance in human nutrition. That steroid is cholesterol, a large steroid alcohol (sterol) with the molecular formula $C_{27}H_{46}O$.

CHOLESTEROL

Cholesterol is the principal sterol in higher animals and is an indispensable constituent of all cells and fluids of the body. It comprises from 10 to 50 percent of cell membrane lipids, where its function is related to membrane flexibility. In addition to its own vital biochemical and physiological functions, cholesterol is the starting point (precursor) for the biosynthesis of several groups of very important steroid derivatives. Biochemicals synthesized from cholesterol include male and female sex hormones, metabolic steroid hormones, vitamin D, and bile acids.

Cholesterol exists in the body either as free cholesterol or as esters of cholesterol, which are combinations of cholesterol with fatty acids. Cholesterol esters are the preferred form for delivery of cholesterol to cells, where it is either used immediately or stored for future use. Cholesterol and its esters are transported in the blood plasma in combination with special proteins known as apolipoproteins. This combination forms lipid-protein molecules of varying density, hence the familiar LDL and HDL cholesterols (low-density and high-density lipoproteins) that are routinely measured in medical examinations.

Unfortunately, the LDL and HDL forms of cholesterol have been inappropriately and erroneously named "bad" cholesterol and "good" cholesterol, respectively. Actually, they are neither bad nor good; both forms of cholesterol are necessary and perform vital functions. In general, LDL is the form in which cholesterol is synthesized by the body and delivered to all cells and tissues where it is used either for cellular functions or for synthesis of cholesterol derivatives such as vitamin D. HDL is the form in which spent or excess cholesterol is removed from cells and tissues for delivery to the liver and excretion in the bile (1). The belief of the nutrition establishment that cholesterol is a "major determinant" of heart disease (2) is probably the basis for the LDL and HDL characterizations; cholesterol that is delivered to cells is "bad," and, by contrast, cholesterol that is removed from cells is "good."

Dietary cholesterol, which is present only in foods from animal sources, is poorly absorbed from the intestines. Cholesterol that is absorbed does not cause a significant increase in the normal level in the blood. This has been demonstrated by numerous studies that have shown that blood cholesterol is independent of dietary cholesterol (3). Despite the fact that it has long been known that dietary cholesterol intakes have little impact on blood cholesterol (4), most doctors, dietitians, and governmental agencies continue to stress elimination of cholesterol-containing foods from the diet.

The reason that dietary cholesterol has little impact on blood cholesterol levels is because of the frugality of biological systems. Biological frugality applies to many biochemicals that the body normally makes for itself, including cholesterol; if a biochemical is supplied in the diet, the body will use the dietary supply and reduce the amount it synthesizes by the amount it receives. Thus if the diet supplies 100 milligrams of cholesterol, the body saves the energy required to make 100 milligrams by using the dietary source and synthesizing only the difference between 100 milligrams and the amount it would normally make. The human body is a very energy-saving machine in most aspects of its biochemistry, not just in cholesterol synthesis. It does not waste energy in making what is provided by an outside source. Healthy individuals maintain relatively constant levels of blood cholesterol regardless of the quantity of cholesterol in the diet.

CHOLESTEROL METABOLISM: The first step in cholesterol synthesis is the condensation of three molecules of acetyl CoA, followed by numerous and complex reactions that ultimately yield cholesterol (see Figure 6-4). Active synthesis of cholesterol occurs in virtually all cells of the body, including the walls of arteries (1), but the major portion is synthesized by liver cells. The biosynthesis of cholesterol is controlled by mechanisms that turn the process on and off, depending on the body's need for cholesterol. Under normal circumstances, the body produces no more cholesterol than its life processes require. Excess or expended cholesterol is excreted from the body by the liver, via the gallbladder, into the small intestine and eliminated with the feces.

Even though dietary cholesterol does not cause a significant increase in normal cholesterol level, imbalances of other nutrients in the diet, such as an excess of carbohydrates, can force the body to synthesize more cholesterol than it requires. Such imbalances can override the cholesterol-synthesizing control mechanisms and cause the body itself to overproduce cholesterol. This excess production of cholesterol results in an abnormal increase in blood cholesterol. Hypercholesterolemia (excess cholesterol in the blood) has been designated a risk factor for heart disease by the medical profession because the two conditions are often found in association with each other.

NORMAL BLOOD CHOLESTEROL VALUES: For many decades, normal cholesterol values were considered to be from 100 to 320 milligrams of total cholesterol per 100 milliliters of blood. Normal values can increase by as much as 10 to 30 percent in some individuals as they advance in age (5). In recent years, medically acceptable values for blood cholesterol have been gradually lowered; now anyone with blood cholesterol level of more than 200 milligrams percent is considered a prospective heart attack victim.

Despite the public campaign warning of the dangers of high blood cholesterol levels, there are data in the literature indicating that low blood cholesterol levels also carry with them a danger. A paper presented at the American Heart Association's annual stroke conference reported that the risk of hemorrhagic stroke was twice that in people with blood cholesterol levels less than 180 as compared with people whose blood cholesterol levels were 230 or greater (6).

Hypercholesterolemia: As explained in the chapter on carbohydrates, acetyl CoA in excess of the body's energy requirements is directed by insulin to the synthesis of body fat and cholesterol. The dietary components primarily responsible for insulin release are carbohydrates. A significant fraction of the carbohydrate in the modern diet is ordinary table sugar (sucrose) plus its monosaccharide fructose, which is found in fruits and in sweeteners such as high fructose corn syrup. Breakdown of sucrose yields equal quantities of glucose and fructose. Dietary fructose does little to stimulate insulin release, but it contributes significantly to the formation of excess acetyl CoA.

As shown in Figures 4-1 and 6-1, dietary fructose, either free in the diet or released from sucrose, bypasses glycolysis and goes directly to pyruvate, which, in turn, goes to acetyl CoA. A rapid buildup of pyruvate acts as a brake on glycolysis and keeps the rate of conversion of glucose to pyruvate in check; however, fructose catabolism bypasses this important control of glycolysis. As a result, the pool of acetyl CoA from fructose increases quickly and exceeds the amount required for energy. The excess acetyl CoA produced from fructose is converted to body fat and cholesterol.

Controlled feeding studies in humans conducted by Milton Winitz and colleagues in the 1960's and 1970's and reported by Pauling (7, p. 42) support the adverse effect of fructose on cholesterol levels. Subjects with moderately elevated cholesterol levels were placed on a rigorously controlled, low-carbohydrate diet in which glucose was the sole carbohydrate. Their cholesterol levels gradually dropped to normal levels. After four weeks on the diet, one quarter of the glucose was replaced with sucrose. Within one week, cholesterol levels rose to pre-experiment levels.

It is extremely important for people who have high cholesterol levels to understand that most cholesterol in blood is manufactured by their own body's biochemistry. It is excess sugar and refined carbohydrates in the diet, not saturated fat or cholesterol content of food, that are the major causes of high cholesterol levels in the blood. Interestingly, statin drugs administered to reduce blood cholesterol levels work by inhibiting the first committed step in a multistep pathway to synthesis of cholesterol, namely the conversion of 3-hydroxy-3-methylglutaryl CoA (HMG CoA) to mevalonate (see Figure 6-4).

Mevalonic acid is a precursor of coenzyme Q_{10} (CoQ). A deficiency of CoQ causes congestive heart failure. Thus, an unintended consequence of statin drug therapy and its concomitant inhibition of the synthesis of CoQ is congestive heart failure. CoQ is a very important biochemical that serves as a coenzyme in energy production (electron transport reactions).

Statin drugs not only inhibit the biosynthesis of cholesterol and CoQ but also all of the other intermediate biochemicals between HMG CoA and cholesterol.

Fatty Acid Subgroups

The fatty acid group of lipids comprises, in addition to the fatty acids and triglycerides, several smaller subgroups of biochemicals known as phospholipids, sphingolipids, and waxes. As a general rule, members of these subgroups that are required by an organism for some structure or function can be synthesized by the organism as the need occurs.

Phospholipids, as the name implies, are lipids that contain a phosphate ester in the form of a phosphatidyl group. Phospholipids have the same structure as triglycerides except that the third fatty acid is replaced by a phosphatidyl group. The most common phosphate ester is phosphatidyl choline, followed by the phosphate esters of inositol and serine. Serine is a nonessential amino acid. Choline and inositol are considered by some authors to be B vitamins; however, because they are nonessential (can be synthesized by the body), they are not officially classed as vitamins.

Despite the similarity in structure, triglyceride lipids and phospholipids differ considerably in physical and biochemical properties. Triglycerides are water insoluble, whereas phospholipids are good emulsifiers. Triglycerides have various functions in the body, but they are not found in membranes. Phospholipids are the most abundant lipids in cell membranes and in nerve tissues and structures.

Phospholipids provide vital structural components for all membranes throughout the body, and they play an essential role in peripheral and central nervous system biochemistry. They are vital to maintaining the integrity of cells and to the active participation of cellular membranes in biochemical reactions.

Perhaps the phospholipid best known to the general public is lecithin. Lecithin is actually a mixture of phospholipids, the majority of which contain phosphatidylcholine. As a result, lecithin is often referred to as phosphatidylcholine. Lecithin is widely distributed in plants and animals. There is considerable evidence that lecithin and other dietary sources of phosphatidylcholine improve brain function, protect against high blood cholesterol levels, and improve memory. Egg yolks are an important dietary source of lecithin. Soybean lecithin is widely used as a food additive and dietary supplement.

Although sphingolipids and waxes are of little importance nutritionally, they serve valuable functions in living organisms. Sphingolipids are second only to phospholipids as the most abundant lipids in plant and animal membranes. In animals, they are major lipids in nervous system tissues and sheaths. Waxes are very large molecules with as many as 50 or 60 carbons in straight or branched chains. They are widely distributed in nature, and serve as protective coatings. Earwax (cerumen) is probably the most familiar of the animal waxes.

Fatty Acids – The True Fats

Of all the lipids, the group that is most familiar to the general public is the true fats – fatty acids and their triglycerides. Well over 95 percent of the lipids in the diet are true fats. The true fats are salad oils, cooking fats, margarines, butter, cream, and fatty parts of animal and vegetable foods. Because these familiar fats form the major lipid fraction of the diet, the word *fat* has become synonymous with *lipid* and, for all practical purposes, has replaced *lipid* in the nutrition vocabulary. As a result, the distinction between the familiar fats and oils and the other smaller and lesser-known members of the dietary lipid complex has been lost.

This loss of distinction would be of little importance if it were not for the active and vigorous campaign that has been waged for the past few decades by the nutrition and medical communities against dietary fats, primarily those of animal origin. This crusade fails to distinguish between the lipids labeled "bad" (saturated fatty acids and cholesterol) and the lipids that are essential for life (fat-soluble vitamins and essential fatty acids). As a result, the general public, with the cooperation of the food industry, has gone to great lengths to eliminate fats, including the essential lipid nutrients, from the daily fare.

COMPOSITION

Fatty acids are chains of carbon atoms with a carboxyl (acid) group at one end. The length of carbon chains varies from 3 to well over 30 carbons, which may be in a straight line or branched. Over 100 fatty acids have been identified in nature, but those that are most important for humans are fatty acids that have an even number of carbons in straight chains of approximately 22-24 carbons or less. Fatty acids are the most abundant lipids in the human body and in the human diet.

The fatty acids most commonly encountered in human biochemistry and nutrition contain 18 carbon atoms. Among the 18-carbon fatty acids, stearic acid and oleic acid are the principal fatty acids in animal products. Oleic acid and linoleic acid are the principal fatty acids in vegetable products. Two other important fatty acids are 16-carbon palmitic acid, found in both plants and animals, and 18-carbon alpha-linolenic acid, found in a few plant species. Table 8-1 lists some basic information on the important dietary fatty acids; Table 8-2 gives the fatty acid composition of raw edible fats and oils before processing.

It is extremely important to emphasize that the data on composition of fats and oils given in Table 8-2 are for raw oils. The composition of raw oils is radically altered during processing so that the omega-3 alpha linolenic acid content is sharply reduced or eliminated (see the section on hydrogenation below). As will be explained in Chapter Nine in the discussion of the nutritional importance of the omega-6 to omega-3 ratio, destruction of alpha-linolenic acid during hydrogenation has a serious, detrimental effect on the nutritional quality of vegetable seed oils.

TABLE 8-1
COMMON FATTY ACIDS

Fatty Acid	Number of Double Bonds	Comments	Number of Carbons in Fatty Acid Molecule
Butyric	0 (saturated)	In butter	4
Capric	0 (saturated)	In coconut, palm oils, and butter	10
Lauric	0 (saturated)	In coconut & palm oils	12
Palmitic	0 (saturated)	In many natural fats	16
Stearic	0 (saturated)	In beef fat	18
Oleic	1 (monounsaturated)	In olive oil	18
Linoleic	2 (polyunsaturated)	An omega-6 essential fatty acid	18
Alpha-linolenic	3 (polyunsaturated)	An omega-3 essential fatty acid	18

FREE FATTY ACIDS: Fatty acids are seldom found in the free state in nature. They are free in the body only when being used for some specific biochemical function. Otherwise they exist as triglycerides. The physical properties of free fatty acids are such that their presence in living tissues in significant concentrations would be very disruptive.

The problem that fatty acids could cause if they were free in the blood stream is due to the fact that the carboxyl group at one end of a fatty acid molecule attracts water and the long carbon tail at the other end repels water; thus, fatty acids act as detergents. If they were present in large concentrations in biological systems, they would emulsify and disrupt cell membranes and fluids.

TRIGLYCERIDES: Triglycerides are not only the storage form for fatty acids but they also are the transport form. A triglyceride molecule is a package of three fatty acids linked to a glycerol molecule by what are called ester linkages. Each alcohol group in the glycerol molecule couples with the carboxyl group of a fatty acid to make an ester link. Triglycerides are E-shaped molecules, with glycerol forming the backbone and the carbon chains of the three fatty acids standing out like legs to form the E. Triglyceride molecules contain at least two and often three different fatty acids, one of which is usually an unsaturated fatty acid.

TABLE 8-2

COMPOSITION OF COMMON RAW EDIBLE FATS AND OILS

Type of Fat or Oil	Linoleic Acid (polyunsat.) Omega-6 Fatty Acid	Alpha-Linolenic Acid (polyunsat.) Omega-3 Fatty Acid	Oleic Acid (monounsaturated)	Saturated Fat (saturated)
Beef Tallow (a)	02%	01%	49%	48%
Butterfat (a)	03%	01%	28%	68%
Canola Oil (a)	21%	11%	61%	07%
Coconut Oil (a)	02%	00%	07%	91%
Corn Oil (a)	57%	01%	29%	13%
Cottonseed Oil (a)	54%	trace	19%	27%
Flax Seed Oil (b)	14%	58%	19%	09%
Lard (a)	09%	01%	47%	43%
Olive Oil (c)	08%	02%	75%	15%
Palm Oil (a)	10%	trace	39%	51%
Peanut Oil (a)	33%	trace	48%	19%
Safflower Oil (a)	76%	trace	14%	10%
Soybean Oil (a)	54%	08%	23%	15%
Sunflower Oil (a)	71%	01%	16%	12%

(a) Canola Oil Council of Canada, www.canola-council.org/
(b) Murray MT, Beutler J. *Understanding Fats and Oils*. Encinitas, CA: Progressive Health, 1996.
(c) Simopoulos, A.P. *The Omega Plan*. New York, NY: HarperCollins Publishers, 1999

The physical properties of triglycerides are quite different from those of their component fatty acids. This difference is of tremendous physiological importance; triglycerides do not possess detergent action because the water-attracting carboxyl groups of the fatty acids are tied up in ester bonds. Hence, triglycerides are neutral fats. Nature wisely devised triglycerides as a means of neutralizing fatty acids and keeping them from doing damage until they are required in free form.

CHEMISTRY

Organic chemistry came late to the laboratory benches of the chemical sciences because it was viewed as a phenomenon unique to living organisms; it was the province of the Creator and, as such, was not to be understood by mere humans. This view was reinforced by the great structural complexity of the chemicals isolated from living tissues, which, in turn, was due to the distinctive structure of the carbon atom.

Eventually, a few simple organic chemicals such as oxalic acid and urea, which originally were thought to be made only by living creatures, were synthesized in the laboratory. Only then did it become generally accepted that organic chemistry was identical to the chemistry of carbon, the twelfth element in Group IV of the Periodic Table. Although this discovery brought organic chemistry into the material world of science, the "organic" label was never changed; organic chemistry just became a synonym for carbon chemistry.

STRUCTURE

One of the difficulties early chemists faced in integrating organic chemistry into the well established chemical sciences related to carbon's bonding properties. Elements in Group IV, with four electrons in their outermost shells, are unlike the elements in all other groups. They are neither acidic (electron donors), like Groups I, II and III, nor basic (electron acceptors) like Groups V, VI, and VII. Thus, they do not form ions (electrically charged atoms or groups of atoms) or salts. Instead, they prefer to share their four electrons in covalent bonding with other elements.

CARBON-CARBON BONDING: A carbon atom can bond with four other atoms (four single bonds), three other atoms (two single bonds and one double bond), or two other atoms (one single bond and one triple bond – one carbon atom cannot hold two double bonds). Thus, carbon atoms can combine not only with other elements, but also with each other to make a great variety of molecules including very large, complex compounds with chains that are straight, branched, or cross-linked. It has been estimated that the number of known organic chemicals exceeds ten million. This unusual nature of carbon bonding is of special importance in the chemistry of long chains of carbons such as occur in the fatty acids. More complete information on the chemistry, biochemistry, and structures of fatty acids, including illustrations of structural formulae, can be found on the website of the American Oil Chemists Society (8).

Bonds between carbon atoms linked together in long chains, as is the case with fatty acids, are primarily of two kinds – single bonds or double bonds. Single bonds (-C-C-C-C-) are called saturated and double bonds (-C-C=C-C-) are called unsaturated. Saturation/unsaturation in fatty-acid nomenclature refers to the degree of hydrogenation of the carbon chain. Double bonds cannot occur sequentially in a chain, but must be separated by at least one single bond (-C=C-C=C-). Triple bonds cannot occur within a chain but only at an end carbon. Triple bonds are uncommon, very reactive, and have short lives.

Single (Saturated) Bonds: Saturated fatty acids contain all of the hydrogen they are capable of holding. All of the links between carbon atoms are single links (bonds) and, with the exception of the carboxyl carbon at the beginning of a carbon chain and the terminal carbon at the end, each carbon in the chain bonds to two hydrogen atoms. The molecules are fully saturated with hydrogen. In fatty acid chains, the carbon bonds are either all single bonds or mostly single with one to several double bonds.

Double (Unsaturated) Bonds: Unsaturated fatty acids do not contain their full complement of hydrogen. A double bond is formed from a single bond by removing a hydrogen atom from each of two adjacent carbons and joining the two vacated links to each other to form the second bond between the two carbons. Unsaturated fatty acids are classified as mono-unsaturated, with one double bond, or polyunsaturated, with two or more double bonds in the chain.

The biochemistry of vertebrate animals does not permit synthesis of double bonds in fatty acids beyond the ninth carbon from the carboxyl end of the chain. Oleic acid, the mono-unsaturated 18-carbon fatty acid component of oils from both plant and animal species, has its one double bond between carbon-9 and carbon-10. The polyunsaturated fatty acids linoleic acid and alpha-linolenic acid, which have double bonds beyond the double bond at the ninth carbon, for a total of two and three double bonds, respectively, are required by but cannot be synthesized by vertebrate species. Thus, these fatty acids and their metabolites are labeled essential fatty acids (EFAs).

The Omega System for Essential Fatty Acids: EFAs are identified on food labels and in dietary recommendations by the location of the double bonds in their chains, with descriptions such as *omega-3* and *omega-6*. Such omega descriptions are usually puzzling to scientists trained in organic chemistry or biochemistry because they are schooled in the chemical nomenclature of the International Union of Pure and Applied Chemistry (IUPAC), more familiarly known as the Geneva system. The Geneva system for identifying positions of double bonds in long chain fatty acids is quite different from the omega scheme used in nutritional sciences. In the Geneva system, the location of a double bond in a fatty acid is counted from the carboxyl end of the chain with the carboxyl carbon labeled as carbon-1. In nutritional sciences, counting starts from the terminal carbon, which is at the opposite end of the chain from the carboxyl group. The terminal carbon is named the omega carbon because *omega*, the last letter of the Greek alphabet, has come to mean *end* or *last* in English. Count is then made from the terminal end with the omega carbon labeled carbon-1. The Geneva and omega numbering systems for carbon atoms in 18- and 20-carbon fatty acid chains are shown in Figure 8-1.

Nutritional scientists created the omega system for the very important reason that the nutritional properties of EFAs are dependent *only* on the location of the last double bond in the carbon chain, *independent* of chain length. In 1963, after almost four decades of struggling with the Geneva system, Ralph T. Holman proposed the omega system for classifying EFAs by the location of their last double bonds (9).

The omega system was an effort to organize the volumes of data on the function and metabolism of polyunsaturated fatty acids that had been developed since the discovery in 1929

FIGURE 8-1
POLYUNSATURATED FATTY ACID NOMENCLATURE

Numbering System

18-Carbon Fatty Acid
IUPAC Number --- 18 17 16 15 14 13 12 11 10 9 8 7 6 5 4 3 2 1
C – C – C – C – C – C – C – C – C – C – C – C– C – C – C – C – C – COOH
Omega Number --- 1   2   3   4   5   6   7   8   9 10 11 12 13 14 15 16 17 18

20-Carbon Fatty Acid
IUPAC Number - 20 19 18 17 16 15 14 13 12 11 10 9 8 7 6 5 4 3 2 1
C – C – C – C – C – C – C – C – C – C – C – C – C – C – C – C – C – C – C – COOH
Omega Number - 1   2   3   4   5   6   7   8   9 10 11 12 13 14 15 16 17 18 19 20

Examples

Omega-6 Family   **Omega-3 Family**
18-Carbon Fatty Acid

Common Name:	linoleic acid	alpha-linolenic acid
Geneva Name:	9,12-octadecadienoic acid	9,12,15-octatrienoic acid
Omega Name:	6,9-octadecadienoic acid	3,6,9-octatrienoic acid
Shorthand: *	C18:2n6	C18:3n3

20-Carbon Fatty Acid

Common Name:	arachidonic acid	EPA
Geneva Name	5,8,11,14-eicosatetraenoic acid	5,8,11,14,17-eicosapentanenoic acid
Omega Name	6,9,12,15-eicosatetraenoic acid	3,6,9,12,15-eicosapentanenoic acid
Shorthand: *	C20:4n6	C20:5n3

C—C—C—C—C—C—C—C—C=C—C—C—C—C—C—C—C—COOH
1   2   3   4   5   6   7   8   9   10   11   12   13   14   15   16   17   18
Omega-9 oleic acid (octadecamonoenoic acid)

C—C—C—C—C—C—C—C—C=C—C—C=C—C—C=C—C—C—C—COOH
1   2   3   4   5   6   7   8   9   10   11   12   13   14   15 16   17   18   19 20
Omega-9 Mead acid (eicosatrienoic acid)

Note: octadeca- = 18; eicosa- = 20;
monoenoic, dienoic, trienoic, tetraenoic, pentaenoic = 1, 2, 3,4, 5.
* In some older reports, the omega symbol is used. The more recent convention is to use the letter "n" for the omega symbol.

that they were essential nutrients. By 1963, it was known that EFAs were not of all one kind nutritionally, but rather of two major types (families). However, because of the complexity of polyunsaturated fatty acid structure and chemistry and because the two families each produce a cascade of metabolites using the same pathway and the same enzyme systems, it was difficult to sort out which metabolites belonged to which family.

In both EFA families, when using the Geneva system, each step in the metabolic cascade yielded a product with a different pattern of double bond location numbers. Examination of the double bond locations in all EFA metabolites revealed that the terminal double bond in a chain always occurred either between carbons 3 and 4 or carbons 6 and 7 from the terminal end of the chain, *not* the carboxyl end. It was also discovered that all metabolites within a family had their terminal double bonds in the same position, either 3 or 6, independent of chain length or degree of unsaturation. Thus, the omega system identified the nutritional family to which the EFA belonged, 3 or 6, whereas the Geneva system made no such distinction.

The problem with the Geneva system is made evident in Figure 8-1 by examining the Geneva designations of the omega-6 and omega-3 members. The conversions of omega-6 linoleic acid to arachidonic acid and omega-3 alpha-linolenic acid to EPA each involve the addition of two carbon atoms and two double bonds. As can be seen in Figure 8-1, the Geneva numbering designation changes with the length of the carbon chain and is independent of nutritional properties.

The omega numbering system eliminates this problem; the first double bond always carries the number of the family, either 6 or 3 as shown in Figure 8-1. The omega system is invaluable for study and practical application of the nutritional properties of the EFAs, as will become obvious in Chapter Nine, in which the EFA metabolic cascades will be discussed in detail.

Cis/Trans Double Bonds: Double bonds can exist either as *cis* or *trans* isomers. Isomers are molecules that have the exact same chemical formula but differ only in the spatial arrangement of their atoms. Enzyme systems can recognize the difference between isomers of the same chemical. Almost without exception, naturally occurring unsaturated fatty acids are *cis* isomers. Biochemical reactions actively select the *cis* form and reject the *trans* form. *Trans* isomers of fatty acids are uncommon in nature, but are easily and inadvertently formed in the hydrogenation process, discussed below, which is used to refine salad oils and to manufacture deep frying oils, shortenings, and margarines.

Two unique properties of double bonds are responsible for the occurrence of *cis* and *trans* forms of fatty acids. One is that a double bond is shorter than a single bond. This shortened bond produces a kink in the carbon chain at the site where it occurs. The other property is that a double bond limits rotation around the kink. In order to picture the differences in rotation between a single bond and a double bond, imagine a toothpick with an olive stuck on each end. You can freely twist one olive around the toothpick axle while holding the other olive stationary.

This same freedom of twist is afforded the carbons on either side of a single bond. Now envision the two olives linked together with two parallel toothpicks. If you hold one olive still, the other olive cannot be rotated. The two olives must rotate together. This same limitation is imposed on carbon atoms that are joined by a double bond.

The kink and limited rotation around double bonds are responsible for the occurrence of isomers. The two isomers of unsaturated fatty acids are shown in Figure 8-2. The *cis*, or boat, isomer has a wide U-shaped bend in the chain at the location of the double bond. The double bond (kink) is at the base of the U and the two sides of the carbon chain are bent out from the kink in the same direction in boat-like fashion. The *trans*, or chair, isomer has a Z-shaped bend, with the double bond at the spine of the Z, and the two sides of the carbon chain are bent away in opposite directions in chair-like fashion.

FIGURE 8-2
Cis AND *Trans* CONFIGURATIONS

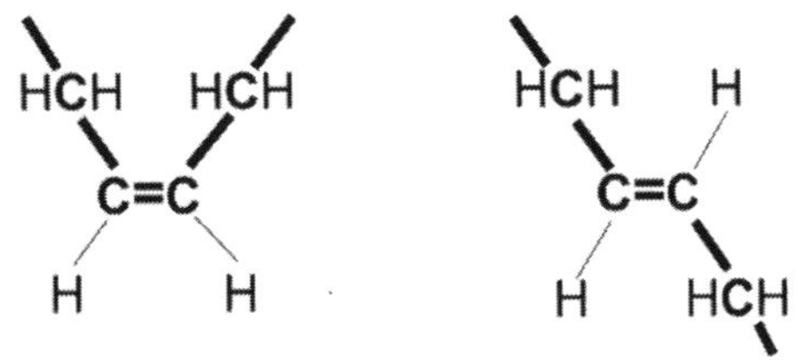

Cis (Boat) Form   *Trans* (Chair) Form

Conjugation: In organic chemistry, the term *conjugation* means alternation of double bonds and single bonds (-C=C-C=C-C=C-). With few exceptions, the double bonds in naturally occurring polyunsaturated fatty acids are not conjugated, but rather have two single bonds between each double bond (-C=C-C-C=C-C-C=C-). Human biochemistry does not make conjugated double bonds in fatty acid chains.

Conjugated Linoleic Acid: A naturally occurring conjugated fatty acid that has come to public attention in recent years is conjugated linoleic acid (CLA), a conjugated form of linoleic acid found primarily in cow's milk. Trace amounts of CLA are said to occur naturally in plant lipids, and it has been isolated from foods derived from ruminant animals. The synonyms of CLA, bovinic acid and rumenic acid, reflect its ruminant connection. CLA found in foods from animal sources (beef, butter, and cheese) is probably not synthesized by the animals themselves but rather produced by their rumen organisms and absorbed into the animals' fatty tissues. Microorganisms other than rumen organisms are also capable of converting linoleic acid to CLA. In addition, the conversion to CLA occurs to a small extent in vegetable oils during hydrogenation and in other high temperature processes.

Interest in CLA was spawned a little over 10 years ago when a substance with anti-cancer activity in animals was isolated from grilled ground beef and identified as CLA (10). Since that time, numerous animal studies have been reported that indicate, in addition to its anticancer effects, CLA may be useful in treating obesity and in inhibiting the development of atherosclerosis. Thus far, CLA is the only conjugated fatty acid that has been subjected to extensive laboratory investigation. A good review of both beneficial and adverse effects of CLA reported in the literature can be found on WebMD (11).

At the present time, clinical studies of CLA in humans are essentially nonexistent. One human study conducted in Norway reported a 20-percent weight loss without a change in diet (12). No mention is made of adverse effects. However, a letter to the editor of a scientific journal from Swedish scientists (13) warned of increased lipid peroxidation in human subjects after three months of supplementation with CLA and stressed the need for further investigation of the effects of CLA in humans.

There are no data to show that conjugated fatty acids serve as nutrients in animal or human nutrition. Data from animal experimentation indicates the toxicity of CLA in the amounts present in foods is low, but there is little information on chronic toxic effects from prolonged use or from higher doses. The warning from the Swedish scientists about lipid peroxidation suggests CLA may have chronic adverse effects. If CLA is shown to be effective in treatment of obesity, cardiovascular disease, or other ailments it should be used only as a drug under medical supervision rather than as a nutritional supplement.

PROPERTIES

The kind of bonding (single or double) affects the properties of fatty acids in two ways. One is in their physical state, which makes for the distinction between fats and oils. For the same carbon-chain length, saturated fatty acids have higher melting points than unsaturated fatty acids; melting points decrease with increasing number of double bonds. Thus, saturated fatty acids tend to be solid (fats) at room temperature, whereas unsaturated fatty acids tend to be liquid (oils). Whether a triglyceride is a fat or oil depends on the degree of saturation or unsaturation in its fatty acids and its ambient temperature. Interestingly, fatty acids in fish tend to be predominantly polyunsaturated, with cold water fish having the greatest degree of unsaturation. This is essential for the flexibility of aquatic animals in cold waters. Saturated fats would solidify under the same conditions.

In addition to affecting physical properties, the kind of bonding also alters chemical properties. Saturated fatty acids are quite stable chemically. Unlike the single bonds of saturated fats, double bonds are chemically reactive and can be converted back to single bonds relatively easily by the addition of hydrogen. They also are easily attacked by oxygen and are unstable in the presence of heat, light, or impurities.

Monounsaturates are relatively stable but polyunsaturates are not, with instability increasing with increasing numbers of double bonds. Polyunsaturates in plant oils usually contain antioxidants, such as tocopherols, that are naturally added by plant biochemistry to protect the integrity of their double bond compounds.

The instability of double bonds causes rancidity in cooking oils. The reaction of double bonds with the oxygen in air creates new, oxidized molecules that have an unpleasant rancid taste and odor. Rancidity is probably more of a problem of esthetics than health; however, little information is available on whether rancid oils have any adverse health effects. Single bonds, on the other hand, are relatively inert and highly resistant to oxidation; thus, rancidity is not a problem with saturated fats that have few or no unsaturated fats in their mixtures.

HYDROGENATION: As the name implies, hydrogenation converts double bonds to single bonds by adding hydrogen atoms to them. Heat, pressure, various catalysts, and hydrogen are used in the procedure, which is the single most important process currently employed by the vegetable oil industry (14). It is used to increase the shelf life of salad oils by making them resistant to rancidity, resistant to high temperatures, and resistant to smoking during frying. Hydrogenation is also used to convert vegetable oils into low-cost fats such as the shortenings and margarines that take the place of lard and butter.

The amount of hydrogen added during hydrogenation depends upon how many double bonds are to be eliminated (converted to single bonds), which in turn depends on what the process is intended to achieve, either reduce rancidity and smoking or increase the melting point. The amount of hydrogen used is always partial because full hydrogenation would produce a saturated fat that would be so hard it would have no commercial value.

Partial hydrogenation converts double bonds, which are naturally in the *cis* form, either to single bonds or to *trans* double bonds. The conversion of *cis* double bonds to the *trans* configuration is the result of hydrogenation being only partial. During the hydrogenation process, all or most of the double bonds are opened. The amount of hydrogen added is that which is required to convert the desired number of double bonds to single bonds. At the end of the process, the opened double bonds that have not received hydrogen close back to their former double bond state. When they reform their double bonds, most do so in the *trans* configuration. This is because it is easier to do; the amount of energy that is required to make a *trans* bond is a great deal less than that required to form a *cis* bond.

Light partial hydrogenation is used primarily to extend the consumer acceptance and shelf life of salad and cooking oils. It attacks the most vulnerable double bonds, primarily those in polyunsaturated fatty acids with three double bonds, which are the fatty acids most responsible for rancidity. Unfortunately, these particular double bonds are the more fragile omega-3 EFA bonds. The selective destruction by hydrogenation of omega-3 EFAs in salad oils produces an unhealthful ratio of omega-6/omega-3 EFAs (15; 16).

Heavier partial hydrogenation is used to make soft spreads and margarine. The severity of hydrogenation is adjusted so that more double bonds are converted to single bonds and, coincidentally, to *trans* isomers, both of which increase the melting point (hardness) of the product. These products are relatively high in *trans* fats.

Apart from their real and potential adverse health effects, *trans* fatty acids taste, look, and feel the same as *cis* fatty acids made by nature. *Trans* fats do not cause upset stomach, diarrhea, or other acute symptoms. Like every other chemical, the potential damage to health posed by *trans* fatty acids depends on how much, how often, and for how long exposure exists. A very small amount every day is probably not harmful.

Fatty Acid Digestion

As mentioned above, fatty acids present in the diet are in the form of triglycerides. Dietary triglycerides must be broken down to their component parts before they can cross the intestinal wall and be absorbed into the body. Digestive enzymes break two of the three ester bonds of a triglyceride to yield two free fatty acids and a monoglyceride. Fatty acids and monoglyceride molecules are small enough to pass through the intestinal wall, whereas triglycerides are not. Fatty acids and monoglycerides are transported across the intestinal wall by a series of complicated reactions involving bile salts and specialized proteins.

Once through the intestinal wall, long chain fatty acids (>12 carbons) are reassembled as triglycerides and transported by the lymph system to the heart and then to the general circulation. Short chain fatty acids (< 8 carbons), like water-soluble nutrients, are transported individually via the hepatic portal vein to the liver. Medium chain fatty acids (9-11 carbons) can go either as triglycerides by lymph or free by the hepatic portal vein.

Fatty Acid Metabolism

The metabolism of fatty acids centers on the biochemical acetyl CoA. Figure 4-1 shows that acetyl CoA is a vital and pivotal endpoint for the breakdown (catabolism) of carbohydrate, protein, and lipid macronutrients. Interestingly, for fatty acids other than essential fatty acids, which cannot be synthesized by mammalian biochemistry, it is not only the endpoint of catabolism but also the starting point for their synthesis (anabolism).

ACETYL CO A

The metabolic fate of acetyl CoA is controlled in large part by the carbohydrate fraction of the diet. Figure 6-4 shows that a high-carbohydrate diet stimulates production of insulin, which, in turn, sends acetyl CoA on pathways that make body fat or cholesterol. Figure 6-5 shows that a low-carbohydrate diet removes fat from body fat stores, converts it to acetyl CoA, and directs acetyl CoA to production of ketone bodies. The major source of acetyl CoA from high-carbohydrate diets is glucose provided by the diet, and the major source from low-carbohydrate diets is fatty acids provided by mobilization from body fat stores.

ANABOLISM: The first step in fatty acid synthesis is combination of acetyl CoA with CO_2 (carboxylation) to form the 3-carbon unit malonyl CoA. The 3-carbon unit starts the building of a fatty acid chain by condensing with another acetyl CoA to form a 5-carbon unit. It then splits off the CO2 group to form a 4-carbon unit. The four-carbon unit can either leave the sequence to yield butyric acid, the smallest of the fatty acids, or it can condense with another malonyl CoA, split off the CO2 group, and repeat the sequence of adding two carbons at a time until a fatty acid of the desired chain length is achieved.

The product formed at each step can leave the sequence or continue further buildup; however, it is usual for the sequence to continue to completion. The most common final product of fatty acid synthesis is palmitic acid (16 carbons), but, because many cells need longer chains or unsaturated chains, they have enzyme systems required to make them as needed. However, recall from above that, in human biochemistry, desaturation reactions (formation of double bonds from single bonds) cannot occur further away from the carboxyl group than carbon-9. After synthesis, fatty acids are combined with glycerol to form triglycerides and transported to adipose tissues in various locations for storage.

CATABOLISM: Unlike most biochemicals, which use only one pathway reversibly for both synthesis and degradation, the synthesis and degradation of fatty acids use entirely separate pathways. The metabolic pathway that predominates is largely under the control of the insulin/glucagon balance, which is determined by the dietary carbohydrate content.

Unlike the anabolism of fatty acids, which requires 3-carbon units, fatty acid degradation uses a different pathway to produce 2-carbon units. Fatty acids are mobilized from storage sites by a multistep process and transported into cells where they undergo catabolism by an energy-producing reaction known as β-oxidation. This reaction provides the energy normally provided by catabolism of glucose through the Krebs cycle (see Figure 4-1). The reaction is called β-oxidation because it results in oxidation of the single bond between the α- and β-carbons of a fatty acid chain. The Greek letters, α and β, are the designations for the first and second carbons, respectively, after the carboxyl group of a fatty acid.

After β-oxidation, the double bond that is formed is cleaved to yield two molecules. One molecule is a 2-carbon unit made from the carboxyl carbon and the α-carbon of the fatty acid. This 2-carbon unit then forms acetyl CoA by combining with coenzyme A. The other molecule is a new fatty acid that is two carbons shorter than is its parent. The β-carbon of the parent fatty acid is now the carboxyl carbon of the new fatty acid. This new fatty acid is now ready to undergo further β-oxidation. Thus, fatty acids are broken down, two carbons at a time, until the parent fatty acid is completely converted to acetyl CoA molecules. Because all mammalian fatty acids have an even number of carbons, there are no odd pieces left over.

Unsaturated fatty acids, including EFAs, undergo β-oxidation in the same manner as satu-rated fatty acids with the exception that when a double bond is reached, another set of enzymes come into play to rearrange the position of the double bond by moving it further toward the end of the chain. The reactions of β-oxidation then resume until the next double bond is reached, and so on until the fatty acid is completely broken down. All two-carbon units formed by β-oxidation are added to the pool of acetyl CoA.

INTERMEDIARY METABOLISM: As mentioned in Chapter Four, intermediary metabo-lism is the term used to describe the sequence of reactions that occur between a biochemi-cal precursor and its final biochemical product. For example, the intermediary metabolism of acetyl CoA going to CO_2+H_2O+energy is described by the sequence of intermediary reactions known as the Krebs cycle.

The intermediary metabolism in both fatty acid anabolism and catabolism, as described above, is fairly simple. Both involve numerous steps, but the steps are merely repetitions of the same reaction, which are malonyl CoA condensation in anabolism and β-oxidation in catabolism. EFAs, on the other hand, have their own intricate and interdependent inter-mediary metabolism between absorption and ultimate synthesis of their final end products known as eicosanoids, which will be the subject of Chapter Nine.

Metabolic Energy Control

In normal individuals, the insulin/glucagon ratio is the most important determinant of the relative contribution of the two major sources of fuel to the body's energy needs. When the ratio is large, glucose is the major fuel; when the ratio is small, it is fatty acids. The insulin/ glucagon ratio can vary almost a 100-fold depending on nutritional state and/or glucose availability. It can be from as high as 30 immediately after eating to as low as 0.5 several hours later or after fasting, (17, p.715).

Despite the fact that glucose serves as the usual and ready source of energy for meta-bolic functions, fatty acids are a much more efficient fuel than glucose. For example, palmitic acid (16 carbons) yields about 25 percent more energy than glucose (6 car-bons) on a carbon-for-carbon basis. Fatty acids are also a much more efficient form for storage of fuel. Triglycerides, the storage form of fatty acids, require less space for storage than glycogen, the storage form of glucose. In addition, triglycerides have an almost endless supply of adipose tissue storage depots throughout the human body whereas glycogen has a limited number of depots, the largest and most important of which is in the liver.

A brief outline of the metabolic events that occur with switching the energy source from glucose to fatty acids is as follows: When blood glucose falls to low or below normal levels, the rate of glycolysis slows; This decreases the amount of pyruvate formed; The decrease in quantity of pyruvate results in a deficiency of oxaloacetic acid, which is made from pyruvate (see Figure 4-1). The deficiency of oxaloacetic acid then slows the Krebs cycle, because oxaloacetic acid is required to keep the cycle going by combining with acetyl CoA to make citric acid; This reduction in energy production by the Krebs cycle creates the demand for a source of energy other than glucose, which is met by an increased mobilization of fat from storage depots and degradation of fatty acids. The energy produced by β-oxidation replaces that normally provided by glucose.

Most of the acetyl CoA produced by increased mobilization and degradation of fatty acids cannot enter the Krebs cycle for further conversion to CO_2 and energy because of the insufficiency of oxaloacetic acid, described above, resulting from the slowing of the rate of glycolysis. Thus, acetyl CoA must be diverted to a catabolic pathway other than the Krebs cycle. This alternate pathway, via HMG CoA (see Figure 6-5) is called ketogenesis – the production of ketone bodies. Because the public has been so badly misinformed about the significance of ketone body production, it is important to explain more fully what ketone bodies are and how and why they are formed.

KETONE BODIES AND KETOSIS

Ketones are organic chemicals in which an interior carbon in a molecule forms a double bond with an oxygen molecule. Acetone, a familiar chemical, is the smallest ketone possible. It is composed of three carbons, with the double bond to oxygen on the middle carbon. Biological ketone bodies include acetone, larger ketones, and biochemicals that can become ketones. The most important of the ketone bodies are hydroxybutyrate and acetoacetate, both of which are formed from condensation of two acetyl CoA molecules. Acetone is formed from a nonenzymatic decarboxylation of acetoacetate.

Ketone bodies are fuel molecules that can be used for energy by all organs of the body except the liver. The production of ketone bodies is a normal, natural, and important biochemical pathway in animal biochemistry (17, p. 577). Small quantities of ketone bodies are *always* present in the blood, with the quantity increasing as hours without food increase. During fasting or carbohydrate deprivation, larger amounts of ketone bodies are produced to provide the energy that is normally provided by glucose.

Excessive levels of circulating ketone bodies can result in ketosis, a condition in which the quantity of circulating ketone bodies is greater than the quantity the organs and tissues of the body need for energy. People who go on extremely low-carbohydrate diets to lose a large excess of body fat usually go into a mild ketosis that moderates as weight is lost. There is no scientific evidence that a low-carbohydrate diet is capable of producing sufficient ketone bodies to be harmful.

Excess ketone bodies are excreted by the kidneys and lungs. Exhaled acetone gives the breath a characteristic, sweetish odor. If ketosis is maintained for prolonged periods, as can occur in untreated type-1 diabetes (insulin-dependent diabetes), the blood can become very acidic. This is a life-threatening disorder is known as ketoacidosis.

Ketone bodies that are excreted in the urine and the breath carry with them the calories they contain. These are calories that were counted in the diet but were made unavailable to the body by being excreted before being used. In effect, the body actually receives fewer calories than the amount calculated. Thus, for individuals with normal pancreatic function, a ketogenic (low-carbohydrate) diet containing a given number of calories will result in greater weight loss than a nonketogenic diet (high-carbohydrate) containing the same number of calories. This difference in apparent caloric content between low-carbohydrate and high-carbohydrate diet plans has given rise to the observation that ketogenic diets have a metabolic advantage over nonketogenic diets with regard to weight loss.

DIETETIC VERSUS DIABETIC KETOSIS: The nutrition community has fostered the popular misconception that ketone-body production, *per se*, is an undesirable metabolic circumstance. It has warned that the formation of ketone bodies is a dangerous consequence of low-carbohydrate diets in an effort to discredit any recommendations that deviate from official dietary recommendations. As a result, the public has come to view formation of ketone bodies as a symptom of a pathological condition rather than a normal attempt by the body to satisfy its demands for energy when glucose supplies are short. This unfortunate misunderstanding stems from allegations that brief periods of dietary ketosis from diets low in carbohydrates have the same medical significance as diabetic ketosis. These allegations are foundationless and grossly in error.

There is no question that the ketosis of type-1 diabetes is undesirable and dangerous. In type-1 diabetes, the ability of the pancreas to make insulin is either diminished or absent. The mechanism by which ketone bodies are formed in type-1 diabetes is similar to that which occurs with a low-carbohydrate diet, as diagrammed in Figure 6-5. In the absence of insulin, fatty acids are mobilized and degraded, excess acetyl CoA is produced, and the excess is directed to HMG CoA and ketone bodies and potentially to ketoacidosis.

Diabetic ketosis is the body's plaintive call for insulin administration. It is a warning signal that insulin levels have been permitted to fall too low and blood sugar levels are too high and out of control. This is a medical emergency. If insulin is not promptly administered and blood glucose brought under control, the insufficiency of insulin could lead to life-threatening physiologic responses, one of which is ketoacidosis.

Dietary ketosis is an entirely different condition because it occurs in people with sound pancreatic function with an ample supply of insulin. If glucose is not supplied by the diet, blood glucose levels drop. As a result of low blood glucose, insulin drops to a lower level and its counterpart hormone, glucagon, assumes control.

To spare glucose by providing a substitute energy source, glucagon stimulates the degradation of fatty acids and the conversion of surplus acetyl CoA to ketone bodies (Figure 6-5). It is only when glucose sources are severely restricted that excess ketone bodies are produced and the acetone odor in the breath becomes noticeable.

Dietary ketosis is the body's request not for insulin but for more glucose. It is a signal that the glucose supply is insufficient and, as a result, the body is burning fatty acids mobilized from fat storage sites for energy. If glucose sources are not supplied, mobilization and degradation of fatty acids continue. In a starvation situation, this is a serious matter. However, for healthy people on low-carbohydrate diets, the only result of ketone body production is loss of body fat. In summary, diabetic ketosis is a call for more insulin because the blood glucose level is dangerously high. Dietary ketosis, on the other hand, is a call for more glucose because the blood glucose level is becoming low.

Nutritional Requirements for Lipids

There are no known nutritional requirements for any lipids other than the very small component known as the essential fatty acids (EFAs). However, that does not lessen the nutritional importance of the lipid fraction of the diet. The official recommendation to avoid dietary lipids, primarily saturated fats and cholesterol from animal sources, constitutes an unwarranted impediment to public health and chronic disease prevention.

SATURATED FATTY ACIDS

The Dietary Guidelines' proscription against saturated fats is based on the allegation that elevated blood cholesterol levels are caused by excess dietary saturated fats. The nutritional biochemistry that refutes this contention is described in Chapter Six. Despite the fact that saturated fats have been indiscriminately labeled as harmful foods with no redeeming value, scientific corroboration of an adverse effect of saturated fats on health are lacking (18; 19; 20). To the contrary, numerous studies demonstrate their benefits. For example, saturated and monounsaturated fats but not omega-6 polyunsaturated fatty acids protected the liver against acetaminophen-induced liver damage (21); diets rich in saturated fatty acids (not unsaturated) have been found to reverse alcoholic liver damage (22).

There are also considerable data that one or more saturated fatty acids provide health benefits over and beyond their basic nutrient properties. Such nutrients are classed as functional foods (23). Lauric acid, a 12-carbon-chain saturated fatty acid, and its monoglyceride monolaurin are examples. They have long been known to possess antiviral, antibacterial, antiprotozoal, and antifungal properties. In recent years, other medium- chain saturated fatty acids such as 10-carbon capric acid have been found to possess similar activity. In addition to antibiotic activity, oils whose major saturated fat is lauric acid (lauric oils) have been shown to promote conversion of omega-3 alpha-linolenic acid to EPA and DHA and improve the immune system's anti-inflammatory response (23).

The major sources of lauric oils are the tropical oils, especially coconut and palm kernel oils. Approximately 50 percent of coconut oil is lauric acid. Minor amounts are present in the oils of numerous plants (23). Interestingly, about 3 percent of milk fat is lauric acid (15, p. 255). Butter and milk fats are the only animal sources of lauric acid. The lauric acid component of mothers' milk is credited with protection of human infants from viral and bacterial infections (15, p. 215).

Since the publication of Ravnskov's pioneering book, *The Cholesterol Myths* (24), a number of other scholarly works have appeared that fully document the scientific basis for Ravnskov's charge that saturated fat and cholesterol are not the cause of heart disease (25; 26). In addition, a tremendous expenditure of time and money in the past several decades in the conduct of many long-term studies has failed to confirm an association, much less causal relationship, between saturated fat and chronic disease (18; 19; 26).

MONOUNSATURATED FATTY ACIDS (OLEIC ACID)

Oleic acid is an 18-carbon fatty acid with one double bond in the omega-9 position. It takes its name from olive oil, of which it is a major component. There is very little information available about a dietary need for monounsaturated oleic acid. This probably is because the human body is capable of synthesizing it. Like cholesterol and many other nutrients the body can make for itself, it may use the oleic acid provided in the diet and then only make as much oleic acid *de novo* as it requires.

Epidemiological studies suggest that dietary olive oil is an important contributor to the health benefits associated with dietary patterns found in Mediterranean countries. Olive oil is used in Mediterranean cuisines in place of common vegetable oils, which have high proportions of omega-6 EFAs. Olive oil is about 75-percent oleic acid and contains only small, but balanced amounts of omega-6 and omega-3 fatty acids. Is the benefit conferred by olive oil due to the oleic acid component or to the acceptable ratio of omega-6 to omega-3 oils (about 4:1)? A few laboratory and clinical studies have suggested that oleic acid itself may indeed have beneficial effects; however, with the exception of a reduction in LDL/HDL ratio, thus far none have been described by the nutrition community.

MEAD ACID: An interesting biochemical use of oleic acid is the attempt by the body to use it to make substitutes for EFAs when they are deficient in the diet. In the metabolic pathway to the eicosanoids (see Figure 9-1) linoleic and alpha-linolenic acids are desaturated and elongated in alternating steps. The products, arachidonic acid and EPA, each have two carbons and two double bonds more than its respective parent. The new double bonds in arachidonic acid and EPA are in the C-12 and C-15 positions.

When the diet is inadequate in EFAs, the body makes Mead's acid. In a desperate attempt to make up for the EFA deficiency, the body tries to make omega-3 and/or omega-6 EFAs from oleic acid. It adds two more carbons to oleic acid to make a 20-carbon omega-9 acid, and then it desaturates the single bonds at C-12 and C-15 to make the double bonds it normally makes in linoleic and alpha-linolenic acids. The result, Mead acid, is a biochemical marker of EFA deficiency in humans (see Figure 8-1).

Mead acid cannot substitute for either arachidonic acid or EPA. Thus, it cannot correct a deficiency of either. It has the potential to interfere with the body's metabolic processes; however, little is known about it other than that it accumulates in people whose diets are deficient in EFAs. The synthesis of Mead acid is an eloquent example of the body's unceasing drive to maintain wellbeing despite deprivation and abuse.

POLYUNSATURATED FATTY ACIDS (ESSENTIAL FATTY ACIDS)

Two of the polyunsaturated fatty acids known to be essential are linoleic acid (LA), an omega-6 fatty acid with 18-carbons and two double bonds, and alpha-linolenic acid (ALA), an omega-3 fatty acid with 18-carbons and three double bonds. These two EFA's provide the starting points for two families of polyunsaturated fatty acids; the omega-6 family and the omega-3 family (see Figure 9-1). Some biochemistry texts also list arachidonic acid (AA) as essential for humans.

Arachidonic acid is a 20-carbon member of the omega-6 family, with four double bonds. It is synthesized *in vivo* from linoleic acid by the addition of two more carbons and two more double bonds (see Figure 9-1). The fact that the body can synthesize arachidonic acid from linoleic acid may be the reason for the question about its being essential.

Regardless of its classification, there are considerable clinical data that show, in combination with omega-3 docosahexaenoic acid (DHA), arachidonic acid is essential for fetal and neonatal growth and development (27; 28). Considerable evidence also exists that it not only played an essential role, along with DHA, in brain evolution but also that its absence would have been a constraint on further evolution of the primate brain (29). The logical conclusion is that even though arachidonic acid may not fit the biochemical definition of essential it is *de facto* essential because it cannot be biosynthesized in sufficient quantity to serve the needs for it.

Like any other dietary fats, EFAs can be used for energy if needed. However, the EFAs have unique and much more important biological roles than energy production. First, they provide flexibility, selective permeability, and self-sealing properties to individual cells throughout the body, and they are key building blocks for brain, nerve, and eye tissue. The most common fatty acid in nervous system tissues and brain is DHA (27).

Probably more important than their own structural and functional roles in living systems, is the fact that they are the precursors of vitally important omega-3 and omega-6 lipid mediators known as eicosanoids, which will be discussed in Chapter Nine.

Dietary Recommendations for Lipids

The official nutrition policy of the United States, the *Dietary Guidelines for Americans*, is revised and reissued jointly every five years by the U. S. Departments of Agriculture and Health and Human Services (30). To date, these agencies have not established estimated average requirements (EARs) or recommended daily requirements (RDAs) for any dietary lipids (30; 31). In addition, neither daily adequate intakes (AIs) nor tolerable upper limits of intakes (ULs) are given for total fats, ostensibly because data are insufficient to determine the minimum amount of total fat necessary for health and the maximum amount that will not cause cardiovascular disease (30).

TOTAL FATS AND CHOLESTEROL

The nutrition and medical communities decided decades ago that dietary fat and cholesterol are major risk factors for cardiovascular disease. This decision was based primarily on population studies in countries for which heart disease mortality was associated with average fat consumption (see Chapter Three). The acceptance of this association as a causal relationship has been labeled as "probably one of the greatest and most harmful misconceptions in the history of medicine" (25, p. *x*).

The recommended upper daily limits in the 2005 Dietary Guidelines was 30 percent or less of calories from dietary fats and 300 milligrams or less of cholesterol (2; 31). The more recent guide, *Dietary Reference Intakes* (DRI), recommends that total fat represent 25 to 35 percent of calories and that saturated fats, trans fats, and cholesterol "remain as low as possible" (2; 30). The National Cholesterol Education Program, sponsored by the National Heart, Lung, and Blood Institute, issues its own recommendation of a daily maximum for blood cholesterol of 200 milligrams and less than 7 percent of total calories as saturated fat for people whose blood cholesterol is greater than acceptable (32).

The reluctance to set dietary standards for fats is due to official acceptance of the proposition that, beyond the absolute minimum intake possible, "any incremental increase in intake [of fat] increases the risk of CHD [coronary heart disease]" (2; 30, p. 124). The foods to be avoided are all animal-based foods plus coconut and palm oils. Although the dietary guidelines do not specifically recommend low-fat diets, they do state that there is no "strong" evidence "that low-fat diets predispose to chronic disease" (2; 30, p.133).

POLYUNSATURATED FATS - ESSENTIAL FATTY ACIDS

Despite decades of promoting the use of polyunsaturated vegetable seed oils in the heart healthy diet, the nutritional importance of these oils was largely ignored. In 2005, linoleic and alpha-linolenic acids were included in the table titled Nutrients in Proposed Food Intake Patterns of the 2005 Dietary Guidelines. This addition apparently was in response to a request from the administration urging inclusion of information about the importance of omega-3 EFAs for public health (33).

To date, very little information of worth is presented in the guidelines to support the requirement for polyunsaturated fatty acids other than to say they are essential and that they are used for eicosanoid synthesis (2; 30). Even the average intakes (AIs) recommended for linoleic and alpha-linolenic acids are not based on scientific data but rather on the median dietary intakes of these two EFAs in current dietary patterns.

Nutrition academia has long known of a dietary requirement for EFAs, but it is still virtually silent on the distinction between the omega-6 and omega-3 families of fatty acids and the importance of a balance between them. Despite the large volume of scientific data showing the vital importance of EFAs, the official recommendations of the government and nutrition communities pay scant attention to them and provide little guidance to the public about their requirements or importance.

The guidelines do acknowledge that low-fat diets might present an EFA deficiency problem, but they discount the possibility by claiming that such a deficiency is very rare. As ill-advised as is such a conclusion, the statement that EFA deficiency is "nonexistent in healthy individuals" (30, p.124) is a gross misstatement that contradicts a wealth of scientific evidence to the contrary. Study of the scientific literature makes it apparent that the only well-founded information on health effects and probable human requirements of EFAs has come not from the government or academia but from scientists working in the fields of biochemistry and human nutrition.

Heart-Healthy Diet Plans

As mentioned above, the position that excess dietary fat presents a significant risk of CVD is a long-standing government nutrition policy. This many-decade long official sponsorship of the dietary regime founded on the lipid hypothesis developed from misguided epidemiology by Ancel Key and colleagues (26) has fostered an awe-inspiring growth in the heart-health and weight-loss diet industries. Diet programs are widely promoted by the news media, as well as by direct mail, mass market media, books, and newsletters. With a few exceptions, these dietary regimes all seem to follow the low-fat model that restricts fat and cholesterol and promotes vegetable seed oils and carbohydrates (30; 31).

LOW-FAT DIET PLANS

Low-fat diets are those that may contain up to 35 percent, but preferably 20 percent or less, of calories from the fat component of the diet. They are based on the premise that dietary fats, *per se*, make body fat and cholesterol. That this premise is faulty is detailed in the section on metabolism of fatty acids, above. Biochemical truths notwithstanding, the low-fat fad has many dedicated proponents.

If anyone must be credited with popularizing the low-fat diet, it would have to be Nathan Pritikin (34). Pritikin, a survivor of cardiovascular disease, credited his recovery to a non-fat diet and exercise program that he devised for himself, without benefit of a medical or nutrition counsel. By the mid-1970's, his Pritikin Longevity Centers were models for the burgeoning health spa industry. They were also the training grounds for a new generation of weight-loss treatment centers.

Today, the name in low-fat diets is Ornish (35). The Ornish Life Choice Diet is not only low in fat but is also vegetarian. The foods it avoids include meats of all kinds, oils of all kinds, avocados, nuts and seeds, all but nonfat dairy products, and any commercially prepared food containing more than 2 grams of fat per serving (36).

There is considerable controversy in the public media today about whether low-fat diets are effective. Ornish claims his diet can reverse heart disease (37), yet others say his data are not convincing (24, p. 214ff). Many of Ornish's cardiac patients feel they have benefited from his low-fat diet. It is quite logical that such patients actually have had some benefit, at least in the short term. The Ornish diet is a very low calorie diet, despite its high carbohydrate component. If a body has no calories in excess of daily requirements, regardless of macronutrient source, it will not have excess calories to divert to cholesterol or fatty acid synthesis. Further, because the body is always in a state of dynamic equilibrium, cessation of the production of excess cholesterol theoretically could cause a reversal of cholesterol deposition and pull some cholesterol out of arterial plaques.

Regardless of whether the Ornish diet is of benefit for some cardiac patients, the very real problems associated with low-fat diets do not bode well for its adherents. The human body is very forgiving. It will suffer for a long time, even years, before finally giving up. But it will give up eventually.

NUTRITIONAL IMPACT OF LOW-FAT DIET: Apart from their exceptional nutritional roles, essential fatty acids are fats; they behave physically and chemically like all true fats. They occur, albeit in small amounts, mixed together with all the other components of a diet's total fat. Any circumstance that affects total fat affects its components.

EFA Deficiency: Perhaps the most important nutritional impact of low-fat diets is the potential for EFA deficiency. Because the composition of fat varies considerably among food groups, both in kind and quantity, the contribution by a food to an EFA requirement depends not only on its EFA content but also on its total fat. It has also been shown that the EFA content of population food supplies varies widely with geography and population ethnicity (38). The American diet is excessively high in omega-6 linoleic acid as a result of heavy use of vegetable seed oils.

Gallstones: In addition to the problem of EFA deficiency, diets low in total fat are associated with gallstones. The presence of fatty foods in the diet stimulates contraction of the gallbladder and the emptying of its content of bile into the intestines. This periodic and frequent emptying of the gallbladder prevents the bile solids from aggregating to form crystals and, ultimately, stones. Low-fat diets often do not provide the necessary stimulation for gallbladder contraction and emptying. The bile remains undisturbed for long periods, allowing time for bile contents, including cholesterol, to crystallize.

A chance observation that people who have had their gall bladders removed appear to have a higher incidence of pancreatic cancer begs for an answer to the question of whether biliary disturbances disrupt the digestive functions of the pancreas.

Lipid Soluble vitamins: Low-fat diets can also contribute to deficiencies of the lipid vitamins A, D, E, and K. They are fat-soluble and require the presence of fats in the intestines to stimulate release of bile from the gallbladder. These vitamins require bile for absorption into the body.

Other Effects: Further evidence that low-fat diets, over the long term, may be detrimental to health is gradually coming forth. Interestingly, much of these data are coming from research institutions that themselves have long advocated, and still advocate, avoidance of dietary saturated fats and cholesterol. For example, a recent report that concludes that low intakes of saturated fat and animal protein are associated with hemorrhagic stroke in women (39) is only one of many scientific papers citing a positive role for saturated fats that are now coming forth from the Department of Nutrition of the Harvard School of Public Health, which has long supported and continues to support the proscription against the use of butter because of its saturated fat content (40, p. 75).

It is apparent that the medical and nutrition communities should be far more concerned about the quality of the fat in a diet rather than the quantity. Their concern should be that, regardless of percent fat in the diet, sufficient care is exercised in food selection to insure that the diet includes adequate balance of EFAs and other healthful fats.

IF NOT LOW FAT, HOW MUCH FAT?

If low-fat diets present a serious problem of EFA deficiency and high fat diets pose a serious risk of CVD, a logical question is what quantity of fat in the diet might be the proper amount? The answer in *Protein Power* is most sensible and helpful (41, p. 91ff).

> Don't worry about fat, but choose healthy fats: olive oil, avocados, and butter (yes!). Your body can and will use incoming fat as fuel. [As long as you keep a] weather eye on your carbohydrate – *don't worry about counting fat grams*.

In essence, do not be troubled about the fat content of foods but do be concerned about their source. It is the fats that are added to foods as spreads or dressings that are the fats that must be selected with care. These are primarily fats and oils derived from plant sources. Coconut oil and olive oil are exceptions. Avoid vegetable seed oils. They have high concentrations of omega-6 EFAs (see Table 8-2). To reduce intake of *trans* fats, avoid any product that has been partially hydrogenated. Use only butter and lard, whole fat dairy products, and meats with good marbling. As shown in Chapter Six, it is excess carbohydrates in the diet, not fat, that makes body fat.

An unforeseen benefit of dietary fat is that it produces a profound feeling of satiety when dietary carbohydrates are restricted. This is demonstrated by a comparison of diets of equal calories but different in fat content, which shows that those higher in fat provide longer hunger-free periods between meals (42). This helps prevent overindulgence.

A note of caution about diets that severely restrict carbohydrates: They *must* have an alternate source of fuel. Sufficient fat must be included in the diet to provide for energy needs. Protein foods are not capable of providing energy on a sustained basis. A possible but not probable result of a diet that is lacking in both carbohydrate and fat is a condition known to early explorers as rabbit starvation (43).

IF DIETARY FAT DOES NOT MAKE BODY FAT, WHERE DOES IT GO?
This is a very important, frequently asked question. People who eat a diet very low in carbohydrates seem to be able to consume large amounts of dietary fat without gaining weight. Where does excess fat go if it is not stored in fat depots? Biochemists will understand and enjoy the rather complex biochemistry that provides the answer (44).

Very simply, part goes to replace glucose as an energy source and part goes to provide energy to convert nonessential amino acids and glycerol, from protein and triglycerides, respectively, to glucose in the amount needed to maintain the normal blood glucose level.

The amount of fat in excess of what is required to serve the body's needs is not deposited as body fat in the low-insulin environment characteristic of low-carbohydrate diets. Instead the body directs the excess fat to one or more of a number of what might be called "futile" cycles, cycles that require energy but make no net change (44; 45, p. 398). An example of a futile cycle would be the act of turning the ignition of an automobile on, letting the car idle for a while, then turning the engine off. It uses a lot of fuel without doing any work (no net change). Some of these cycles could also be likened to many make-work housekeeping activities; for example, an equation for a rerun of a dish washing cycle could be expressed as *clean dishes + energy = clean dishes.*

The Chronicle of the Essential Fatty Acids
The medical community has paid scant attention to the fact that essential fatty acids are strongly related to both health and disease. Few doctors, for example, inquire about their patients' dietary intake of essential fatty acids or recommend EFA supplementation. One

reason may be that, until recently, little was known about EFA biochemistry. It was not until laboratory methods developed after World War II made it possible to identify them chemically that the roles of the EFAs and their metabolites began to be revealed. Nonetheless, prior to that time, their existence had long been suspected.

THE CULTURAL SYMBOLISM OF THE FISH

From symbolism in scriptural stories to incarnations of gods, fish is commonly portrayed as a pure, frequently profoundly sacred, food. Fish and gods are often entwined in mythology and religious symbolism....Over several millennia, as people devoted to religion and spirituality made this identification through careful observation of how dietary practices altered their internal states, they simultaneously crafted the traditions, symbolism, and rituals of their religions, into which they codified their beliefs (46).

Throughout recorded history, the fish has not only found meaning in religious and spiritual life but also in the healing arts. Ancient Chinese medicine instructed that the doctor attend first to sleep and diet before turning to drugs. The fish symbol, as Westerners call the familiar Taoist yin-yang icon, has long represented internal balance. All through the ancient world, food was the primary treatment for physical and mental ailments (46). The use of food as medicine continued to be an important if not only tool in the physician's instrument bag until the advent of modern medicine and pharmacology in the 20th Century.

A review of the religions of the world reveals that the recognition of fish as a sacred food or sign appears to be ubiquitous. In Judaism, the importance of fish is stressed in religious books; no matter how difficult to procure, fish is always a part of Sabbath meals in orthodox homes. In Islam, Allah was been said to have declared fish of all kinds to be clean and acceptable for pious Muslims. In Christianity, fish was not only considered pure and sacred but also was used as a symbolic representation of Jesus that predates that of the crucifix (46).

"It is remarkable that symbols associated with fish are at the core of the world's major religions and have endured for so long" (46). It is also remarkable that primitive cultures throughout the world and throughout the ages had the intuitive knowledge that food from the sea was essential for health and especially for reproductive success. There are many anecdotal tales of ancient tribes making yearly treks to the sea to obtain foods for their young women of reproductive age. Weston Price, in his study of nutrition in primitive cultures, wrote about natives travelling long distances to gather special sea foods used for production of a healthy child. One story told of a tribe living high in the Andean Sierras:

> It was, accordingly, a matter of great interest to discover that these Indians
> regularly used dried fish eggs from the sea. Commerce in these dried foods
> is carried on today as it no doubt has been carried on for centuries. When

I inquired of them why they used this material they explained that it was necessary to maintain the fertility of their women. I was informed also that every exchange depot and market carried these dried fish eggs so that they were always available (47, p. 265).

A story contemporaneous with that of the fish, although with little or none of its cultural or spiritual relevance, is the story of flax oil, which, along with cod liver oil, became one of the ancient healing oils.

THE HEALING OILS

Flax is one of the oldest fiber crops known to man. It was cultivated in ancient Egypt and India and areas bordering the Mediterranean. Throughout recorded history, flax has provided fiber for linen and both seeds and oil for medicine. The ancient Greek physicians used the seeds of flax for their laxative properties and the oil, along with cod liver oil, for a variety of ills.

Early European medical practitioners also noticed the health benefits of flax and cod liver oils, even though the specific chemical constituents involved were not known. Historically, as far back as the 17th century, flax oil and cod liver oil were mentioned as folk remedies. They were used at that time for chronic rheumatism (probably arthritis), scrofula (a form of tuberculosis), and lung diseases. In the early 20th century, cod liver oil was used for rickets, arthritis pain, as a daily tonic for children, and was recognized as a source of vitamins A and D (48, p. 102).

By this time, health scientists were learning about the different fatty acids in vegetable and animal fats and the fact that some of these fats were essential for human health. However, analytical chemistry had not yet evolved to the point where chemists had the tools to separate individual fatty acids from each other, identify them, or reveal the details of their very complex structures. This was the state of the art in the period after World War II, as scientists returned to their laboratories and their interests in peaceful pursuits.

JOHANNA BUDWIG: One such scientist was Johanna Budwig. In 1959, and later in her long career, Dr. Budwig, a German research biochemist and physician, talked and wrote about the value of a mixture of flax oil and cottage cheese in extending the life and ameliorating the suffering of patients with arthritis, cardiovascular disease, and cancer. It was her conviction that certain unsaturated fats in the flax oil, together with the proteins found in milk, were easily absorbed and of benefit to people suffering with these diseases (49).

In addition, Dr. Budwig argued that the process of hydrogenating oils to thicken them and to increase their shelf life destroyed important double bonds in the unsaturated fats that naturally occurred in the raw oils. Her work led her to believe that dietary deficiencies of the highly unsaturated fats found in flax oil were related to diabetes and to brain and nerve function. Over the years, Dr. Budwig accumulated evidence that these highly unsaturated fats (today recognized as the omega-3 family, alpha-linolenic acid and its metabolites) were also important in the prevention of heart attacks, liver and gallbladder disease, atherosclerosis, and tumorous growths.

Few doctors paid attention to Dr. Budwig's findings. In Germany, she was prosecuted by the medical establishment for malpractice for using flax oil to help patients with untreatable cancers. She was taken to court numerous times, and each time she was acquitted. In each instance, the courts exonerated her because case histories supported the benefits of her treatment methods (49, p. 43).

THE SLOW DISCOVERY OF THE IMPORTANCE OF OMEGA-3 EFAS

The first demonstration that one or more polyunsaturated fatty acids, such as alpha-linolenic or linoleic acids, were essential was made by the Drs. Burr in 1929 at the University of Minnesota Medical School (9; 16). At that time, "essentiality" meant promotion of growth and prevention of the eczema produced by a fat-free diet in laboratory mice. Although linoleic and alpha-linolenic acids had been produced in quantity by early German chemists decades before, analytic methods were still not available to separate them from mixtures or to identify individual fatty acids in small biological samples. Thus, EFA research proceeded slowly.

In general, the medical profession agreed that the Burr's research demonstrated that polyunsaturated fatty acids were essential – for mice, but not for humans. Despite lack of approval by the medical profession, the physicians in the Burr's medical school were not skeptical. They used lard, with great success, as a treatment for cases of intractable eczema in children that came to their clinic (9).

Over succeeding years, as work progressed and the individual fatty acids in biological samples were isolated and identified, it became obvious to the researchers that they were dealing with two separate families of EFAs. By the early 1960's, it was recognized that the two families differed from each other only by the position of the terminal double bond in their molecules. The development of a new numbering system to separate the two kinds of EFAs into the omega-6 and omega-3 families, as explained earlier in this chapter, greatly facilitated EFA research. However, despite voluminous scientific data on the health effects of EFA deficiency, the acceptance that linoleic and alpha-linolenic acid were essential for humans did not occur until the latter part of the 20th Century when EFAs were added to total parenteral (intravenous) nutrition preparations (TPN), thereby eliminating the deadly outcomes that plagued fat-free TNP (9).

Today we know a great deal about the EFAs, the differences between their two families, their requirements for good health, and the many effects of their deficiencies. Today we know that both flax oil and cod liver oil contain members of the omega-3 family of fatty acids and that this group of fatty acids was the most likely reason for the positive health effects observed by early medical practitioners. Today we know why fish is an important food and why its symbol has generated such reverence throughout recorded history.

Prevention of the modern nutritional diseases would take a major leap forward if the ancient wisdom that gave us the healing oils supplanted the physician's *materia medica*.

References

1.) Cantarow, A, Trumper M. *Clinical Biochemistry.* Philadelphia, PA: W. B. Saunders Co., 1962.

2.) http://www.cnpp.usda.gov/Publications/DietaryGuidelines/2010/DGAC/Report/D-3-FattyAcidsCholesterol.pdf/ Accessed Sept. 28, 2012.

3.) Ravnskov U. *Fats and Cholesterol are Good for You.* Sweden: GB Publishing, 2009.

4.) Keys A, et al. Human blood cholesterol and diet. *Science.* 1950; **112**: 79.

5.) Keys A. *Cholesterol.* XIX International Physiology Congress. 1953: 512.

6.) Faloon W. Inside the Foundation's Laboratory. *Life Extension Magazine.* October 1999: 7-9.

7.) Pauling L. *How to Live Longer and Feel Better.* New York, NY: W. H. Freeman and Co., 1986.

8.) http://lipidlibrary.aocs.org/ Accessed Sept. 28, 2012.

9.) Holman RT. The slow discovery of the importance of 3 essential fatty acids in human health. *The Journal of Nutrition.* 1998; **128**(2): 427S-433S.

10.) Pariza MW, et al. Conjugated linoleic acid and the control of cancer and obesity. *Toxicological Science (Supplement).* 1999; **52**: 107-110.

11.) http://www.webmd.com/ Accessed Sept. 28, 2012.

12.) Greenwell I. Lose the fat: Keep the muscle. *Life Extension Magazine.* February 2000: 96-100.

13.) Basu S. Conjugated linoleic acid induces lipid peroxidation in humans. *FEBS Letters.* 2000; **468**: 33.

14.) Fuller G. Animal and vegetable oils, fats, and waxes. *Riegel's Handbook of Industrial Chemistry, Eighth Edition,* Kent JA, editor. New York, NY: Van Nostrand Reinhold, 1983.

15.) Enig MG. *Know Your Fats.* Silver Spring, MD: Bethesda Press, 2000.

16.) Allport S. The Queen of Fats. Berkeley, CA: University of California Press, 2006.

17.) Rhoades RA, Tanner GA. *Medical Physiology.* Boston, MA: Little, Brown, 1995.

18.) Kuipers RS, et al. Saturated fats, carbohydrates and cardiovascular disease. *Netherland Journal of Medicine.* 2011;69(9). http://www.ncbi.nlm.nih.gov/pubmed/21978979/ Accessed Sept. 28, 2012.

19.) Siri-Tarion P, et al. Meta-analysis of prospective cohort studies evaluating the association of saturated fat with cardiovascular disease. *American Journal of Clinical Nutrition.* 2010; **91**(3):535-546.

20.) Ramsden CE, et al. Dietary fat quality and coronary heart disease: A unified theory based on evolutionary, historical, global, and modern perspectives. *Current Treatment Options in Cardiovascular Medicine.* 2009; **11**: 289-301.

21.) Hwang J. Diets with corn oil and/or low protein increase acute acetaminophen hepatotoxicity compared to diets with beef tallow. *Nutritional Research and Practice.* 2009; **3**(2): 95-101.

22.) Nanji AA, et al. Dietary saturated fatty acids: a novel treatment for alcoholic liver disease. *Gastroenterology.* 1995; **109**: 547-554.

23.) http://coconutoil.com/coconut_oil_21st_century/ (Enig MG. Address to the 36th Session of Asian Pacific Coconut Community. Coconut) Accessed Sept. 28, 2012.

24.) Ravnskov U. *The Cholesterol Myth: Exposing the Fallacy that Saturated Fat and Cholesterol Cause Heart Disease.* Washington, DC: NewTrends Publishing Inc., 2000.

25.) Colpo A. *The Great Cholesterol Con.* http://www.Lulu.com/ 2006.

26.) Taubes G. *Good Calories, Bad Calories.* New York, NY: Alfred A. Knopf, 2007.

27.) Crawford MA, Sinclair AJ. Nutritional influences in the evolution of the mammalian brain. In: *Lipids, Malnutrition and Developing Brain.* A Ciba Foundation Symposium. Amsterdam: Elsevier, 1972, p. 267ff.

28.) Hornstra G. Essential fatty acids in mothers and their neonates. *American Journal of Clinical Nutrition.* 2000; **7**(5): 1262-1269S.

29.) Williams G, Crawford MA. Comparison of the fatty acid component in structural lipids from dolphins, zebra, and giraffe: possible evolutionary implications. *Journal of Zoology, London.* 1987: **213**; 673-84.

30.) *Dietary Reference Intakes: The Essential Guide to Nutrient Requirements.* Washington, DC: The National Academies Press, 2006.

31.) http://health.gov/dietaryguidelines/ Accessed Sept. 28, 2012.

32.) http://www.nhlbi.nih.gov/guidelines/cholesterol/atglance.pdf/ Accessed Sept. 28, 2012.

33.) Press release 2003-13. May 28, 2003. Executive Office of the President; Office of Management and Budget. To Save Lives, OMB Urges Revising Dietary Guidelines: New information on reducing heart disease risk encourages.

34.) Pritikin N. *The Pritikin Program for Diet and Exercise.* New York, NY: Grosset and Dunlap, 1979.

35.) Ornish D. *Eat More, Weigh Less.* New York, NY: Harper Mass Market Paperbacks, 1997.

36.) http://www.fatfree.com/diets/ornish.html/ Accessed Sept. 28, 2012

37.) Ornish D. Reversing heart disease through diet, exercise and stress management. *Journal of the American Dietetic Association.* 1991; **91**: 162-165.

38.) Hibbeln JR, et al. Healthy intakes of n-3 and n-6 fatty acids: estimations considering world wide diversity. *American Journal of Clinical Nutrition.* 2006; **8**(3 supp.): 1483S-93S.

39.) Iso H, et al. Prospective study of fat and protein intake and risk of intraparenchymal hemorrhage in women. *Circulation.* 2000; **103**(6): 856-863.

40.) Willett WC. *Eat, Drink, and Be Healthy: the Harvard Medical School Guide to Healthy Eating.* New York, NY: Free Press, 2001.

41.) Eades MR, Eades MD. *Protein Power, Paperback Edition.* New York, NY: Bantam Books, 1999.

42.) Atkins RC. *Dr. Atkins' New Diet Revolution.* New York, NY: Avon Books, Inc. 1999.

43.) Cordain L, et al. Plant-animal subsistence ratios and macronutrient energy estimations in worldwide hunter-gatherer diets. *American Journal of Clinical Nutrition.* 2000; **71**: 682-692.

44.) http://www.proteinpower.com/drmike/metabolic-advantage/thermodynamics-and-the-metabolic-advantage/ Accessed Sept. 28, 2012.

45.) Horton H, et al. *Principles of Biochemistry, Second Ed.* Upper Saddle River, NJ: Prentice Hall, 1996.

46.) Reis LC, Hibbeln JR. Cultural symbolism of fish and the psychotropic properties of omega-3 fatty ac-ids. *Prostaglandins, Leukotrienes, Essential Fatty Acids*. 2006; **75**: 227.

47.) Price WA. *Nutrition and Physical Degeneration*. Los Angeles, CA: Keats Publishing, 1998.

48.) Sollmann T. *A Manual of Pharmacology, Eighth Edition*. Philadelphia, PA: W.B. Saunders Co, 1957.

49.) Budwig J. *Flax Oil as a True Aid against Arthritis, Heart Infarction, Cancer, and Other Diseases*. Vancouver, BC, Canada: Apple Publishing Company Ltd, 1994.

Chapter Nine

Essential Fatty Acids and Eicosanoids

The miracle of life is revealed in the study of its workings. Anon. - All works of Nature are miracles, and nothing makes them appear otherwise but our familiarity with them. **Samuel Butler (1).**

Essential Fatty Acids.

The essential fatty acids (EFAs) are true fats. They are exactly like their saturated and monounsaturated relatives described in Chapter Eight in that they are all straight chains of carbon atoms with a carboxyl carbon at one end. When provided in the diet, they are mixed with their fatty acid brethren to travel throughout the body and store with them as triglycerides. Like all true fats, they are little different in their metabolism from their fatty acid relatives; they can be broken down, two carbons at a time by β-oxidation, to provide energy when they are in excess of the body's need for them.

However, unlike their saturated and monounsaturated relatives, EFAs cannot be made *de novo* by human biochemistry. Thus, they are classed nutritionally as essential. Also unlike the true fat family, which is comprised of innumerable members, they occur only in long chains of from 18 to 24 carbon atoms with from 2 to 6 double bonds. The essential category has traditionally been considered to contain only three EFAs; linoleic acid (LA 18:2n6), alpha-linolenic acid (ALA 18:3n3), and arachidonic acid (AA 20:4n6). Recent scientific studies have concluded that eicosapentaenoic acid (EPA 20:5n3) and docosahexaenoic acid (DHA 22:6n3) are also essential. Although all other metabolites of this unique group (see Figure 9-1) may be provided by diet, their main source is biosynthesis.

Note that each box in Figure 9-1 includes a form of shorthand that shows how each product is modified at each step in the cascade. For example, the omega-6 fatty acid (LA) entering at the top right of the diagram is described by this shorthand as 18:2n6. The 18 means the fatty acid carbon chain contains 18 carbon atoms. The 2n6 means that the fatty acid chain contains 2 double bonds and that the terminal double bond occurs on the number 6 carbon counting from the omega carbon of the fatty acid molecule. The omega carbon is the carbon at the end opposite the carboxyl group of the fatty acid molecule. These shorthand symbols will be useful in following the discussion below of the changes that occur with each reaction.

The double bonds of EFAs, both in number and location, confer on them very special and important nutritional and biochemical roles. EFAs and their metabolites not only have their own functions in lipid metabolism and membrane biochemistry but they also provide the raw materials for synthesis of the vital hormone-like cellular messenger and regulator biochemicals grouped together under the label of eicosanoids.

NUTRITIONAL REQUIREMENTS FOR ESSENTIAL FATTY ACIDS

After the discovery in the early 1960s that essential fatty acids (EFAs) were not all of a single kind but rather were comprised of two types (2; 3), one with the terminal double bond between carbons 6 and 7 from the carbon at the end of the carbon chain (omega 6) and the other with the terminal double bond between carbons 3 and 4 from the end carbon (omega-3), the question of how much of each kind of EFA should be included in a healthful diet became a matter of nutritional concern.

During the same period, analyses of food oils provided data showing that omega-6 EFAs were primarily of plant origin, whereas oils/fats from fish and other animals were the major source for omega-3 EFAs. These data made it apparent that the typical American diet (large consumption of vegetable seed oils and low consumption of fish and animal fats) provided much more omega-6 than omega-3 EFAs. This finding that the American diet was more than ample in omega-6 EFAs combined with considerable evidence that the proinflammatory actions of the omega-6 family were inhibited or modified by omega-3 compounds led to greater interest in nutritional requirements for omega-3 EFAs.

A review of the early literature on omega-3 fatty acid intake indicated that 4 to 8 grams of omega-3 fatty acids a day, with a minimum of 1 gram of eicosapentaenoic acid (EPA) plus docosahexaenoic acid (DHA), was considered adequate and well within safe limits (4). One report recommended that 1 gram of EPA plus DHA and 2 grams of the parent ALA be taken each day, with larger daily amounts of ALA if the diet contained no fish or fish oil because it takes the body about 10 grams of ALA to make 1 gram of EPA (5). Research showing that conversion of ALA (18:3n3) to DHA (22:6n3) is severely restricted in humans supported a daily intake of 1.25 grams EPA plus DHA (6).

The fact that the ratio of omega-6 to omega-3 EFAs is at least as important as their totals in the diet has long been assumed. The scientific literature offers several recommendations for the proper omega-6 to omega-3 ratio. One is that it should be about 5:1 (7). Other researchers suggest a ratio ranging from 1:1 to 4:1 (8; 9; 10), and still others advise a maximum ratio of 3:1 (6).

The important point here is that all available scientific evidence indicates that, whatever the ratio, it should be considerably less than the 16:1 to 20:1 ratio currently estimated to be in the American diet (10). Taking together all of the data on recommended ratios, a reasonable estimate of the requirement for omega-3 fatty acids was 2 grams of ALA plus 1 gram of EPA and DHA combined, for a daily total of 3 grams of the omega-3 family.

A striking example of an association between the modern nutritional diseases and an imbalance of the EFAs was reported by Yam (11). Israel was considered to have the highest incidence in the world of cardiovascular diseases, hypertension, adult-onset diabetes, obesity, and cancer. It also had one of the highest dietary omega-6 fatty acid intakes in the world, roughly 8 to 12 percent higher than in America or Europe. In 1984, analyses of fat tissues from a small sample of Israelis found ranges of 20.3 to 32.3 percent of omega-6 LA and 1.0 to 1.8 percent of omega-3 ALA in body fat. These data translate to an omega-6 to omega-3 ratio of roughly 20-to-1. As a matter of interest, the range of *trans* fats in the tissue samples from Israelis was 1.9 to 6.6 percent, which is similar to that found in the United States and Britain (7).

A recent study by Hibbeln et al. of the worldwide diversity of omega-6 and omega-3 intakes and their relationship to attributable burden of chronic diseases (12) brings significant insight and refinement to estimation of the nutritional requirements for both omega-6 and omega-3 families. It shows that not only is the ratio important but also is the absolute value of dietary LA (linoleic acid).

For example, countries with very low omega-6/omega-3 ratios plus very low intakes of LA (Greenland, Iceland, Philippines) had the lowest burdens of chronic diseases (12). The United States was found to have the highest average intake of LA of all countries; approximately 9 grams of LA per day. In addition, ALA intake was one gram per day, which amounts to a LA/ALA ratio of about 9:1. Excellent counsel for people interested in healthful nutrition is contained in a conclusion of the study.

> … a healthy dietary allowance for n-3 LCFAs [long chain fatty acids] for current US diets was estimated at 3.5 g/d [grams/day] for a 2000 kcal diet. This allowance for n-3 LCFAs can likely be reduced to one-tenth that amount by consuming fewer n-6 [omega-6] fats (12).

THE ESSENTIAL FATTY ACID CASCADE

Figure 9-1 is a simplified diagram of the biochemical reactions that convert the two parent essential fatty acids, alpha-linolenic acid (omega-3 ALA) and linoleic acid (omega-6 LA), through a succession of steps to their respective eicosanoid end-products The eicosanoid end-products are shown in bold-outlined boxes. Prostaglandins PGs), prostacyclins, leukotrienes (LTs) and thromboxanes (TXs) are names of major eicosanoids. The first eicosanoids discovered were found in prostate tissues, which accounts for the name prostaglandin.

The two parent essential fatty acids, ALA and LA, and the products formed from them in each biochemical reaction in the cascade are shown in boxes drawn with solid lines. The enzymes responsible for each reaction are shown in dotted-line boxes.

FIGURE 9-1
METABOLISM OF THE ESSENTIAL FATTY ACIDS

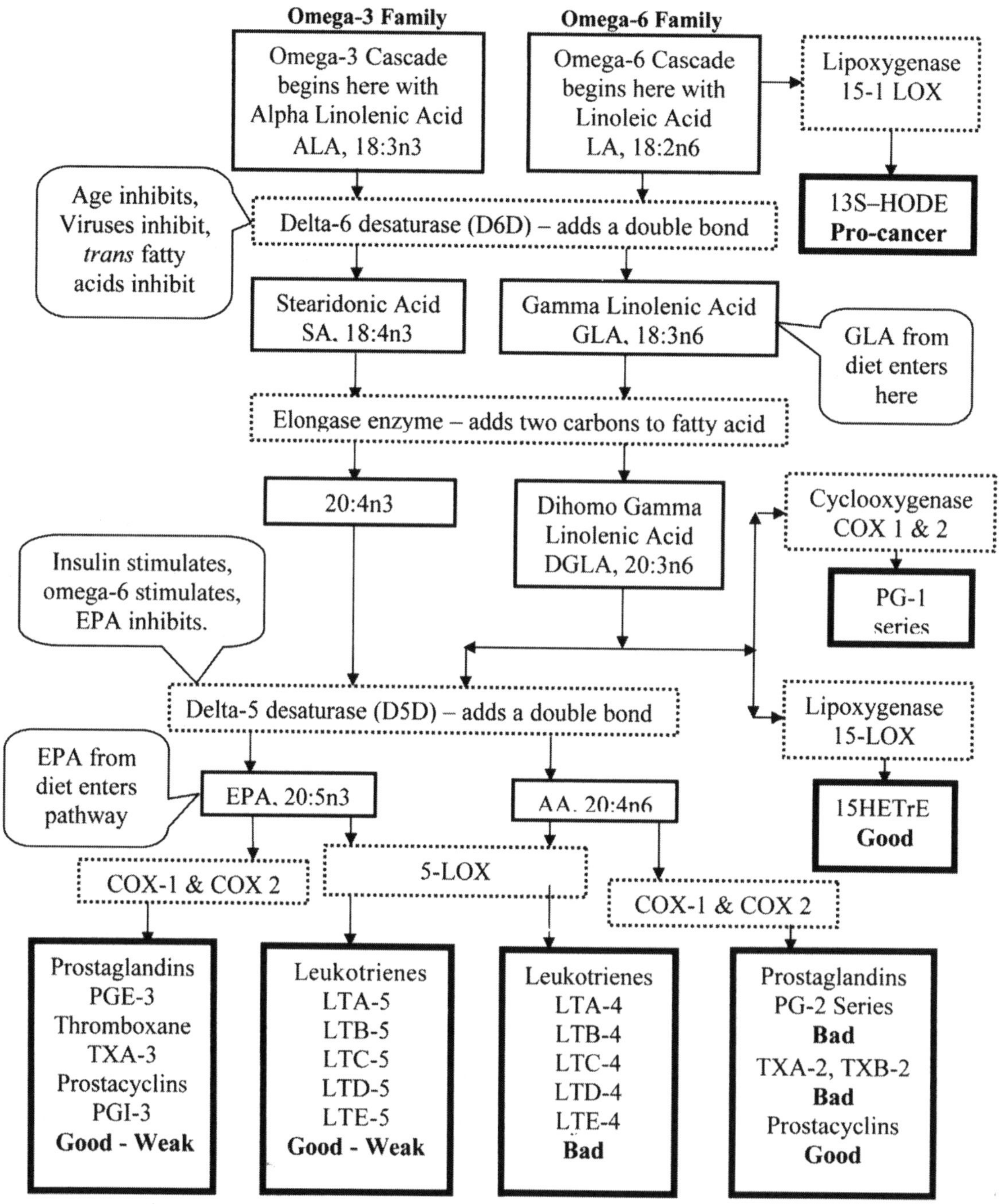

Omega-3 Family

Omega-3 Cascade begins here with Alpha Linolenic Acid ALA, 18:3n3

Omega-6 Family

Omega-6 Cascade begins here with Linoleic Acid LA, 18:2n6

Lipoxygenase 15-1 LOX

13S–HODE **Pro-cancer**

Age inhibits, Viruses inhibit, *trans* fatty acids inhibit

Delta-6 desaturase (D6D) – adds a double bond

Stearidonic Acid SA, 18:4n3

Gamma Linolenic Acid GLA, 18:3n6

GLA from diet enters here

Elongase enzyme – adds two carbons to fatty acid

20:4n3

Dihomo Gamma Linolenic Acid DGLA, 20:3n6

Cyclooxygenase COX 1 & 2

PG-1 series

Insulin stimulates, omega-6 stimulates, EPA inhibits.

Delta-5 desaturase (D5D) – adds a double bond

Lipoxygenase 15-LOX

EPA from diet enters pathway

EPA, 20:5n3

AA, 20:4n6

15HETrE **Good**

COX-1 & COX 2

5-LOX

COX-1 & COX 2

Prostaglandins PGE-3 Thromboxane TXA-3 Prostacyclins PGI-3 **Good - Weak**

Leukotrienes LTA-5 LTB-5 LTC-5 LTD-5 LTE-5 **Good - Weak**

Leukotrienes LTA-4 LTB-4 LTC-4 LTD-4 LTE-4 **Bad**

Prostaglandins PG-2 Series **Bad** TXA-2, TXB-2 **Bad** Prostacyclins **Good**

In studying Figure 9-1, keep in mind that at each step the same enzyme system is utilized by both the omega-3 and the omega-6 families in their metabolism. As a result, the omega-3 and omega-6 fatty acids must compete with each other to serve as substrates for each enzyme. Recall from Chapter Four on how enzymes work that when two substrates compete for the same enzyme, there are two possible outcomes: If one of the substrates is preferred by the enzyme, it will be metabolized preferentially. But, if the preferred substrate is not present in sufficient amounts, the enzyme will metabolize the substrate that is present in greater quantity. These facts help explain why the ratio of omega-6 to omega-3 in the diet is of critical importance to the balance of the eicosanoids that are produced from them.

Beginning at the top of Figure 9-1, follow the omega-3 and the omega-6 fatty acids downward. The first biochemical reaction that both undergo is catalyzed by the same enzyme, delta-6 desaturase (note that most enzymes have names that end in -ase). Delta-6 desaturase (D6D) adds a double bond to the 18-carbon fatty acid by converting a single bond to a double bond. This forms stearidonic acid (SA 18:4n3) in the omega-3 cascade and gamma linolenic acid (GLA 18:3n6) in the omega-6 cascade. However, note that LA has another pathway available to it – the 15-LOX-1 enzyme. The significance of 15-LOX-1 in cancer formation is discussed below in the eicosanoid section.

It is important to note here that there is a report in the scientific literature that dietary saturated fatty acids inhibit D6D and, thus, disrupt a healthful eicosanoid balance by interfering with the flow of LA and ALA to GLA and SA, respectively. This finding was published as an hypothesis over thirty years ago (13), and despite a lack of scientific corroboration since that time, the claim that saturated fatty acids inhibit D6D is reported as fact in some well-respected diet books. However, recent biochemical studies using radioisotopes demonstrated that diets high in saturated fatty acids do not *inhibit* but greatly *enhance* conversion of ALA to EPA and DHA (14).

As will be discussed later in the section on eicosanoids, there are a number of factors that can inhibit D6D. Inhibition of D6D has very important consequences. For example, Figure 9-1 shows that inhibition would prevent both ALA and LA from being metabolized and going further down their cascades. As a consequence, ALA would remain unchanged and LA would be directed to the 15-1 LOX pro-cancer pathway.

The next step in the cascade after the D6D enzyme is performed by an elongase enzyme, which adds two carbons to the 18-carbon fatty acid to make a 20-carbon compound. The compound formed in the omega-3 cascade is 20:4n3 (unnamed); the corresponding omega-6 compound is dihomo gamma linolenic acid (DGLA 20:3n6). At this point, on the omega-6 side, the cascade branches. One branch sends DGLA, via cyclooxygenase (COX) or lipoxygenase (LOX) enzymes, to a group of important eicosanoids, including the PG-1 series of prostaglandins. The other branch sends DGLA to arachidonic acid (AA 20:4n6) via the delta-5 desaturase (D5D) enzyme, which adds another double bond to DGLA. This branch is of great significance because it determines whether the result will be anti-inflammatory or proinflammatory.

As shown on Figure 9-1, AA leads to two groups of eicosanoids, PG-2 series of prostaglandins via the COX enzymes and the LT-4 series of leukotrienes via the LOX enzyme. On the omega-3 side of Figure 9-1, the product from the elongase enzyme goes via D5D enzyme, where one double bond is added, to form eicosapentaenoic acid (EPA 20:5n3), a fatty acid with 20 carbons. EPA is converted to PG-3 series prostaglandins via the COX enzymes and to the LT-5 series leukotrienes via the same lipoxygenase enzyme that produces the LT-4 leukotrienes.

EPA IS ALSO A PRECURSOR OF DHA

In addition to being a precursor of PG-3 and LT-4 eicosanoids, EPA is also a precursor of docosahexaenoic acid (DHA 22:6n3), an important member of the omega-3 family that is a major component of brain and neural tissue. DHA is not shown in the omega-3 cascade of Figure 9-1 because it is formed from EPA, all or in part, by a side reaction from the cascade, referred to by some researchers as Sprecher's Shunt (15).

In the proposed shunt reaction (see Figure 9-2), EPA is elongated to 22 carbon docosapentaenoic acid (DPA 22:6n3), which in turn enters Sprecher's Shunt. In the shunt, DPA is further elongated to compound 24:5n3 and desaturated by D6D to yield compound 24:6n3. The resulting 24-carbon product is the longest carbon chain fatty acid that has thus far been identified in the omega-3 series. The 24-carbon compound is then shortened to DHA via the removal of a 2-carbon unit by β-oxidation. Figure 9-2 shows that DHA can be retro-converted to EPA.

Because DHA is biosynthesized by a side reaction from the cascade, one may question why Nature would devise an elaborate shunt system to create it. Is it because the conversion of EPA to DHA is not adequate to supply the body's needs for DHA? A thoughtful observation by Heiby stating that Nature does not create worthless entities merits consideration (16, p. 188).

The logical answer can be found in the tremendous importance of DHA for construction and function of brain, eyes and other nervous system structures and tissues. This need is probably much greater than could be supplied by EPA from the cascade. The shunt would provide a storage mechanism for DHA (15). An ample quantity of DHA precursor, stored in the shunt's 24-carbon pool, would supply DHA as needed without disrupting the pathway to the eicosanoids by draining off EPA.

FIGURE 9-2
DOCOSAHEXAENOIC ACID BIOSYNTHESIS

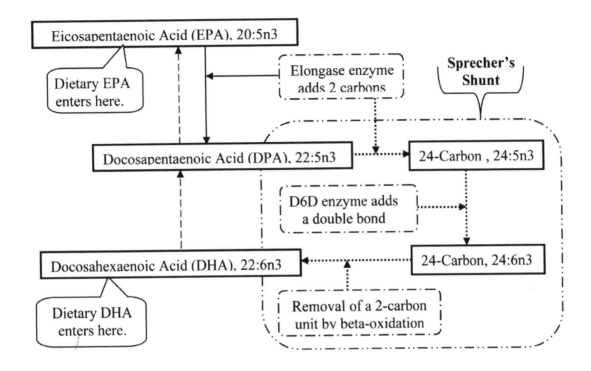

Eicosanoids

The scientific history of the eicosanoids is short; they were essentially unknown and unstudied until about 1980. Their very brief lives, low concentrations in living tissues, and complex chemical structures make them difficult to study and to understand. An unfortunate result has been that eicosanoids and their great value in understanding and preventing chronic diseases still remain a mystery to most nutritionists and medical professionals

The authors recognize that the biochemistry that follows here is not easy to understand. However, biochemistry holds enormously valuable lessons because it is a hard science. It draws a line between fact and fiction. It eliminates confusion as to the true impacts of dietary sugar, vegetable oils, and the essential fatty acids on human health. Importantly, this biochemistry illuminates the path to dependable, scientifically-based prevention of the chronic inflammatory diseases that plague this nation.

WHAT ARE EICOSANOIDS?

The word eicosanoid comes from the Greek word for number 20 (*eicosa*) because most of the eicosanoids are derived from 20-carbon essential fatty acids. Eicosanoids are short lived, biologically active messenger chemicals that are biosynthesized in all mammalian cells except red blood cells (erythrocytes). Eicosanoids are very potent and cause physiological effects at minimal levels. They consist of two major groups, omega 6 and 3.

The omega-6 group is mostly inflammatory and the omega-3 group is anti-inflammatory. Eicosanoids from these two groups tug against one-another to form a net signal, the strength of which depends on their relative concentrations in a given cell or tissue. Common practice has been to label these as "bad" and "good" eicosanoids despite the fact that both are necessary components of the eicosanoid control system.

TWO VITAL TASKS ARE PERFORMED BY EICOSANOIDS: One task is to respond to injuries and infections and to manage the repair and healing processes. The other task is to constantly monitor and adjust internal functions to maintain normal bodily stability (homeostasis). The former task is brought into play in emergency situations; the second is an indispensable ongoing maintenance function.

A good example of emergency response to an injury is a cut finger. The pain, clotting, and healing that automatically occur with such an injury do not happen by magic or by chance. Eicosanoids are released in the proper sequence to cause immediate pain, followed by inflammation (redness, warmth, and swelling). Blood clotting soon stops the bleeding. Then, at the appropriate time, inflammation ends, dead cells and other debris are removed from the wound, and healing is initiated and completed.

Eicosanoids also maintain physiological stability by controlling a large number of body functions. Some examples are regulation of blood pressure, gastric mucosal secretion, and gestation and parturition in pregnancy. Eicosanoid imbalance is implicated in a number of chronic inflammatory diseases, including cardiovascular diseases (10).

THE EICOSANOID CONTROL SYSTEM

Most people are unaware of the automatic control systems that continually work to keep their bodies functioning smoothly. Body temperature remains constant through summers and winters, eyes automatically adjust to light intensity, and breathing rates increase or slow down depending on physical activity. These systems work so well that we tend to believe that our bodies will always operate properly without any effort on our part. The eicosanoid control system however, is critically affected by diet and cannot function properly on the modern American diet.

During good health, the anti-inflammatory (good) eicosanoids offset and balance the proinflammatory (bad) eicosanoids. However, the current American diet distorts this natural state of balance so that the bad eicosanoids outnumber the good eicosanoids. Such distortion occurs when high insulin levels caused by excess dietary sugar and starch and/or high omega-6 to omega-3 ratios, instruct the body to produce a surplus of bad eicosanoids. The result is low level inflammation. When continued over a long period of time, the condition becomes chronic inflammation, and the consequences are the chronic diseases (17) at issue in this book.

The eicosanoid control system can be likened to the thermostat in your home heating system. When you move the set point on the thermostat in the direction of a higher temperature, the furnace turns on and the house warms up. The eicosanoid system is similar in that the modern American diet moves the eicosanoid set point toward increased systemic inflammation. What happens biochemically is that the American diet moves the eicosanoid set point upward by stimulating the delta-5 desaturase enzyme. This increases the biosynthesis of proinflammatory eicosanoids. Such long term inflammation is recognized as a central feature in the pathogenesis of many inflammatory diseases that include obesity, heart disease, stroke, cancer, asthma, autoimmune diseases, Alzheimer's disease, and type-2 diabetes.

The EFAs and their Eicosanoids

Because of the complexity of the biochemistry of the eicosanoids, brief summaries entitled "Biochemical Lessons" will appear periodically in the balance of this chapter to help highlight the significance of previous paragraphs.

In review, Figure 9-1 shows the sequence of biochemical reactions that transform essential fatty acids into their eicosanoid end products. The two dietary essential fatty acids, alpha-linolenic acid (ALA 18:3n3) and linoleic acid (LA 18:2n6), shown at the top of the diagram, are the parent compounds, or starting materials, for the omega-3 and the omega-6 eicosanoid families, respectively. As the metabolites of these parent compounds move downward in the diagram, they are converted by a series of enzymatic biochemical reactions that ultimately transform them into eicosanoid end products (eicosanoids are shown in bold-outlined boxes). The biochemical reactions involved take place at the cellular level and, generally speaking, the ratios of the two fatty acid families in the diet determine their ratios at the cellular level (18).

LINOLEIC ACID IS A CAUSE OF CANCER

Studies reviewed earlier show that people who regularly consume vegetable fats and oils, which contain large amounts of omega-6 fatty acids, have an increased risk of cancer. It is also known that cancer rates increase in populations when their intakes of vegetable fats and oils increase (18).

There are several biochemical routes to cancer that involve the omega-6 fatty acids. One such route to cancer is illustrated at the top right of Figure 9-1. Other routes to cancer are covered later. Note here that excess LA, prior to entering the omega-6 cascade will be metabolized by 15-LOX-1 enzyme to the mitogen 13S-HODE (13S-hydroxyoctadecadienoic acid). A mitogen is a substance that encourages excessive cell division, a cause of cancer. In animal and human studies, 13S-HODE has been associated with increased rates of tumor development. Such tumors reported in humans include cancers of the breast, prostate, liver, and colon (19; 20; 21).

Additional research, has shown that dietary supplementation with the omega-3 eicosapentaenoic (EPA), is associated with a significant decline in these tumor rates. The biochemical reason for this is that EPA strongly competes for the 15-LOX-1 enzyme (see top right of Figure 9-1) and prevents LA from being converted to the carcinogenic mitogen, 13S-HODE. At the same time, the biochemical product of EPA's reaction with 15-LOX-1 is 15S-HEPE (15S-hydroxyeicosapentaenoic acid), a compound shown to have antitumorigenic properties (19; 21; 22). These data make clear that EPA has a twofold approach to cancer prevention: EPA keeps the 15-LOX-1 enzyme busy and prevents it from converting LA to a carcinogenic mitogen; at the same time, EPA is converted by the 15-LOX-1 enzyme to an anticancer compound.

EXCESS DIETARY LA IS A MAJOR PROBLEM: Good health requires an omega-6 to omega-3 ratio of roughly one to one (10). The current ratio of about ten to one, and perhaps higher, is primarily due to large increases in the consumption of vegetable fats and oils over the past century. Prior to 1900, the production and dietary use of fats and oils derived from vegetable seeds was essentially zero. The traditional fats and oils used at that time were lard, tallow, butter, olive oil, and coconut oil. Total dietary intake of LA was very low, perhaps two percent of total calories (18; 23).

The large increase in LA use in today's diet, among other adverse health effects, has reduced relative human tissue concentrations of EPA and DHA (18). It is important to note that although the reported national average daily intake of LA is about 9 percent of total calories, or about 20 grams per day, the whole country does not eat the same foods. Therefore, some individuals ingest more LA than others. An educated guess is that actual LA consumption probably varies roughly from 2 to 20 percent of daily calories. This suggests that the adverse health impact of LA ranges from no effect to serious illness, depending on each individual's LA dose. The fraction of the population with the very high LA intakes will suffer the highest risk of cancer and other inflammatory diseases.

Excess LA in the diet monopolizes D6D, which slows or stops the conversion of ALA to its most important metabolite EPA. Further, as shown below, D6D is considered an unreliable enzyme that malfunctions in some people. For these reasons, supplemental intake of ALA should not be depended upon to supply adequate amounts of longer chain omega-3 EFAs such as EPA.

BIOCHEMICAL LESSON: Excess LA and the lack of EPA in the American diet, from the biochemical point of view, is a demonstrated cause of several cancers. Aim for a dietary omega-6 to omega-3 ratio of one to one. Do this by limiting dietary intake of vegetable fats and oils, but recognize that this will be difficult because the seed oils (vegetable fats and oils) are almost universally used in restaurants, processed foods, deep frying, candies, and many bakery products. Because LA use in foods is not clearly known or controlled, surplus LA in the average diet probably cannot be reliably reduced to safe levels. However, 4 grams (4 teaspoons) a day of cod liver or fish oil will counter excess LA and reduce the risk of the inflammatory diseases, including cancer (18).

Many people also believe that dietary omega-6 arachidonic acid (AA) is a health problem and try to avoid AA-containing foods such as eggs and red meat. Such avoidance is not warranted in light of the data on the dietary intake of essential fatty acids presented by Hibbeln (18). Dietary AA consumption has not changed significantly over the years and the amount of AA in food is relatively small. However, consumption of LA has increased tremendously; surplus dietary LA is the problem. The excess AA that is causing health problems is not from the diet but rather derived from the bioconversion of surplus LA via the omega-6 cascade.

THE DELTA-6 DESATURASE ENZYME (D6D)

Note in Figure 9-1 that the first biochemical reaction in the omega-6 cascade is catalyzed by the D6D enzyme. This enzyme transforms LA (18:2n6) to GLA (gamma linolenic acid 18:3n6) by inserting a double bond in the omega-9 position of LA. This chemical transformation is called desaturation. GLA occurs naturally in organ meats and some plant seeds. It is a natural component of human milk; the D6D enzyme is not active in infants younger than about six months of age. GLA is essential for good health because it is the precursor of DGLA (dihomo gamma linolenic acid 20:3n6) and the anti-inflammatory metabolites derived from DGLA further down in the omega-6 cascade. In the omega-3 chain, the D6D enzyme desaturates ALA (alpha linolenic acid 18:3n3) and converts it to SA (stearidonic acid 18:4n3).

As mentioned earlier, LA is known to increase the risk of cancer. Interestingly, GLA, a direct metabolite of LA, when added to the diet in the form of a supplement causes no such cancer risk. Studies in laboratory animals show that GLA inhibits tumor cell growth in breast, pancreatic, and bladder cancer models. In a rat glioma (brain cancer), GLA inhibited tumor growth in a dose dependent manner (19). Other studies show that elongation products of GLA and DGLA suppress chronic inflammation and inhibit small cell proliferation associated with the formation of atherosclerotic plaque (24).

EPA CONVERSION TO DHA BY D6D: Until recently, the literature has indicated that LA and ALA alone competed with one another for a finite amount of D6D enzyme space. However, it is now known that human biochemistry requires the same D6D enzyme to desaturate two more biochemicals; 24:4n-6 in the omega-6 family and 24:5n-3 in the omega-3 family (25). Little known about them except that 24:4n-6 is formed from AA. and 24;5n-3 is an intermediate in the pathway that converts EPA to DHA (Figure 9-2).

DHA is required for the construction and maintenance of brains, eyes and nerves. DHA deficiency in pregnant women results in post partum depression. Such deficiency in pregnant women results in infants with smaller brains. Some will grow up with attention deficit hyperactivity disorder (26). Adults with DHA deficiency are at high risk for neurodegenerative diseases such as Alzheimer's, Parkinson's, and macular degeneration. From a practical point of view, populations at risk due to these problems are comprised of individuals who do not supplement their diets with fish oil or other sources of DHA.

DHA is not in the omega-3 cascade, but rather produced by a side reaction from EPA, as shown above in Figure 9-2. The omega-3 cascade, under current dietary conditions of an LA to ALA ratio of ten or more to one cannot produce a meaningful amount of EPA or DHA via Sprecher's shunt because the D6D enzyme is monopolized by an overload of LA. And, as indicated in the next section, dietary supplementation with EPA alone cannot produce the amount of DHA required for good health in an individual with a nonfunctional D6D enzyme.

D6D MALFUNCTION: There is evidence that the D6D enzyme does not always function properly. Some individuals are born with a genetically nonfunctional D6D and cannot convert LA to GLA. In other individuals, a malfunctioning D6D may be caused by dietary *trans* fats, advancing age, excess alcohol use, and diets that lack adequate vitamins and minerals. D6D malfunctions have been associated with diabetes, alcoholism, atopic dermatitis, premenstrual syndrome, rheumatoid arthritis, cardiovascular disease, cancer, poor pituitary or thyroid functions, irritable bowel syndrome, and the immune system disorder Sjogren's syndrome (24; 27). It would appear that a significant fraction of the general population is affected by malfunctioning D6D enzymes.

Four biochemicals must compete for a limited amount of D6D space. These are, LA, ALA, and the two biochemicals, 24:4n-6, and 24:5n-3, which are formed in the Sprecher's shunt (Figure 9-2). When D6D is malfunctioning or monopolized by LA, EPA cannot be converted to DHA. Thus, the diseases that have been attributed to a deficiency of GLA should be reconsidered in the light of the potential impact of a DHA deficiency.

In light of today's excessive intake of LA, it is difficult to be certain if D6D malfunctions are due to failure of the enzyme or to the monopolization of the enzyme by excess dietary levels of LA. In view of this LA problem, a logical way to measure the viability of the D6D enzyme would be to analyze both red cells and plasma for DGLA. Little or no DGLA would indicate poor D6D activity.

From the biochemical point of view, a malfunctioning D6D enzyme can result in several undesirable outcomes. One, already mentioned, is that dietary LA is unable to transit the malfunctioning D6D enzyme and is diverted to the 15-1 LOX enzyme where it is converted to the pro-cancer 13-S HODE. A second problematic result is that malfunctioning D6D obstructs conversion of LA to GLA and prevents the biosynthesis of DGLA, the PG-1 series prostaglandins, and 15 HETrE. All of these are strongly anti-inflammatory and very important for the maintenance of good health. Additionally, if D6D does not function for any reason, the conversion of EPA to DHA stops. When this happens, EPA can only be transformed as far as 24:5n-3, as shown in Figure 9-2. The fate of 24:5n-3 is not known at this time, but it has been suggested that it is a storage reservoir for the precursor of DHA (10; 15). Dietary DHA can be retroconverted to EPA.

BIOCHEMICAL LESSON: D6D malfunction occurs in many individuals due to genetic makeup, increasing age, and other reasons mentioned above. A faulty D6D should be bypassed by taking a GLA supplement. This restores normal flow in the omega-6 cascade. Such GLA supplements have been used for years. They are found in borage, evening primrose and blackcurrant oils. Borage oil seems to be the most available (24).

The faulty D6D should also be bypassed by taking a DHA supplement. From a practical point of view, the failure of D6D to bioconvert ALA to EPA via the omega-3 pathway is not serious because even under ideal circumstances, such conversion is not sufficient to meet current nutritional needs. The scientific literature recommends that both EPA and DHA be considered essential fatty acids (10; 15). Hence, daily dietary supplementation with fish oil to provide the essential fatty acids, EPA and DHA, are required for good health (18). Two to four teaspoons of fish oil daily should ensure ample EPA and DHA intake. If faulty D6D is suspected, pure DHA should be taken in addition to fish oil (28).

D6D MALFUNCTION: SPECULATION

In 1991, Voss reported that the metabolic pathway from EPA to DHA was dependent on the D6D enzyme, not D4D as had been thought (29). However, until recently, the biochemical literature, insofar as D6D was concerned, continued to assume that D6D acted only upon ALA and LA, and that EPA was converted to DHA by the D4D enzyme, which by the way does not exist in humans. The result has been that any diseases that were associated with D6D malfunction were considered to be the result only of a deficiency of eicosanoids derived from LA via GLA and DGLA. The possibility that D6D was also required to convert EPA to DHA appears to have been largely ignored.

The general view was that eicosanoids derived from DGLA were important because they supported the immune system and helped prevent atherosclerosis, heart disease, and respiratory allergies. D6D malfunctions and the resulting lack of DGLA derived eicosanoids were also associated in some way with diabetes, rheumatoid arthritis, cancer, cardiovascular disease, and others. However, now that it is known that D6D malfunctions also affect DHA biosynthesis, the probability that some or all of these health problems involve DHA deficiencies must be considered.

The strong possibility exists that excess dietary LA is, and most likely has been for the last 50 years, monopolizing the D6D enzyme. This means that LA should now be considered as possibly interfering with D6D functions. Are the DHA deficiencies that contribute to the growing numbers of cognitive, retinal, and neural diseases related to excess dietary LA monopolizing D6D? Are differences in the causes of D6D inactivity the reason why some people acquire chronic inflammatory diseases and others do not? How much does dietary LA contribute to these particular health problems? Would control of dietary LA reduce the incidence of these diseases?

The bottom line is that current biochemistry indicates that LA is a major underlying cause of the current epidemics of chronic inflammatory diseases. Yet it continues to be freely sold as an unlabeled component of vegetable fats and oils and an unlabeled component of many processed foods. Decisions or lack of same have consequences.

DGLA AND ITS METABOLITES

GLA is elongated by an enzyme that adds two carbons to the 18-carbon GLA (18:3n6) to form DGLA (20:3n6), a 20-carbon fatty acid with three double bonds. Note in Figure 9-1 that at this point in the omega-6 cascade the DGLA flow splits into two branches. The branch to the right leads to cyclooxygenase-1 (COX-1), cyclooxygenase-2 (COX-2), and 15 lipoxygenase (15-LOX) enzymes. The COX-1 and COX-2 convert DGLA to PGE-1, a highly desirable eicosanoid that inhibits the inflammatory 5-lipoxygenase (5-LOX) metabolites derived from arachidonic acid (AA). PGE-1 is also reported to reduce vascular smooth muscle cell proliferation, a mark of the atherogenic process. Concurrently, 15-LOX converts DGLA to 15HETrE (15-(S)-hydroxy-8,11,13-eicosatrienoic acid), another highly desirable eicosanoid that inhibits harmful, pro-inflammatory leukotrienes derived from AA (24). The branch to the left in the omega-6 pathway sends DGLA via the delta-5 desaturase (D5D) enzyme to AA and its inflammatory metabolites.

THE DELTA-5 DESATURASE ENZYME

The D5D enzyme adds one double bond and converts the DGLA (20:3n6) to AA (20:4n6). AA is the substrate (or feed) for the COX-1, COX-2, and the 5-LOX enzymes that produce many harmful eicosanoids.

The position of the D5D enzyme in the flow of the omega-6 cascade is of vital importance because it acts as a valve that directs DGLA either toward anti-inflammatory eicosanoids or proinflammatory eicosanoids. When this valve is open (the enzyme is stimulated), DGLA is transformed to AA, the precursor of a large number of proinflammatory eicosanoids. At the same time, DGLA is diverted away from the production of anti-inflammatory eicosanoids PGE-1 and HETrE. When the valve is closed very little DGLA is converted to proinflammatory AA but rather is directed toward the production of the good anti-inflammatory eicosanoids, PGE-1 and HETrE.

The D5D enzyme is opened (stimulated) by two dietary factors. One stimulating factor is high blood insulin levels caused by dietary sugar and starch (high glycemic carbohydrates). The other stimulating factor is high omega-6 to omega-3 ratios in the circulating blood, also caused by diet. Such stimulation of D5D over a period of years by sugar, starch, and/or high omega-6 to omega-3 ratios is a major underlying cause of chronic inflammation and the diseases discussed in this book. The D5D enzyme is closed (inhibited) by a healthful diet, namely one low in high glycemic carbohydrates, low in LA, and adequate in EPA.

When D5D is not stimulated by diet but is inhibited by EPA, surplus DGLA is not converted to AA and its harmful metabolites. Instead, it accumulates in the body tissues and increases the DGLA to AA ratio in these tissues. This stored DGLA competes with AA for access to the 5-LOX enzyme and reduces the amount of AA that can be converted to inflammatory leukotrienes (24; 30). Accordingly, EPA (and DHA) should be considered necessary dietary supplements (10; 15).

BIOCHEMICAL LESSON: The significant point is that good health depends on regulating the D5D enzyme. High insulin levels due to dietary sugar and starch and high dietary omega-6 to omega-3 ratios, stimulate the D5D enzyme, and move the biochemical set point away from normal and toward inflammation. On the other hand, control of dietary sugar and starch, reduction of LA in the diet, and a daily supplement of fish oil to provide EPA will inhibit the D5D enzyme so that the appropriate amounts of both proinflammatory and anti-inflammatory eicosanoids are produced. Keep in mind that all of the eicosanoids, both the so-called good and bad, are important. The body is designed to use eicosanoids with opposing effects to control vital functions. In a state of optimum health, the good and the bad eicosanoids balance one another.

THE CYCLOOXYGENASE ENZYMES

The cyclooxygenase enzymes occur in two isoforms, COX-1 and COX-2. They are similar in many, but not all respects. Each has two catalytic sites. The first active site converts AA to the prostaglandin PGG-2. The second active site in these enzymes changes the PGG-2 to PGH-2. The product, PGH-2, is further processed by specific isomerases that generate three eicosanoid groups; prostaglandins, thromboxanes, and prostacyclins. Note that the series numbers on the eicosanoids in boxes at the bottom of Figure 9-1, such as the 2 in PGE-2 in the omega-6 cascade, indicate the number of double bonds in that particular eicosanoid (31).

COX-1 is the smaller of the two enzymes in both size and eicosanoid production capacity. COX-1 can process only AA. It exists primarily in what is called the constitutive form. This means COX-1 is constantly present and active in most tissues. COX-1 has been called the housekeeping enzyme because it does its work by continually releasing small amounts of eicosanoids as required to regulate normal cell activity (32).

The prostacyclins biosynthesized by COX-1 are generally protective. For example, they are antithrombotic (prevent clotting) when released in the endothelium, the layer of cells that line the inside of blood vessels, the heart, and some other closed cavities. They are cytoprotective when released by the gastric mucosa, the thin lining of the stomach that secretes a protective slimy substance called mucin.

COX-2 exists primarily in inducible form. This means that COX-2 is not detectable in most healthy, resting cells. COX-2 is induced and made active by increased levels of its substrate, AA, and by inflammatory stimuli, such as cytokines and trauma. Cytokines are a group of biochemicals that trigger inflammation by recruiting other eicosanoids and immune cells to fight infectious organisms and foreign bodies including cancer cells. COX-2 can process a wider range of fatty acids than COX-1, including AA, DGLA, EPA, and other lipids (31). The eicosanoid thromboxane TXA-2 derived from AA, is involved in the causation of diseases when biosynthesized in excess (32). TXA-2 leads to lymphocyte proliferation and bronchoconstriction, and also causes platelet aggregation, an underlying cause of cardiovascular diseases.

5-LIPOXYGENASE ENZYMES AND THE LEUKOTRIENES

The leukotrienes are eicosanoids that are biosynthesized from both AA and EPA by the 5-lipoxygenase enzyme (5-LOX). As a group, the leukotrienes produced from AA in the omega-6 cascade tend to be highly inflammatory when overproduced. In a healthy person, the leukotrienes derived from AA are released to cause the acute inflammation required to help the body cope with injuries and infections. The overproduction of the leukotrienes derived from AA however, is involved with the causation of arthritic pains in older adults and a host of other inflammatory diseases.

The leukotrienes derived from EPA via 5-LOX s are either anti-inflammatory or neutral and do not cause inflammation or diseases. They have been largely ignored because research interest has been in the causation of diseases. Later thinking however, noted that when sufficient EPA was present in the diet, it monopolized the 5-LOX enzyme and produced anti-inflammatory or neutral eicosanoids. This prevented the conversion of AA to inflammatory eicosanoids. Ample dietary EPA provides an important health benefit.

BIOCHEMICAL LESSON: The series-4 leukotrienes derived from AA in the omega-6 cascade, via the 5-LOX enzyme, are highly inflammatory and undesirable (see Figure 9-1). When ample dietary EPA is available, it will dominate the 5-LOX enzyme; stop the processing of AA; and use EPA to produce non-inflammatory series 3 leukotrienes.

EOXINS, PROINFLAMMATORY METABOLITES

The eoxins (EXs) are pro-inflammatory metabolites of AA produced via the 15-LOX-1 pathway, primarily in human eosinophils and mast cells. The EXs are potent proinflammatory eicosanoids that increase the vascular permeability that leads to plasma leakage. The EXs may also be involved with malignancies. A laboratory study of a Hodgkin lymphoma cell line showed a high expression of 15-LOX-1 and also showed that these cells readily converted AA to EXs (33). Another research study found that EXs are significant factors in the causation of asthma, allergies, rhinitis, and chronic obstructive pulmonary disease (COPD). Eosinophils and airway epithelial cells in asthmatic individuals were found to contain large amounts of 15-LOX-1. These cells, using endogenous AA, are believed to be the main producers of the inflammatory EXs seen in connection with asthma and other airway diseases (34).

Ample EPA will prevent the biosyntheses of the EXs and their adverse effects because EPA competes with AA for the 15-LOX-1 enzyme. This competition prevents the conversion of AA to the harmful EXs. Instead, the 15-LOX-1 transforms the competing EPA to 15S-HETE, a metabolite with anti-inflammatory properties.

BIOCHEMICAL LESSON: Ample dietary EPA will prevent many of the health problems caused by chronic inflammation. EPA also competes with AA for the COX-2 and the 5-LOX enzymes and is converted to non-inflammatory eicosanoids instead of the inflammatory eicosanoids derived from AA in the omega-6 cascade. Finally, as mentioned earlier, EPA competes with LA for the 15-LOX-1 enzyme. This results in the biosynthesis of anti-tumorigenic 15S-HEPE (15S-hydroxyeicosapentaenoic acid) and prevents the conversion of LA to the pro-cancer 1S-HODE (35).

Even though the biochemical story of the eicosanoids involves many details that are hard to understand, the bottom line is becoming clear: If the battle for good health is to be won, the diet must contain ample quantities of the omega-3 fatty acids, EPA and DHA.

Eicosanoids That Heal

Once thought to be a passive process, the resolution of inflammation is now shown to involve active biochemical programmes that enable inflamed tissues to return to homeostasis (36).

In the 1990s, a new group of anti-inflammatory, pain-moderating, and pro-healing eicosanoids began to be discovered and described. These were new pro-resolving lipid eicosanoids. As a group, they are referred to as lipid autacoids or lipid mediators, and are individually identified as lipoxins (LXs), derived from AA, and resolvins (RvEs and RvDs), protectins (PDs), and maresins (MaRs), derived from EPA and DHA. These discoveries are tremendously important because they elucidate the biochemical processes that end inflammation, initiate healing, protect involved tissues, control pain, and return damaged tissues to homeostasis (37; 38).

Uncontrolled inflammation and failure to heal are characteristics of the many chronic inflammatory diseases that currently affect older adults. In these cases, the lack of dietary essential fatty acids, primarily EPA and DHA, limit the biosynthesis of the lipid mediators necessary to resolve inflammation and promote healing (36). In fact, more recent research has discovered that high dietary levels of LA caused by the wide use of vegetable seed oils totally annul the ability of the omega-3 lipid mediators, resolvins, protectins, and maresins, to protect against atherosclerosis (39).

THE LIPOXINS (LX)

The biochemical originators of acute inflammation and pain are the inflammatory eicosanoids derived from AA via the COX-2 and LOX-5 pathways (See Figure 9-1). The LXs are biosynthesized from AA by three different routes. In the first route, the LOX-5 pathway is closed. This stops the biosynthesis of inflammatory series-4 leukotrienes derived from AA. AA then becomes the substrate for the 15 LOX -1 enzyme. The LOX 15-1 converts the AA to intermediates (15-HpETE or 15S-HETE) that, in turn, are converted by the LOX-5 enzyme, followed by hydrolase enzymes, to LXA-4 and LXB-4. These (LXA-4 and LXB-4) are vasodilators and down-regulators of inflammation. They are found to be protective against atherosclerosis in animal studies and are believed to be important in tissues during inflammation and its resolution (40).

LX Formation, Second Route: Here, LTA-4, an inflammatory leukotriene derived from AA via LOX-5 in the omega-6 cascade, is instantly converted by 12-LOX to LXA-4 and LXB-4. This reaction occurs between cell types in the vascular system and in the blood where LOX-5 in neutrophils converts AA to LTA-4 and 12-LOX in platelets convert the LTA-4 to LXA-4 and LXB-4. As part of the immune system, leukocytes (blood cells that lack hemoglobin) protect the body against foreign particles and microorganisms. Platelets (thrombocytes) are small tiny bits of living substance (irregular-shaped anuclear cells) that cause blood clotting.

LX Formation, Third Route: This route is a method of storing a precursor of LXs for later use. 15S-HETE, mentioned earlier as being formed from AA by 15-LOX-1, is stored in phospholipids within neutrophil membranes. It is released when needed and converted to LXA-4 and LXB-4. Neutrophils are phagocytic white blood cells that ingest and destroy bad cells, microorganisms, and other foreign matter in the blood and tissues.

ASPIRIN-TRIGGERED LIPID MEDIATORS

Aspirin was invented in 1897 by a chemist working at the Bayer Company in Germany. By the early 1900s, aspirin had become the most widely used medicine in the world. Today, in the United States alone, about 30 billion aspirin tablets are used annually (41). Why has aspirin been so widely used for so many years? The answer a century ago was that aspirin satisfied people's needs for relief from pain. In the mid 20th century, the American Heart Association advised the daily use of "baby" aspirin (81 milligrams) because regular use had been found to prevent heart attacks, stroke, and unstable angina.

Fifty years later, in the years near the turn of the 21st Century, biochemists discovered why aspirin was so highly effective. Aspirin is a unique drug. There is no other drug known that can do what aspirin does. It triggers the biosynthesis of lipid mediators inside the body that are biochemically similar and slightly more potent than the naturally-formed lipid mediators known as lipoxins, resolvins, protectins, and maresins. In brief, aspirin "jump-starts" the endogenous (within the body) pathways of resolution and healing by triggering the biosynthesis of pro-resolving lipid mediators (42).

ASPIRIN TRIGGERED LIPOXINS (ATLX): Biochemically, aspirin works by acetylating and blocking both of the two active catalytic sites in the COX-1 enzyme and blocking one of the two active catalytic sites in the COX-2 enzyme. COX-1, when disabled by aspirin, benefits individuals with cardiovascular diseases because the COX-1 enzyme can no longer produce anything, including thromboxane, and other inflammatory eicosanoids.

The single site that remains active on the acetylated COX-2 enzyme causes COX-2 to produce 15R-HETE from AA instead of the usual inflammatory PGE-2 series prostaglandins, thromboxanes, and prostacyclins. This 15R-HETE is immediately transformed by 15-LOX-1 to 15-epi-lipoxin A4, also called aspirin-triggered lipoxin A4 or ATLXA4.

Aspirin literally forces the COX-2 enzyme to produce anti-inflammatory eicosanoids from AA, which normally is a major source of proinflammatory compounds.

Recall that 15S-HETE was mentioned earlier as an intermediate in the production of natural lipoxins (LXs) from AA. 15S-HETE and 15R-HETE are chemically the same except that the stereo chemistry of 15S-HETE is slightly different. The difference is that an alcohol moiety (OH) is connected to carbon number 15 at an unusual angle in the aspirin- triggered 15R-HETE. This dissimilarity does not materially change the effectiveness of the ATLXs except that the ATLXs remain biologically active in the human body for a longer time and are more potent than the naturally formed LXs (38).

As mentioned earlier, COX-2 is not normally expressed (not active) in the body. However, it is constitutive (always expressed) in blood vessels due to the fluid motion of blood flow. During chronic inflammation, this active COX-2 within the vascular system is constantly converting AA to inflammatory PGE-2 series prostaglandins and thromboxanes. This is an important cause of cardiovascular diseases. But, when COX-2 is acetylated by aspirin, this damage cannot occur because acetylated COX-2 transforms AA to 12R-HETE that is further converted within the vascular system to pro-resolving ATLXs.

A further benefit is that this AA is no longer available to be converted in the omega-6 cascade to inflammatory eicosanoids. This particular biochemical pathway modification is a clear example of why the regular use of aspirin is associated with the prevention of cardiovascular diseases (40).

Lipoxins and aspirin-triggered 15-epi-lipoxins are the first lipid mediators of endogenous anti-inflammation and resolution to be discovered. According to a number of studies in animal models, a low ratio of LX and/or ATLX to leukotrienes (LTA-4 and others) derived from AA via the omega-6 cascade, appears to be connected with many human diseases. These include cardiovascular disease, asthma, kidney inflammation, cystic fibrosis, gastrointestinal problems, and periodontal disease (38).

BIOCHEMICAL LESSON: Aspirin alone, without the long chain essential fatty acids, will not produce maximum health benefits. Dietary AA is usually ample, but dietary supplementation with EPA and DHA is also required for aspirin to do its work.

RESOLVINS AND PROTECTINS

Resolvins and protectins are a group of highly beneficial lipid mediators derived from EPA and DHA. Those derived from EPA are termed E-series resolvins, RvE1 and RvE2. Those derived from DHA are referred to as D-series resolvins, RvD1, 2, 3, and 4 and protectin, PD1. Protectin, PD1 is referred to as neuroprotectin NPD1 when it is generated by neural cells because of its extremely potent tissue-protective behavior in brain and retinal cells (43).

RESOLVINS RVE-1 AND RVE-2: The research literature indicates that the resolvins are formed by both natural and aspirin-triggered biochemical pathways. Interestingly, these pathways are generally the same as those described earlier with regard to the lipoxins (LX). In the natural pathway, LOX 15-1 converts EPA to an intermediate that is further changed by 5-LOX to other intermediates that form RvE1 and RvE2. The aspirin-triggered pathway begins with acetylated COX-2 that transforms EPA to intermediates that are further converted to ATRvE1 and ATRvE2 (37). In general, RvE1, RvE2, and their aspirin-triggered homologues reduce inflammation and pain, and promote resolution. In animal models, they have been shown to improve survival against colitis, control peritonitis, stop tissue and bone loss in the oral disease, periodontitis, and protect against osteoclast-mediated bone destruction (37).

RESOLVINS DERIVED FROM DHA

The D-series resolvins are derived from DHA. The finding that EPA could be converted to a proresolving lipid mediator by aspirin-acetylated COX-2 caused researchers to investigate the possibility that DHA might be transformed in the same way. Testing showed that, as was the case with EPA, aspirin-acetylated COX-2 followed by 5-LOX created four new, potent lipid mediators. These were named the D-series resolvins, ATRvD1, 2, 3, and 4. Later the naturally-formed versions of this group of resolvins were discovered. In animal studies, the D-series resolvins exhibit strong anti-inflammatory and proresolving effects against periodontitis and kidney injury. In a study involving harmful bacteria, these resolvins resulted in survival of animals that otherwise would have perished (43).

PROTECTIN NPD1/PD1 AND AT-NPD1/PD1

Both the natural and aspirin-triggered versions of this lipid mediator are derived from DHA, and both have powerful anti-inflammatory and tissue-protective effects. PD1 is naturally biosynthesized by several enzymatic steps. It was originally called PD1 but because it was found to provide such potent protection to the brain, retina, and other neural tissues it is now being identified as PD1/NPD1. In forming the natural version, LOX 15-1 converts DHA to an intermediate that undergoes further modification by enzymes that lead to PD1/NPD1. PD1/NPD1 and its aspirin-triggered version have been found to reduce experimental periodontitis and kidney injury in animal studies.

Importantly, PD1/NPD1 is now known to prevent the excess growth of new blood vessels in the layer of tissue directly under the retina of the human eye, the cause of macular degeneration. This is a significant discovery because macular degeneration, also known as wet AMD, is a cause of blindness in older adults (43).

MARESIN, MAR1

Maresin, MaR1, was only recently discovered. DHA is converted to an intermediate by 12-LOX, which is converted to MaR1 by enzymatic oxidation. When compared against RvE1 derived from EPA and PD1/NPD1 from DHA, MaR1 was equally potent. It is believed that that MaR1 is important in bacterial particle containment, removal of dead cells, shortening of resolution time, controlling inflammation, healing of wounds, and the return to normal functions (44). Although aspirin-triggered forms of all resolvins have now been discovered, an aspirin-triggered form of MaR1 has not yet been found (45).

BIOCHEMICAL LESSON: The above biochemistry tells us that the plague of chronic inflammatory diseases that besets this country can be prevented by utilizing dietary adjustments to properly balance the biosynthesis of eicosanoids.

EICOSANOIDS DERIVED BY NONENZYMATIC REACTIONS

A significant number of eicosanoid-like compounds are produced in the body as a result of oxidative stress caused by oxygen free radicals, also referred to as reactive oxygen species (ROS). These eicosanoids are called isoprostanes, a group of non-enzymatically-derived eicosanoids. The biosynthesis of isoprostanes is not catalyzed by enzymes; the oxygen free radicals in the body simply react with any fatty acids having three or more double bonds. The reaction products tend to be harmful bioactive chemicals that are found in body tissues, blood plasma, and urine. The cause of oxidative stress is dietary deficiency of anti-oxidants (46).

HEALTH EFFECTS OF ISOPROSTANES

The isoprostanes of interest in terms of human health tend to be derived from arachidonic acid (AA), eicosapentaenoic acid (EPA), and docosahexaenoic acid (DHA). Isoprostanes derived from AA and those derived from DHA (termed neuroprostanes) are increased in diseased regions of brains of individuals who have died of advanced Alzheimer's disease and Parkinson's disease. These levels are also increased in the cerebrospinal fluid in the early stages of Alzheimer's disease and Huntington's disease.

In these cases, it is not clear if the isoprostanes are the cause of the diseases or if the isoprostanes are simply the product of oxidative stress in the diseased patients. Curiously, isoprostane levels in plasma and tissues are highest during fetal and neonatal life compared to adults. Is this a normal physiological state? This raises questions about the possible role of oxidative stress in causation of autism and attention deficit/hyperactivity disorder in children (31).

LABORATORY TESTS: Isoprostane levels determined by an inexpensive urine test are considered a reliable indicator of oxidative stress in humans. Normal levels in healthy individuals have been accurately defined so that the degree of oxidative stress in patients can be reliably measured. Increased isoprostane levels have been associated with smoking, alcoholism, and cirrhosis of the liver. Using this urine test, oxidative stress has been implicated in brain degeneration, kidney diseases, atherosclerosis, and type-2 diabetes. Urinary F2-isoprostanes provide an independent marker of coronary heart disease that has been linked to high concentrations of this isoprostane in atherosclerotic plaques (31).

BIOCHEMICAL LESSON: Oxidative stress is an important consideration in the causation and the prevention inflammatory diseases. Oxidative stress is harmful and also produces harmful isoprostanes that destroy AA, EPA and DHA. Isoprostanes in the urine however, are of great value when used as a simple, low cost way to measure oxidative stress (31; 46). The ability to measure isoprostanes means that simple tests can be used to warn of oxidative stress early enough to take the following preventive action: Assess total diet; increase dietary intake of antioxidants; and reduce isoprostanes to a safe level. The biochemistry of the eicosanoids is a road map to good health and long life.

Eicosanoids in the Skin

Skin is the organ that forms the great protective envelope that covers the entire body. It holds all the parts together and protects them from all sorts of environmental exposures, infectious and toxic agents, and bumps and scrapes. It also serves to protect its precious contents against drying out with an oily/waxy coating called sebum that forms a barrier that controls water loss (47).

Skin is composed of two layers; the outer epidermis and the inner dermis. The epidermis is composed mostly of cells called keratinocytes. These cells originate at the bottom of the epidermis where they continuously multiply and move upward toward the surface of the skin. As these basal keratinocytes move upward, they are transformed into the tough, leather-like skin surface that requires constant replacement to overcome wear and tear.

The dermis, located below the epidermis, physically and functionally supports the epidermis with necessary nutrients from the body's circulating blood. It also contains sebaceous glands that provide sebum, hair follicles, sweat glands, nerve fibers, and other essential skin components (48).

ARE THERE EICOSANOIDS IN THE SKIN?

Eicosanoids are not only present in the skin but are actively involved in the maintenance of skin health. The essential fatty acid cascade (EFA) in skin is the same as that shown in Figure 9-1 for the whole organism with the exception that both the D6D and the D5D enzymes are not active.

FATTY ACID COMPOSITION: The fatty acid composition of the skin, absent topical applications, is determined by diet (48). Hence, it is reasonable to assume that if the evolutionary diet was proper for primitive man's health, it must also have been proper for primitive man's skin.

LINOLEIC ACID (LA): LA (18:2n-6) makes up about 12% of epidermal fatty acids and is the most plentiful polyunsaturated fatty acid in the epidermis. LA is extremely important in skin because it is used by the sebaceous glands in the dermis to form the long chain wax-like waterproofing molecules that constitute the sebum. Laboratory animals deficient in LA have scaly skins (termed cutaneous hyper-proliferation) and display increased transdermal water losses. Feeding LA to these animals reverses these symptoms (49). When LA is deficient in the skin the body uses oleic acid (an omega-9 fatty acid) in the production of sebum. This causes skin irritation and acne (48).

ARACHIDONIC ACID (AA): AA (20:4n-6), at about 9% of total fatty acids, is the second most prevalent polyunsaturated fatty acid in skin epidermis; hence it is abundantly available to serve as a substrate for the biosynthesis of inflammatory eicosanoids via activated COX-2 enzymes.

SPECIAL BENEFITS OF CERTAIN VITAMINS

The relationships between eicosanoid activity and vitamins C, D, and E have not been fully clarified. It appears that these and perhaps others do play an important part in skin health. Also unclear are the interactions, if any, among these three vitamins and the proresolving lipid mediators, the lipoxins, protectins, resolvins, and maresins.

VITAMIN C: Vitamin C is a normal constituent of skin. It is a powerful anti-oxidant and is required for collagen synthesis. To an extent, dietary vitamin C prevents sunburn. In animal studies, it reduced the risk of skin cancers. Importantly, vitamin C prevents scurvy, a potentially fatal systemic disease that causes severe skin damage. Signs of scurvy in skin are spots of subcutaneous bleeding, slow healing, and failure to heal (50).

VITAMIN D: Cells in the skin utilize the UVR (ultra violet radiation) from sunlight to biosynthesize vitamin D3. Vitamin D3 suppresses tumors, controls hair follicle activity, and regulates proliferation and differentiation of keratinocytes (skin cells). Vitamin D3 also modulates inflammation and is probably involved in wound healing (51).

VITAMIN E: Vitamin E is the common name for a family of antioxidants that consist of eight different tocopherols and tocotrienols. Vitamin E acts as a free radical scavenger. It is required for skin health because it protects against the oxidant free radicals generated by sunlight. Studies show that vitamin E works best when taken as a dietary supplement along with vitamin C. Some research has been done on the topical use of vitamin E on skin, but there are no clear recommendations for general use (52).

THE INACTIVE DESATURASES, D6D AND D5D

The desaturases are enzymes that remove two hydrogen atoms from adjacent carbons that form a single bond and replace them with a double bond. The D6D and D5D enzymes are not active in skin. Reactions catalyzed by these desaturases do not occur in the skin.

D6D: Inactivity of D6D means that in skin, LA (18:2n-6) cannot be converted to GLA (18:3n-6) and EPA (20:5n-3) cannot be converted to DHA (22:6n-3). The fact that ALA (18:3n-3) cannot be converted to stearidonic acid (SA, 18:4n-3) does not appear to be important because of the insignificant amount of ALA currently in the American diet.

BIOCHEMICAL LESSON: Considering that the metabolic pathways for the EFAs that exist in skin were created by evolution to build healthy humans with the best possible skin, it is reasonable to postulate that the D6D enzyme was rendered inactive in skin to conserve LA by preventing its entry to the EFA cascade. Apparently, in evolutionary times, LA was not in great surplus as it is today, and LA had to be conserved to form the skin's water barrier. Furthermore, in evolutionary times, the inability of the skin to convert LA to GLA and EPA to DHA was not important because GLA and DHA were amply available in the Paleolithic diet.

Today, the large excess LA in the American diet is a major cause of systemic inflammation and is far more than what is required to maintain the skin's water barrier. For good health LA and the other fatty acids in the diet must be in sufficient quantity and properly balanced to supply the body's needs. Excess dietary LA is not required or healthful and should be avoided.

D5D: The inactive D5D means that DGLA (20:3n-6) in the omega-6 cascade cannot be converted to AA (20:4n-6) and that eicosatetraenoic acid (20:4n-3) in the omega-3 cascade cannot be converted to EPA (20:5n-3). It is important to note that even though GLA, DHA, AA, and EPA cannot be biosynthesized in skin; these fatty acids are provided to the dermis by the body's circulating blood and transferred to the epidermis via the dermis interface. Because the elongase enzymes remain active, GLA (18:3n-6) transferred from the body can be transformed to DGLA. However, note that this DGLA cannot be converted to AA because of the lack of D5D. The net effect is that all of the important fatty acids, AA, EPA, DHA, GLA, and DGLA are available to the skin from the circulating blood via the dermis interface (51; 52; 53).

THE SKIN'S BLOOD SUPPLY

The inability of the skin to biosynthesize three important fatty acids, GLA, AA, and DHA would appear to increase the complexity of understanding the metabolism of the essential fatty acids in skin. But the scientific literature indicates that the missing fatty acids, GLA, EPA, and AA are automatically supplied to the skin from the body's circulating blood (48). Thus it is important to recall that the fatty acid levels in circulating blood reflect the fatty acid levels in the diet. Today's modern American diet underlies the chronic disease epidemics in today's America, hence today's skin is supplied with the same circulating blood. As reviewed earlier, this blood is very likely to contain an overabundance of LA and AA, and a deficiency of GLA, EPA, and DHA.

INFLAMMATORY SKIN DISEASES

Inflammation, as in the case of chronic systemic diseases, also appears to be a major underlying cause of skin disorders. These include atopic dermatitis, psoriasis, sunburn, and skin cancers (53). Due to lack of D5D in epidermis, AA is supplied from the body. The cyclooxygenase enzymes (COX 1&2) transform the AA to pro-inflammatory PGE-2 prostaglandins. Such eicosanoid-induced inflammation is involved with a number of skin diseases that include psoriasis, atopic dermatitis, disorders resulting from over-exposure to sunlight, and skin cancers. Importantly, EPA is also supplied to the epidermis by the body. When ample, EPA will utilize the COX enzymes to produce anti-inflammatory PGE-3 prostaglandins instead of the inflammatory PGE-2 prostaglandins.

ATOPIC DERMATITIS: Atopic dermatitis is described as a chronic allergic inflammatory disease, although the precise cause is not clear. Epidermal keratinocytes appear to respond to allergenic and inflammatory stimulators by releasing excess amounts of arachidonic acid (AA). This AA increases the biosynthesis of inflammatory PGE-2 prostaglandins via the COX enzymes. Laboratory studies suggest that increased dietary GLA and DHA might be beneficial against atopic dermatitis (53).

In a clinical study, Kawamura found that epidermal hyper-proliferation caused high trans-epidermal water loss that resulted in dry skin and mild atopic dermatitis (54). Dietary supplementation with GLA-rich oil tended to normalize epidermal hyper-proliferation and reduced inflammatory symptoms. A literature review suggests that not much biochemical research has been devoted to atopic dermatitis.

PSORIASIS: Psoriasis is a common chronic inflammatory skin disease that results in a red, scaly rash on elbows, knees, scalp, ears, navel, genitals and buttocks (55). It has been considered to be an immunological disease that combines dermal inflammation and epidermal hyperplasia (the proliferation of normal cells). The cause is uncertain, but thought to be interaction of the immune system, genes, and environmental factors (56).

In recent years, an epidemiological association between psoriasis and metabolic syndrome has been discovered. Metabolic syndrome is defined as having any three of the following conditions: abdominal obesity; hypertriglyceridemia; low levels of HDL cholesterol; high blood pressure; and high fasting glucose. Patients with psoriasis have a high prevalence of metabolic syndrome. These patients also have higher rates of morbidity and mortality (57).

An interesting hypothesis by Balbas (56) is that psoriasis is associated with metabolic syndrome due to a shared inflammation mechanism. In other words, the chronic inflammation that is the cause of the metabolic syndrome may also be the underlying cause of psoriasis. Several studies have shown that C-reactive protein is elevated in psoriasis patients. Additionally, dietary EPA and DHA reduce symptoms in psoriasis and other skin diseases (56).

A review by Nicolaou (53) suggests that diets rich in EPA/DHA, and GLA (the precursor of anti-inflammatory DGLA) would counteract the inflammation caused by the metabolites derived from AA. A study of patients with psoriasis found that EPA, DHA, vitamin D, and anti-oxidants significantly reduced the symptoms of this disease (56).

BIOCHEMICAL LESSON: The underlying cause of psoriasis is likely to be chronic inflammation caused by the modern American diet. The strong association of psoriasis with metabolic syndrome, mentioned above, supports this idea.

SKIN CANCER: Non-melanoma cancers of the skin make up the largest group of malignancies in America (58). Estimated attack rates for 1994 were 900.000 to 1,200,000. By the year 2006, attack rates of non-melanoma skin cancers had tripled to approximately 3,507,000 cases. These cancers appear mostly on sun-exposed parts of the body; face, neck, and arms. Ultra violet radiation (UVR) primarily from the sun is the cause. The increasing incidence of these cancers is thought to be due to the combined influences of an aging population and higher levels of solar UV brought about by ozone depletion in the upper atmosphere. National guidance on avoiding skin cancer, namely stay out of the sun, wear a hat and long sleeves, and use sunscreen has not been effective in controlling these cancers (59).

Role of Sunburn: Overexposure to sun causes sunburn, an acute inflammatory response in skin to the UVR in sunlight. Symptoms are redness, swelling, and pain. The biochemistry is as follows: Inflammation is induced by the appearance of cytokines, the influx of inflammatory cells such as macrophages and lymphocytes, and the activation of the normally dormant COX-2 enzyme. When activated, the COX-2 enzyme transforms arachidonic acid (AA) to inflammatory PGE-2 and other inflammatory eicosanoids in the PG-2-series prostaglandins (60).

Chronic high levels PGE-2 and other eicosanoids in the 2-series derived from arachidonic acid, have been shown to possess intrinsic tumor promoting activity (61). Mice specially bred with no COX-2 enzymes are resistant to skin cancer caused by either UVR or carcinogenic chemicals (62).

Meeram looked at the impact of chronic UVR exposure to the skin of mice fed either a high-fat or a low-fat diet. The high- and low-fat diets included linoleic acid, saturated fatty acids, monounsaturated fatty acid, alpha linoleic acid, and small amounts of fats termed omega-3. The high fat diet contained approximately four times more of each fat than the control diet. The findings of this study were as follows: UVR induced epidermal COX-2 expression and PGE-2 production with both diets. However, the high fat diet exacerbated COX-2 expression, PGE-2 production, and inflammation. The authors concluded that this study suggested that the high fat diet exacerbated UVR-induced inflammation and that this may lead to higher risk of inflammation-associated skin diseases, including the possible risk of UVR-induced skin cancers (63).

BIOCHEMICAL QUESTIONS: The above paper described an excellent piece of scientific research. The findings that the high-fat diet exacerbated COX-2 expression, PGE-2 production, and inflammation become quite meaningful when the following question is asked: What fat was the probable underlying cause of the exacerbated PGE-2 production and the subsequent inflammation? Biochemically, the only possible precursor of PGE-2, via the COX-2 enzyme, was arachidonic acid. Further, this arachidonic acid had to come from systemic blood because the skin, lacking the D6D enzyme, could not biosynthesize it. Thus, the AA in the systemic blood had to come from diet, or more likely from the excess LA in the diet transformed to AA via the omega-6 cascade.

Diets high in LA and AA and deficient in EPA and DHA inhibit the body's ability to end inflammation, repair damaged tissue, and return to homeostasis. As reviewed earlier, these essential fatty acids must be present in the proper balance for the biochemistry of the body to produce the eicosanoids that heal, namely the lipoxins, resolvins, protectins, neuro-protectins, and maresins (36).

A Fitting Close to this Chapter

In recent years it has become widely appreciated that, in addition to the classic diseases associated with inflammation such as psoriasis, periodontal disease and arthritis, uncontrolled inflammation governs the pathogenesis of many other prevalent diseases including cardiovascular and cerebrovascu-lar disease, cancer, obesity and Alzheimer's disease. Serhan CN, Yacoubian S, Yang R. Anti-inflammatory and pro-resolving lipid mediators. Annual Review of Pathology. 2008; 3: 279-312

References

1.)   Evans P. Dead as I'll Ever Be. London, ON, Canada, Shavian Publishing, 2002.

2.)   Holman RT. The slow discovery of the importance of 3 essential fatty acids in human health. The Journal of Nutrition. 1998; 128(2): 427S-433S.

3.)   Allport S. The Queen of Fats. Berkeley, CA: University of California Press, 2006.

4.)   Felix C. All About Omega-3 Oils. Garden City Park, NY: Avery Publishing Group, 1998.

5.)   Simopoulos AP, Robinson J. The Omega Diet. New York, NY: HarperPerennial, 1999.

6.)   Gerster H. Can adults adequately convert alpha-linolenic acid (18:3n-3) to eicosapentaenoic acid (20:n5-3) and docosahexaenoic acid (22:6n-3)? International Journal of Vitamin Nutrition Research.1998; 68(3): 159-173.

7.)   Wander R. A primer on dietary fat: The good, the bad, and the unknown. The Linus Pauling Institute Newsletter. Fall/Winter 1998: 8-10.

8.)   Simopoulos AP. The importance of the ratio of omega-6/omega-3 essential fatty acids. Biomedicine and Pharmacotherapy. 2002; 56(8): 365-379.

9.)   Murray MT, Beutler J. Understanding Fats and Oils. Encinitas, CA: Progressive Health, 1996.

10.) Simopoulos AP. The importance of the omega-6/omega-3 fatty acid ratio in cardiovascular and other chronic diseases. Experimental Biology and Medicine. 2008; 233: 674-688.

11.) Yam, D, et al. Diet and disease – the Israeli paradox: possible dangers of a high omega-6 polyunsatu-rated fatty acid diet. Israeli Journal of Medical Science. 1996; 32(11): 1134-43.

12.) Hibbeln JR, et al. Healthy intakes of n-3 and n-6 fatty acids: estimations considering world wide di-versity. American Journal of Clinical Nutrition. 2006; 8(3 supp.): 1483S-93S.

13.) Horrobin, D.F. et. al. Medical Hypothesis. 1979; 5: 969-985.

14.) Disease Prevention and Treatment Protocols. 2n Ed (1998). Life Extension Foundation. Published by Life Extension Media, Hollywood, FL.

15.) De Caterina R, Basta G. n-3 Fatty acids and the inflammatory response-biological background. European Heart Journal Supplements. 2001; 3 (Supplement D): D42–D49.

16.) Heiby WA. The Reverse Effect: How Vitamins and Minerals Promote Health and Cause Disease. Deerfield, IL: MediScience Publishers, 1988.

17.) Sears B. The Anti-inflammation Zone. New York, NY: Regan Books/Harper Collins, 2005.

18.) Hibbeln JR, et al. Healthy intakes of n-3 and n-6 fatty acids: estimations considering worldwide diversity. American Journal of Clinical Nutrition. 2006; 83(suppl): 1483S-94S.

19.) Colquhoun A, Miyake JA, Benadiba M. Fatty acids, eicosanoids, and cancer. Nutritional Therapy and Metabolism. 2009; 37(3): 105-112.

20.) Spindler SA, et al. Production of 13-hydroxyoctadecadienoic acid (13-HODE) by prostate tumors and cell lines. Biochemical and Biophysical Research Communications. 1997; 239(3):775-81.

21.) Sauer LA, et al. Eicosapentaenoic acid suppresses cell proliferation in MCF-7 human breast cancer xenografts in nude rats via a pertussis toxin-sensitive signal transduction pathway. Journal of Nutrition, 2005, September 135: 2124-2129.

22.) Kelavkar UP, et al. Prostate tumor growth and recurrence can be modulated by the omega-6:omega-3 ratio in the diet. Neoplasia; 8(2):112-124.

23.) Blasbalg TL, et al. Changes in consumption of omega-3 and omega-6 fatty acids in the United States during the 20th century. American Journal of Clinical Nutrition. 2011; 93(5): 950-962.

24.) Fan Y, Chapkin RS. Importance of dietary gamma-linolenic acid in human health and nutrition. Journal of Nutrition. 1998; 128: 1411-1414.

25.) deAntueno RJ, et al. Activity of human Delta5 and Delta6 desaturases on multiple n-3 and n-6 polyunsaturated fatty acids. FEBS Journal Letters. 2001; 509(1): 77-80.

26.) Hashimoto M, Hossain S. Neuroprotective and ameliorative actions of polyunsaturated fatty acids against neuronal diseases. Journal of Pharmacological Sciences. 2011; 116: 150-162.

27.) Enig, M, Fallon S. Health Topics (2000). http://www.westonaprice.org/know-your-fats/tripping-lightly-down-the-prostaglandin-pathways/ Accessed Sept. 28, 2012.

28.) Berquin IM, et al. Multi-targeted therapy of cancer by omega-3 fatty acids. NIH Public Access, Cancer Letters. 2008; 269(2): 363-377.

29.) Voss A, et al. The metabolism of 7,10,13,16,19-docosapentaenoic acid to 4,7,10,13,16,19- docosahexaenoic acid in rat livers independent of a 4-desaturase. The Journal of Biological Chemistry. 1991; 266(30): 19995-20000.

30.) Chilton FH, et al. Mechanisms by which botanical lipids affect inflammatory disorders. American Journal of Clinical Nutrition. 2008; 87(suppl): 498S-503S.

31.) Christie WW. Eicosanoids and Related Compounds, Lipid Library. http://lipidlibrary.aocs.org/Lipids/fa_eic.html/ Accessed Sept. 28, 2012.

32.) Vane JR, Botting RM. Mechanism of action of anti-inflammatory drugs. In: Szczeklik A, Gryglewski RJ, Vane JR, eds. Eicosanoids, Aspirin, and Asthma. New York, NY: Marcel Dekker, Inc., 1998.

33.) Claesson HE, et al. Hodgkin Reed-Sternberg cells express 15 lipoxygenase-1 and are putative producers or eoxins in vivo; novel insight into the inflammatory features of classical Hodgkin lymphoma. FEBS Journal. 2008; 275(16): 4222-4234. Epub 2008 Jul 18 PMID 18647347.

34.) Claesson HE. On the biosynthesis and biological role of eoxins and 15-lipoxygenase-1 in airway inflammation and Hodgkin lymphoma. Prostaglandins Other Lipid Mediators. 2009; 89(3-4): 120-125.

35.) Kelavkar UP, et al. Prostate tumor growth can be modulated by dietarily targeting 15 lipoxygenase1 and cyclooxygenase-2 enzymes. Neoplasia., 2009; 11(7): 692-699.

36.) Serhan CN, Chang N, Van Dyke TE. Resolving inflammation: dual anti-inflammatory and pro-resolution lipid mediators. National Review of Immunology. 2008; 8(5): 348-361.

37.) Serhan CN, Chiang N. Endogenous pro-resolving and anti-inflammatory lipid mediators: a new pharmacologic genus. British Journal of Pharmacology. 2008; 153: S200-S215.

38.) Serhan CN, et al. Anti-inflammatory and pro-resolving lipid mediators. Annual Review of Pathology. 2008; 3: 279-312.

39.) Merched AJ, et al. Nutragenic disruption of inflammation-resolution homeostasis and atherogenesis. Journal of Nutrigenetics and Nutrigenomics. 2011; 4: 12-24.

40.) Serhan CN. Lipoxins and aspirin-triggered 15-epi-lipoxins are the first lipid mediators of endogenous anti-inflammatory and resolution. Prostaglandins, Leukotrienes, and Essential Fatty Acids. 2005; 73: 141.

41.) Lenfant C. Introduction. In: Szczeklik A, Gryglewski RJ, Vane JR, eds. Eicosanoids, Aspirin, and Asthma. New York, NY: Marcel Dekker, Inc., 1998.

42.) Serhan CN. Novel Lipid Mediators and Resolution Mechanisms in Acute Inflammation. American Journal of Pathology, 2010; 177(4) : 1576-1591

43.) Bannenberg GL. Therapeutic applicability of anti-inflammatory and proresolving polyunsaturated fatty acid-derived lipid mediators. The Scientific World Journal. 2010; 10: 676-712. http://www.tswj.com/2010/127407/abs/ Accessed Sept. 28, 2012.

44.) Serhan CN, et al. Maresins: novel macrophage mediators with potent anti-inflammatory and proresolving actions. Journal of Experimental Medicine. 2008; 206(1): 15-23.

45.) Makriyannis A, Nikas SP. Aspirin-triggered metabolites of EFAs. Chemistry & Biology. 2011; 18(10): 1208-9.

46.) Montuschi P, et al. Isoprostanes: markers and mediators of oxidative stress. FASEB Journal. 2004; 18: 1791-1800.

47.) Michels AJ. Micronutrients and Skin Health. Linus Pauling Institute, Oregon State University. September 2011. http://lpi.oregonstate.edu/infocenter/skin.html/ Accessed Sept. 28, 2012.

48.) Angelo G. Essential Fatty Acids and Skin Health, Micronutrient Information Center, Linus Pauling Institute, Oregon State University. February 2012. http://lpi.oregonstate.edu/infocenter/skin/EFA/ Accessed Sept. 28, 2012.

49.) Ziboh VA, et al. Metabolism of polyunsaturated fatty acids by skin epidermal enzymes. *American Journal of Clinical Nutrition.* 2000;71 (Supplement): 361S-6S..

50.) Michels AJ. Vitamin C and Skin Health, Micronutrient Information Center, Linus Pauling Institute, Oregon State University, September 2011, http//:lpi.oregonstate.org/infocenter/skin/vitaminC/index,html/ Accessed Sept. 28, 2012.

51.) Drake VJ. Vitamin D and Skin Health, Micronutrient Information Center, Linus Pauling Institute, Oregon State University, November 2011. http//:lpi.oregonstate.org/infocenter/skin/vitaminD/index,html/ Accessed Sept. 28, 2012.

52.) Michels, AJ. Vitamin E and Skin Health, February 2012. Micronutrient Information Center, Linus Pauling Institute, Oregon State University. http//:lpi.oregonstate.org/infocenter/skin/vitaminE/index,html/ Accessed Sept. 28, 2012.

53.) Nicolaou A, Eicosanoids in skin inflammation, *Prostaglandins Leukotrienes Essential Fatty Acids* (2012), in press. http://www.ncbi.nlm.nih.gov/pubmed/22521864/ Accessed Sept. 28, 2012. (abstract)

54.) Kawamura A, et al. Dietary supplementation of gamma-linolenic acid improves skin parameters in subjects with dry skin and mild atopic dermatitis. *J Oleo Sci.* 2011; 60(12): 597-607

55.) Linus Pauling Institute, Psoriasis. http//:infocenter/glossary.html#P/ Accessed Sept. 28, 2012.

56.) Balbas GM, et al. Study on the use of omega-3 fatty acids as a therapeutic supplement in treatment of psoriasis. *Clinical, Cosmetic and Investigational Dermatology* 2011:4 73-77

57.) Thorvardur J L, et al. Prevalence of the Metabolic Syndrome in Psoriasis: Results From the National Health and Nutrition Examination Survey 2003–2006. Archives of Dermatology. 2011; 147(4): 419–424.

58.) Rogers HW, et al. Incidence estimate of nonmelanoma skin cancer in the United States, 2006. http://archderm.jamanetwork.com/article.aspx?articleid=209782/ Accessed Sept. 28, 2012.

59.) Bachelor MA and Owens DM) Squamous cell carcinoma of the skin: Current strategies for treatment and prevention, 2009. Current Cancer Therapy Reviews, 2009; 5: 37-44.

60.) Rundhaug JE, et al. The role of the EP receptors for prostaglandin E-2 in skin and skin cancer. Cancer Metastasis Rev. 2011; 30: 465-480.

61.) Rundhaug JE, et al. The effect of cyclooxygenase-2 overexpression on skin carcinogenesis is context dependent. Molecular Carcinogenesis. 2007; 46(12): 981-992.

62.) Tiano HF, et al (2002). Deficiency of either cyclooxygenase (COX-) or COX-2 alters epidermal differentiation and reduces mouse skin tumorigenesis. *Cancer Research*, **62**(12), 3396-3401.

63.) Meeran SM, Singh T, Nagy TR, Katiyar SK. High fat diet exacerbates ubfkn=annatuib abd cekk survival signals in the skin of ultraviolet B irradiated C57BL/6 mice. *Toxicology and Applied Pharmacology.* 2009; **241**: 303-310.

Part Three

The Solution

It is not sufficient to know the solution; it must be put into service. A solution that is neglected is like a plowed field that is not sown. **Anon**

The task of defining a problem and identifying its cause are of little worth without the final step - the solution. The goal of Part Three is to suggest a feasible final step to alleviating the catastrophic drain on national resources by the uncontrolled epidemics of chronic nutritional diseases.

The information presented in Part Three is based on knowledge that must have been part of primitive man's survival dictum: know what you eat. Chapter Ten describes the practical, current knowledge of the relationship between inflammation – the underlying cause of today's chronic disease epidemics – and flawed nutritional habits.

Chapter Eleven tells of primary prevention - the long lost science of disease prevention that can trace its very beginnings to the dawn of creation when primitive man had to learn to recognize foods that were good and foods that were bad. He prevented illness by eating the former and rejecting the latter. Today, modern man is faced with the same but a bit more exacting challenge; he must not only learn what foods are good and what foods are bad, but how much of the latter is tolerable. The only viable method for controlling the onerous costs of today's chronic nutritional diseases is to practice primary prevention.

It is worth remembering that very few, if any, diseases in history have been eliminated as large-scale threats to human life by curative means alone. Prevention, either by public-health measures or by immunization, has been much more effective than cure (1).

Chapter Twelve offers the reader a strategy, based on the information presented in the first eleven chapters of this book, for creating one's own program for primary prevention of the modern nutritional diseases.

1.) Theodore Dalrymple, War against cancer won't be won soon. *The Wall Street Journal*. June 12, 2000: A30.

Chapter Ten

The Diet–Disease Connection

A disease known is half cured. **Thomas Fuller, MD, Gnomologia (1732).**

The strong association between the modern American diet and the increasing attack rates of chronic diseases leads to the question of whether there is a causal connection between the two. The U.S. government long ago accepted the premise that there is a cause-effect relationship between diet and disease, specifically between heart disease and saturated fat and cholesterol derived from animal fats.

In 1977, the government promulgated an official nutritional policy despite considerable evidence that it was not scientifically supportable (1). Skeptics were ignored, and soon the low fat approach grew into a national movement that claimed not only prevention of heart disease but also benefit for the health of the whole nation. Now, almost 40 years later, advances in nutritional biochemistry reveal that the lack of success of the official premise that diet could prevent heart disease was not due to failure of the premise but rather to failure of the policy (2).

Since the early 1900s, it has been known that nutrient deficiencies could cause disease (3). The classic nutritional diseases of beriberi and pellagra are testimony to that fact. Today, evidence is mounting that deficiencies of some of the more recently discovered essential nutrients are also causing diseases or disorders, as illustrated by reports of the influence of maternal deficiencies of omega-3 essential fatty acids on maternal (4) and fetal health (5). Today, it is clear that what hitherto has been accepted as good nutrition is causing chronic inflammation (6), and chronic inflammation, in turn, underlies many of the chronic diseases that are part of modern life:

> Inflammation is now widely appreciated in the pathogenesis of many human diseases. These extend from the well-known inflammatory diseases such as arthritis and periodontal disease to those not previously linked to aberrant inflammation that today include diseases affecting many individuals such as cancer, cardiovascular diseases, asthma, and Alzheimer's disease (7).

The reality that inflammation is a major factor in the development of essentially all of the chronic diseases that the general public has long come to know and accept as accompaniments of old age may be difficult to believe or accept. Yet the scientific advances made during the last decade in understanding the nature of inflammation and its role in the etiology of chronic diseases presents no other choice.

Inflammation

The early Roman physician and medical writer Aurelius Cornelius Celsus was the first to describe the essential features of inflammation; rubor (redness), calor (heat), tumor (swelling), and dolor (pain) (8). These are the well-known symptoms of the physical reactions to a cut on the finger or a bump on the knee. This is the acute inflammatory process, the body's response to cellular damage by infection or injury. Acute inflammation is a protective mechanism by which the body attempts to rid a threat and recover from the offending event. How is it possible for a mechanism that is essential to protect against life-threatening traumas to turn on its host and set the stage for development of chronic disease? Or are acute inflammation and chronic inflammation separate entities?

TWO TYPES OF INFLAMMATION: ACUTE AND CHRONIC

The answer appears to be that acute and chronic inflammation are of two different kinds. Acute inflammation is triggered by infection or injury. It is intense and lasts only long enough to set the stage for the next step, a healthy healing process. In contrast, chronic inflammation is low level, insidious, and does not have noticeable symptoms, at least not initially, and absent dietary change is unrelenting.

The onset of acute inflammation is rapid, but the onset of chronic inflammation apparently is seldom or never recognized; it does not display features of acute inflammation. Unless remedial action intervenes, chronic inflammation progresses slowly and relentlessly until it finally results in chronic disease. Acute inflammation is a necessary defense mechanism, but chronic inflammation does not seem to have any redeeming value.

CHRONIC INFLAMMATION IS SILENT: Because it is biochemically maintained in the body for prolonged periods at a level below which it is perceived, chronic inflammation has been appropriately labeled *silent inflammation* (6). Its silence is what makes it so dangerous; it gives no signal that something is amiss and must be dealt with. Thus, no effort is made to rein it in. Eventually there may be some inkling of trouble, such as joint swelling or allergic manifestations, but usually there is no clue until the silent inflammation becomes severe enough to manifest itself as pain or perhaps even as a sudden, unanticipated heart attack.

Pain may be either the advanced notice that a chronic disease is in development or, in the case of a heart attack, the announcement of its arrival. In either event, the only remedy is control or elimination of the inflammation. Elimination of dietary factors that lead to chronic inflammation and their substitution with a healthful diet plan is fundamental to prevention of modern nutritional diseases.

C-REACTIVE PROTEIN (CRP): C-reactive protein is a protein produced by the liver that is not normally found in the blood of healthy people. Blood levels can increase several hundred-fold in response to cellular injury or infection and decrease or disappear with resolution of the illness. People who smoke, have high blood pressure, or are obese tend to have elevated levels of CRP.

Blood tests performed during physical examinations usually include a CRP test. Many physicians use the CRP level as part of their evaluation of a patient's cardiovascular status. This is because considerable data have shown an association between CRP level and recurring coronary events in patients who have already had a heart attack. The fact that elevated CRP levels also occur with numerous other conditions suggest that CRP is a nonspecific marker of inflammation. Sears points out that C-reactive protein is a signal that inflammation is present (6).

Eicosanoids and Inflammation

The vital importance of nutrition in eicosanoid metabolism is underscored by the fact that all of the eicosanoids are synthesized from essential fatty acids (EFAs), which, as their name implies, are essential for life and must be provided by the diet: the body cannot make them. The chronic inflammatory process is ultimately the province of the eicosanoid control system.

The eicosanoids are hormone-like biochemical messengers that occur in every cell of the body and control essentially all cellular functions. Some eicosanoids are proinflammatory and some are anti-inflammatory. In normal good health the two balance each other, but when proinflammatory eicosanoids dominate for prolonged periods, chronic inflammation will almost certainly follow.

EICOSANOID BALANCE

In simplest terms, inflammation is the result of an imbalance of eicosanoids. There are two kinds of eicosanoids; the omega-3 eicosanoids synthesized from the omega-3 family of EFAs and the omega-6 eicosanoids synthesized from the omega-6 family of EFAs. The omega-6 and omega-3 eicosanoids balance each other with opposing actions. In general, the actions of omega-6 eicosanoids are proinflammatory and those of omega-3 anti-inflammatory, with the result that the former have been labeled "bad" eicosanoids and the latter "good." Regardless of label, both are necessary. What conditions disrupt a healthful balance of eicosanoids and cause a chronic proinflammatory imbalance?

NUTRITIONAL INFLUENCES ON EICOSANOID BALANCE: The significant dietary factors that adversely affect eicosanoid balance can be grouped into three major categories.

These are imbalances of essential fatty acids and ultimately eicosanoids, excesses of specific nutrients, and deficiencies of vital micronutrients. These categories are not independent but rather can interact either directly or indirectly with each other.

Imbalances of EFAs and/or Eicosanoids: When the opposing actions between the omega-6 and omega-3 families are properly balanced by healthful nutrition, the delicate push-pull between them permits the body to gently fine-tune its responses to the various circumstances it must contend with. Fine-tuning is a prerequisite for optimum health. Without this capability for fine tuning, responses could be excessive or inappropriate and an invitation to chronic inflammation.

In Figure 9-1 it will be noted that the omega-6 and omega-3 EFAs employ the same enzymes and the same metabolic pathway in their stepwise conversion to their respective eicosanoids. As a result, the two families compete with each other for eicosanoid synthesis. An excess of omega-6 over omega-3 overwhelms the ability of the omega-3 EFAs to compete for the metabolic pathway to the eicosanoids and thereby permits synthesis of an excess of proinflammatory eicosanoids. Nature wisely made the omega-3 EFAs better competitors than omega-6; several of the enzymes in the pathway prefer omega-3. However, this advantage can be overcome by nutritional influences that favor synthesis of omega-6 eicosanoids, which sets the stage for inflammation.

Probably the most common nutritional imbalance in today's American diet is an excess of omega-6 over omega-3 EFAs (9). It is generally accepted that the current ratio in the American diet is 10:1 or greater due to the use of vegetable seed oils, which contain essentially no omega-3 and large amounts of the omega-6 family, LA in particular (10). The *Dietary Guidelines for Americans*, the bible for nutritionists and official nutrition policy, suggests a dietary ratio of 10:1 (11). It sets acceptable intakes (AIs) of 11-17 milligrams for linoleic acid (LA) and 1.1- 1.7 for alpha-linolenic acid (ALA).

The *Dietary Guidelines* acknowledge that high intakes of LA (parent of omega-6 family) create a pro-oxidant state (proinflammatory) that may predispose to several chronic diseases and that a growing body of evidence suggests that a higher intake of omega-3 EFAs may offer some protection against cardiovascular disease (11). Despite these concessions, the official recommendations ignore scientific data showing that ratios greater than 4:1 are proinflammatory. The importance of control of the dietary EFA ratio of omega-6: omega-3 is because many disease states are associated with an overproduction of eicosanoids derived from omega-6 EFAs (12).

Excesses of Specific Nutrients: In recent years, studies of the EFA composition of the American diet have revealed that the LA content (10) far exceeds the much smaller amount required for a healthful eicosanoid balance. Today, the average intake of dietary LA is about ten times higher than it should be. Biochemically, LA simply overwhelms the body's ability to prevent inflammatory disease such as atherosclerosis (13). This dietary debacle is the result of substituting vegetable seed oils for animal fats.

To date, the most complete information available on how nutrient excesses influence eicosanoid balance relates to dietary excesses of carbohydrates, notably sugar and starches. A meal high in carbohydrates, with its high glucose content, stimulates secretion of large amounts of the hormone insulin for the purpose of protecting the body from abrupt increases in blood glucose level. In addition to controlling blood glucose level, insulin has a number of other messenger biochemical functions, all of which it performs by influencing enzyme systems.

One of the enzyme systems influenced by insulin is delta-5-desaturase (D5D) in the omega-3/omega-6 metabolic cascade (see Figure 9-1). DGLA (dihomo gamma linolenic acid), the omega-6 metabolite in the cascade from LA, comes to a divide in the pathway just prior to entry of D5D. DGLA can either go to PG1 or 15 HETrE anti-inflammatory eicosanoids or to AA (arachidonic acid), which yields proinflammatory eicosanoids. The controlling factor in which pathway is followed is the enzyme D5D, which is stimulated by insulin. When stimulated, D5D increases the rate of synthesis of arachidonic acid; when not stimulated or when inhibited, synthesis of PG1 or 15 HETrE are favored.

Thus, high insulin levels are detrimental to a healthful eicosanoid balance. Although it is high insulin levels that stimulate the production of arachidonic acid, the dietary component initially responsible for insulin release is a carbohydrate (glucose). Meals that are low in carbohydrate exert little or no effect on insulin release.

Deficiencies of Micronutrients: Although not well explored, it is known that deficiencies of some essential nutrients such as vitamins or minerals can result in disturbances of biochemical pathways that, in turn, disrupt normal biochemical functioning. Any disturbance of normal biochemistry has the potential for creating a proinflammatory environment and eliciting changes in eicosanoid balance.

B Vitamins: Deficiencies of vitamins B_6, B_{12}, and folic acid have been shown to cause disruption of the methyl transfer process and result in high blood homocysteine levels, which have long been known as a risk factor for cardiovascular disease (14). Homocysteine, a normal metabolite of the essential amino acid methionine, has an important role in methyl group metabolism. However, when blood levels of homocysteine are too high, they are inflammatory and damage arterial walls. This proinflammatory effect is presumed to be due to the ability of high levels of homocysteine to cause release of arachidonic acid (AA) from its phospholipid (15).

With B-vitamin deficiency and homocysteine, as with carbohydrates and insulin, the relation between diet and eicosanoid imbalance is indirect. The dietary deficiency influences some aspect of the body's biochemistry, which, in turn, alters the eicosanoid balance. Never-the-less, the dietary defect is an obligatory precondition for the eicosanoid imbalance to occur.

Antioxidants: A deficiency of dietary antioxidants can be very damaging to eicosanoid balance. EFAs with three or more double bonds, primarily AA, EPA, and DHA, are very fragile and subject to oxidation. When antioxidant protection is not available, the fragile EFAs are destroyed by direct oxidation or by a nonenzymatic oxidation reaction to eicosanoid-like chemicals termed isoprostanes. The isoprostanes are associated with diseases of the brain; however, it is not known if there is a causal relationship or whether isoprostanes are merely markers of oxidative stress (16).

The existence of isoprostanes recalls the old adage that life is an oxidative process. An organism takes in food and extracts energy from it in the form of little electrons that are passed around until they are finally eliminated. Oxidized products (chemicals that have lost their electrons) are constantly being formed within us – by our metabolism, by our immune systems in their war on invaders, by the oxygen we breathe, and by the cosmic rays that shoot through us from outer space. All of these oxidized compounds are grouped together under the label of ROS – reactive oxygen species.

ROS must be neutralized or eliminated from the body before they do damage. This is the job of the antioxidants in the diet. Probably the best known of the antioxidants are vitamins C and E, but fruits and most vegetables are packed with antioxidants. Interestingly, those from fruits are usually highly colored. A build-up of ROS in the body does a great deal of damage to a variety of functions and provides an internal oxidizing environment that promotes cancer.

The Diseases

The increasing incidence of obesity over the last few decades, which is now extending to younger and younger age groups, has brought with it the realization that the burden of excess body weight reaches far beyond the physical strain on the lower back, hips, legs, and knees. Although it had been suspected for decades that obesity was associated with other chronic diseases such as diabetes and heart disease, it wasn't until Gerald Reaven gave this group of ailments the name Syndrome X (now known as Metabolic Syndrome) that the cluster became appreciated as having a similar metabolic dysfunction (17).

It is now recognized that obesity is a credible risk factor not only for type-2 diabetes, high blood pressure, coronary heart disease, and stroke but also for certain cancers such as breast, uterine, prostate, and colon cancers. In addition, recent studies indicate that overweight and obesity are also associated with all-cause dementia, Alzheimer's disease, and underlying neurodegenerative changes (18). Overweight nearly doubles the risk of dementia in old age, and, if the overweight is largely abdominal fat, the risk is boosted to 3.6 times that of a normal-weight individual (19). Not all obese persons will develop one or more or the chronic diseases associated with obesity, but most will (20).

This remarkable circumstance of overweight and obesity being a focal point for a wide variety of chronic diseases prompts the question of what is the cause of excess adiposity (body fat tissue). Examination of this question is basic to the study of the diet/disease association because overweight and obesity are directly connected to dietary excess.

The conclusion that a diet that produces obesity is a proinflammatory diet is supported by evidence that shows that adipose tissue is active metabolically and that it produces a series of biochemicals that are inflammatory (21). Thus, the appropriate beginning of a review of the relationship between diet and chronic diseases is obesity and the diet that causes it.

OVERWEIGHT AND OBESITY

Differences in genetic makeup exert an influence on body weight as they do in all other aspects of the human condition. Some people become obese while others, who seemingly eat the same foods, stay slim. The contribution of genetic factors to obesity is estimated to be 30 to 40 percent, while the contribution of diet and physical activity is estimated to be 60 to 70 percent (21). Regardless of the genetic tendencies that govern a person's body weight, the biochemical reactions that direct the deposition of fat in the obese person are the same as those that direct fat deposition in the slim person.

THE BODY MASS INDEX (BMI): The BMI is the official measure of overweight, obesity, and extreme obesity. Normal weight is under 25; overweight is described as a BMI between 25 and 29.9; obesity is a BMI of more of than 30; and extreme obesity is a BMI of 40 or more. Most people have a pretty good idea of whether or not they are obese, but overweight can be a bit more difficult to recognize (or accept). Anyone concerned about health and nutritional status should know his or her BMI. It is a good benchmark for following a few pounds of weight loss or gain. To calculate the BMI in pounds and inches rather than the standard kilograms and meters: multiply body weight in pounds by 704.5 and then divide the product by height in inches squared. Instructions for calculating the BMI are repeated in Chapter Twelve.

THE OBESITY TO DIABETES PROGRESSION

The pathway from normal weight through obesity to diabetes starts with a customary dietary pattern of high carbohydrate intake. The usual sequence is hypoglycemia (unstable blood glucose), insulin resistance, obesity, and ultimately type-2 diabetes.

HYPOGLYCEMIA: Hypoglycemia is the term used to describe blood glucose levels that are at or below the low end of the normal range. The symptoms are hunger, headaches, irritability, lightheadedness, a feeling of cold, and a lack of energy. Symptoms such as these are common complaints today in the United States. They are increasingly the reasons for doctor visits by people who do not feel well.

It is important to note that hypoglycemia may be a symptom of other serious diseases, but those diseases are not usually the cause for most cases of hypoglycemia. Almost all cases of hypoglycemia are the result of excessive levels of insulin in the blood. Thus, the most common cause of hypoglycemia, which is more properly called reactive hypoglycemia, is unhealthful dietary habits (22, p. 459).

A high-carbohydrate snack or meal, particularly one composed largely of sugar and/or refined carbohydrates, triggers a series of events that lead a person down the road toward reactive hypoglycemia. First, the carbohydrate snack is immediately converted to glucose, which causes a rapid rise in blood glucose. Second, the rapid rise in blood glucose prompts the pancreas to respond with secretion of an abnormally high level of insulin in an emergency-like attempt to keep blood glucose levels from rising too high (23, p. 710). Third, within a short period of time, the excess insulin drives the blood glucose levels down to low or below normal levels, thereby causing symptoms of hypoglycemia. At this point, a fork in the road is reached. One path leads to a return to a normal insulin/glucagon balance – the other to reactive hypoglycemia.

A FORK IN THE ROAD: The path that leads to a return to a normal insulin/glucagon balance is one that satisfies hunger with snacks and meals that are balanced in protein, low-glycemic carbohydrates, and fats. The path that leads to reactive hypoglycemia is one that follows an unhealthful dietary habit – repeatedly satisfying hunger with high sugar/starch snacks and soft drinks. Why is the latter an unhealthful dietary habit? Because a high-carbohydrate snack, as explained above, causes a rapid rise in blood glucose followed by a rapid drop, which brings a feeling of hunger and weakness that demands a second snack. The second snack relieves the symptoms briefly by supplying more glucose, but then restarts the hypoglycemic cycle with production of excess insulin. With time, this sort of dietary pattern can cause almost constant vague feelings of irritability, fatigue, and general ill health.

REACTIVE HYPOGLYCEMIA: Reactive hypoglycemia is more appropriately thought of as unstable blood glucose rather than low blood glucose (24, p. 142). This is because the dietary pattern described above results in swings between very high blood glucose (hyperglycemia) followed by very low blood glucose in roller-coaster-like fashion. Reactive hypoglycemia can be prevented by avoiding snacks or meals that are primarily sugars and refined starches – sweet rolls, cookies, cakes, donuts, candy bars, and soft drinks, including diet soft drinks. As seen in the chapter on carbohydrates, the use of artificial sweeteners is no remedy. Sugar substitutes, like sugar, stimulate the secretion of insulin (25; 26). One could speculate that sugar substitutes might be more detrimental than sugar. The addition of insulin to blood in the absence of a dietary glucose source (sugar) could result in even lower blood glucose levels.

Reactive hypoglycemia does not occur in people who routinely restrict refined carbohydrates and sugars in their diets. An occasional high-carbohydrate snack or meal will cause blood insulin levels to rise quickly to cope with the high blood glucose levels. Hunger pangs and drowsiness may occur several hours after eating as the result of lowered blood glucose levels. However, because the pancreas is not abused by repeated unhealthful dietary practices, it does not react with an excessive amount of insulin that remains in the blood long after it is needed. In people with healthy pancreatic function, insulin levels will drop to match the drop in glucose. The drop in insulin levels permits the release of glucagon that, in turn, releases stored glycogen and converts it into glucose to keep blood glucose from dropping further.

INSULIN RESISTANCE: Reactive hypoglycemia typically leads to insulin resistance. Insulin resistance, as the term implies, is a resistance by the cells of the body to the presence of insulin. When insulin resistance occurs, the body's cells fail to permit insulin to transport glucose across their cell membranes. Insulin resistance might be thought of as an inability of cells to let insulin help them obtain the glucose they require for their life functions. The opposite condition, insulin sensitivity, in which the cells of the body are sensitive to insulin and readily accept the glucose that insulin delivers to them, is the normal state in healthy individuals.

How does reactive hypoglycemia, or more precisely unstable blood glucose, pave the way for insulin resistance? As described in the previous section, the up-and-down, roller-coaster swings in blood glucose concentration result in intermittent excessive secretion of insulin by the pancreas. With time and intermittent exposures to excesses of insulin, the mechanisms that enable cells to respond normally to insulin gradually become exhausted. The exact biochemical mechanism for the failure of cells to respond to insulin is not known (23, p. 717) but it is known that the lack of response by cells is not due to lack of insulin. The pancreas makes adequate amounts of insulin, but the cells are just not able to use the insulin efficiently to metabolize glucose.

As cells become more resistant to insulin, the fine-tuning of the relationship between blood glucose levels and the metabolic hormones, insulin and glucagon, is lost. The reduction in use of glucose by the cells and tissues of the body results in a gradual increase in the amount of glucose circulating in the blood, which, in turn, results in further excessive secretion of insulin (hyperinsulinemia) in an attempt to lower the glucose levels. The high-low swings in blood glucose, which are characteristic of reactive hypoglycemia, give way to longer periods of high blood glucose. This hyperglycemia is kept in check for as long as the pancreas is able to secrete adequate insulin.

An additional problem associated with hyperglycemia is the reaction of excessive blood glucose with body proteins to form new, harmful molecules known as advanced glycation end products. The brown skin spots that appear with aging are caused by glycation. Glycation end products are chemicals that hasten the aging process. They are thought to promote degenerative diseases such as Alzheimer's disease. It is also thought that many of the complications associated with diabetes are most likely the result of the combined effects of insulin resistance and advanced glycation end products.

The most obvious symptoms of insulin resistance are weight gain and feelings of fatigue and weakness that are sometimes overwhelming. The feelings of fatigue and weakness are due to what might be called cellular starvation. Cells and tissues cannot transfer sufficient glucose into themselves to provide the energy they require to function properly. Overwhelming fatigue is the result. Insulin resistance is also associated with high blood pressure, obesity, and high blood levels of triglycerides and LDL cholesterol, and low blood levels of HDL cholesterol. It is a final stage before type-2 diabetes.

Note in addition that the continued high insulin levels associated with insulin resistance cause further damage by stimulating the enzyme D5D (see Figure 9-1). D5D stimulation increases chronic inflammation and associated chronic diseases such as cardiovascular diseases, cancer, and senile dementias.

TYPE-2 DIABETES (ADULT-ONSET DIABETES, NIDDM)

The connection between obesity and type-2 diabetes is insulin resistance. As described above, repeated large releases of insulin into the bloodstream in response to high blood glucose levels cause the body's cells to become resistant to the stimulus of insulin. When this happens, the pancreas must secrete larger and larger amounts of insulin in an attempt to lower blood glucose. Fat cells do not become as resistant to insulin as easily as do other body cells; hence, the deposition of fat that is stimulated by insulin continues after other body cells become resistant.

In insulin resistance, despite increased secretion of insulin, blood glucose levels rise above normal because cells and tissues of the body are not able to remove glucose efficiently from the blood. Eventually, the pancreas becomes exhausted and reaches its insulin-production limit. This allows blood glucose to rise to unsafe levels, despite futile attempts by the pancreas to secrete sufficient insulin to lower them. The result is type-2 diabetes, also known as adult-onset or noninsulin dependent diabetes mellitus (NIDDM).

In addition, excessive blood glucose reacts with body proteins to form new, harmful molecules known as advanced glycation end products. The brown skin spots that appear with aging are caused by glycation. Glycation end products are chemicals that hasten the aging process. For example, they are thought to promote degenerative diseases such as those of Alzheimer's disease. It is also thought that many of the complications associated with diabetes are probably the result of the combined effects of insulin resistance and advanced glycation end products.

The progression from insulin resistance to type-2 diabetes is insidious. In many cases dietary change will prevent the disease. Therefore, it would be wise for anyone who is overweight or obese to seek medical assistance to evaluate his or her glucose tolerance status and take corrective action before any of the serious medical problems that are associated with the diabetic condition occur.

The risk of developing diabetes is estimated to increase 4.5 percent for every 2.2 pounds of extra body weight (27). Thus, people who are obese are prime candidates for type-2 diabetes. The long-forgotten name for type-2 diabetes was sugar diabetes, which reveals that early physicians had an intuitive appreciation that diabetes was caused by diet. The frequent association of diabetes and obesity has resulted in the combination of these two terms into the new word *diabesity*. Diabesity is one of the most common problems found in older patients and is a warning sign that the aging process is accelerating (28, p. 69).

In addition to obesity, people with type-2 diabetes often have an unusual craving for sugar and other sweets, which obviously greatly complicates treatment of the disease. In diabetes, the physiological mechanisms that regulate appetite often become deranged and result in a perverse craving for sugar (29, p. 115; see Chromium, Chapter Five). Other classic symptoms of diabetes, such as excessive thirst and frequent urination, may or may not occur in people with type-2 diabetes.

There are considerable data in the scientific literature indicating that there is a genetic component in the development of type-2 diabetes (23, p. 717; 30). Some people are more susceptible than others to dietary abuses that lead to type-2 diabetes. Given the same diet, some people will get this disease and others will not. This is an example of the concept of biochemical individuality (29, p. 115). People are different, not only in susceptibility to diabetes but also in their susceptibility to virtually all chronic diseases.

Despite differences in susceptibility to type-2 diabetes, there is strong clinical and epidemiological evidence that the underlying cause for most victims of the disease is consumption of excessive sugar and starches. Perhaps more convincing evidence that diet is a major cause of type-2 diabetes is that it often can be reversed by simple changes in diet (23, p. 717; 31, p. 46; 32, p. 91). Drs. Fries and Vickery ask, "Is a condition that is remedied with diet and exercise a disease? Or just a bad habit?" (28, p. 68).

An interesting clinical observation reported by Dr Schwarzbein validates the biochemistry showing that inflammation, caused by the flawed nutrition practices endorsed by the Food Guide Pyramid, is responsible for the association between type-2 diabetes and heart disease. Dr. Schwarzbein, an endocrinologist with a large type-2 diabetes practice, noticed that many of her patients had a large scar down the middle of the chest, indicating that they had had heart bypass surgery before they had been diagnosed with type-2 diabetes. The implication suddenly occurred to her:

> After a heart attack, people are told to go on a low fat-diet, high-carbohydrate diet—which increases both their blood-sugar and insulin levels. *The increases in blood sugar and insulin were turning heart patients into diabetics.* The newly created diabetics are then told to continue eating a diet high in carbohydrates, which further elevates their blood-sugar and insulin levels (33, p. xxi).

THE DIET-DISEASE CONNECTION: The known biochemical pathways and regulatory mechanisms that govern synthesis and deposition of body fat, as mentioned in Chapter Six, support the conclusions that today's epidemic of obesity is primarily the result of excessive intake of carbohydrate foods, particularly sugars and starches, and that dietary fat and protein are not issues in the causation of weight gain and obesity. Despite the role that genetic factors play in certain cases of obesity, the nutritional influences that govern eicosanoid balance are the same for the obese person as for the slim person.

Dietary carbohydrates and the hormone insulin are key agents not only in the synthesis and storage of body fat but also in the production of a proinflammatory environment in the body. The foods that bring insulin into play are almost exclusively carbohydrate foods. As described above and in Chapter Nine, the enzyme delta-5-desaturase (D5D) controls whether the omega-6 fatty acid DGLA will follow a proinflammatory or an anti-inflammatory path (Figure 9-1). Insulin stimulates D5D and sends DGLA to proinflammatory eicosanoids via AA. Chronic stimulation of D5D promotes chronic diseases.

NONCARBOHYDRATE PROINFLAMMATORY INFLUENCES: In addition to the well known action of excess sugar and starch in causing proinflammatory eicosanoid imbalance, it appears that other noncarbohydrate dietary components can also have the same effect. Statistics revealed that by 1997 the prevalence of adult-onset diabetes had grown explosively in India in the prior twenty years to the point where India then had the greatest number of cases in the world (34). This increase in diabetes was correlated with the replacement of the traditional dietary fats, coconut oil and clarified butter (ghee), by modern polyunsaturated vegetable oils high in omega-6 fatty acids. In the summary of the original paper, Raheja states that a high omega-6 to omega-3 ratio in the diet appears to be very strongly related to adult-onset diabetes (35).

A study cited by Murray (22, p. 246) showing that omega-3 fatty acids improve insulin action, reduce insulin resistance, and protect against adult-onset diabetes (type-2 diabetes) supports the conclusion of Raheja. Murray also cites a study indicating that high levels of omega-6 metabolites in serum cholesterol significantly predicted the development of adult-onset diabetes. These data indicate that inflammation induced by a high dietary ratio of omega-6/omega-3 EFAs, which is known to be proinflammatory, has a role in the etiology of chronic diseases associated with obesity.

CARDIOVASCULAR DISEASES

Those who make American nutrition policy have claimed for many years that saturated fats are the major cause of cardiovascular diseases despite the conclusion from an extensive, in-depth review of data from dozens of scientific studies from around the world that the data do not support the claim (36). Scientific facts to the contrary, the nutrition establishment apparently will not relinquish its lipid-hypothesis dogma. For instance, the 2005 dietary guidelines recommend that "individuals maintain their saturated fatty acid consumption as low as possible…" (11).

More recently, the minutes of the 2010 Dietary Guideline Advisory Committee meetings state that dietary saturated fat and cholesterol will continue to be considered major risk factors for CHD (coronary heart disease) in the foreseeable future. The minutes also question whether the proscription against saturated fat and cholesterol should be made even more restrictive because the current recommendations do not seem to be stringent enough to reverse the ever-increasing attack rates of heart disease (37). In view of the continuing official support for high blood cholesterol as a risk factor for cardiovascular disease, a brief revisit to the subject of cholesterol is appropriate.

CHOLESTEROL: Contrary to popular belief, cholesterol is a very important and necessary biochemical. It is a precursor of the steroid hormones, including the male and female sex hormones, the adrenal cortical hormones, and vitamin D. Cholesterol also participates in many other life functions. The biochemistry of cholesterol is outlined in Chapter Eight. Its synthesis by the body, stimulated by insulin, is detailed in the sections on glucose, insulin, and glucagon in Chapter Six and diagrammed in Figure 6-3.

With the exception of rare cases of hypercholesterolemia caused by a genetic defect in cholesterol metabolism, referred to as familial hypercholesterolemia, there seems to be little disagreement that high blood cholesterol is a nutritional event. However, there is considerable lack of accord on what nutritional components are responsible. Medical and nutritional groups remain steadfast in their judgment that dietary fats and cholesterol are the culprits, while biochemistry says it is insulin secreted in response to high-glycemic dietary patterns that directs the body to synthesize cholesterol in excess of its needs.

The common atherosclerotic diseases, coronary heart disease, stroke, and hypertension, are associated with high cholesterol levels in the blood. However, the biochemistry of cholesterol supports the view that high blood cholesterol levels are not a cause of atherosclerosis but rather both are symptoms of an unhealthful diet. Medical and nutrition journals are replete with papers demonstrating the association between hypercholesterolemia (high blood cholesterol) and atherosclerosis and between atherosclerosis and cardiovascular diseases. However, there is no scientific proof that high cholesterol causes atherosclerosis or cardiovascular disease (38).

ATHEROSCLEROTIC DISEASES: Atherosclerosis is an advanced form of arteriosclerosis that is characterized by hardened arteries that contain plaques with calcium, fats, blood clots, and deposits of cholesterol within their artery walls. It is generally accepted that the progression from healthy arterial walls to arteriosclerosis begins with inflammation of the cells and tissues of the arteries. With continued inflammation, damage increases and the body attempts to cover and repair the injured areas with new layers of cholesterol; arteriosclerosis accordingly becomes atherosclerosis. Continued thickening of the walls gradually narrows the lumen of arteries and may eventually occlude them.

The uncertainty is not about the sequence of events in the development of atherosclerosis or whether inflammation is the initiating event but rather about what is the trigger that starts the inflammation in arterial walls. In 1969, McCully proposed that deficiencies of vitamins B_6, B_{12}, and folic acid disrupt the methyl transfer cycle (see Figure 7-1) with the result that the amino acid homocysteine builds up to high levels in the blood. High levels of homocysteine damage the cells and tissues of arteries, causing inflammation, arteriosclerosis, and ultimately atherosclerosis (14).

Ravnskov proposed that the initiator of arterial wall inflammation is infection (39). When low density lipoproteins (LDL, with or without cholesterol attached) bind microbial material, their structures change and they tend to aggregate. If an LDL aggregate blocks a capillary in the arterial wall, the part of the wall that is nourished by that capillary may die, enabling the aggregate and its microbial contents to enter into the tissues of the wall and start an inflammation.

At this point a crossroad is reached. A healthy immune system will resolve the problem and heal the breach with a fibrous plaque. A defective immune system may lead to the following scenario: The LDL mass, associated blood, cholesterol, and other debris form a microscopic boil, also known as a vulnerable plaque, on the inner surface of the artery wall. When a plaque bursts, its contents spill into the lumen, a clot forms, and the artery is occluded. The homocysteine theory of McCully and the infection theory of Ravnskov are not incompatible. Both are scientifically plausible. They may merely represent two mechanisms by which the same outcome is achieved.

HYPERTENSION: Since the beginning of modern medicine, normal blood pressure has been defined as 120mm Hg (millimeters, mercury) during heart muscle contractions (systole) and 80mm between contractions (diastole) and hypertension as a sustained increase in blood pressure, usually greater than 140/90mm. However, in recent years, a new category for which medication may be considered has been identified; patients with pressures between 120-139mm and 80-89mm are now labeled prehypertensive (40).

Notwithstanding the arbitrary criteria, the diagnosis of hypertension is often complicated by individual variations of normal in otherwise healthy individuals and by numerous circumstances that can cause a transitory increase. Blood pressures not only tend to show small variations in normal but they also are apt to increase with age (41). However, it is debatable whether the latter is normal or due to pathologies attending the aging process.

When arteriosclerotic arteries become hardened they lose their flexibility. As a result, the heart has to work harder against the resistance in the arteries, causing a rise in blood pressure. The increased blood pressure can put a strain on the heart, forcing it to work harder. For example, a strain on the left ventricle of the heart (the ventricle that delivers blood from the heart to all parts of the body) can cause its muscle to thicken and weaken. Increased blood pressure can also cause a damaged artery to break, precipitating a heart attack or stroke, depending on the location of the break.

Heart Disease: Atherosclerotic disease in which the coronary arteries are affected is called coronary heart disease (CAD). Early symptoms of CAD are squeezing pains in the chest (angina pectoris), usually brought on by exertion. The symptoms are due to limitation of the delivery of oxygen to the myocardium (heart muscle) by one or more of the narrowed or occluded coronary arteries.

Sudden complete occlusion of a coronary artery deprives the area of the myocardium served by that artery of its blood supply. The deprived area becomes necrotic and dies. This is called a myocardial infarction. The outcome of the event depends upon the severity of the infarction. The usual cause of arterial occlusion is clot formation (thrombus) or hemorrhage at the site of atherosclerotic narrowing. It may also be caused by closure of the lumen by proliferation of plaques or by a hemorrhage into the arterial wall.

Stroke: Cerebrovascular accidents or strokes are the names given to events that cause cerebral infarctions. The most common cause of stroke is hemorrhage from a rupture of an atherosclerotic cerebral artery. Cerebral infarctions may also be caused by occlusion of a cerebral artery by an embolus. The symptoms of a stroke are dependent on the area of the brain affected and the extent of the infarction.

CONGESTIVE HEART FAILURE (CHF): Congestive heart failure is the term used to describe the clinical symptoms produced by the inability of the heart to pump sufficient blood to meet the metabolic needs of the body (42). Depending on the reason for the insufficiency, there may be right ventricle failure (delivery to the lungs), left ventricle failure (delivery to the body), or combined failure in later stages of insufficiency.

Right ventricle failure, described as "cor pulmonale, is less common and usually secondary to obstructive lung disease. Left ventricle failure is most commonly due to hypertension, myocardial infections, coronary heart disease, and, to a lesser extent, heart valve defects. The initial response of a ventricle to increased resistance to blood flow is hypertrophy; the heart muscle thickens in an attempt to increase cardiac output. As the output gradually becomes less able to serve the body's needs, the ventricular space becomes larger and the muscle becomes thicker and weaker. This is the pathway to clinical congestive heart failure.

Interestingly, the great increase in cases of CHF closely parallel the increase in sales of statin drugs (see Chapter Two). Statin drugs not only inhibit the biosynthesis of cholesterol but also inhibit the biosynthesis of Q10. The reversal of adverse effects of statin therapy by administration of Q10 is proof that the association between CHF and statin drugs is a causal one (43). This appears to be a situation in which a drug designed to treat one kind of heart disease has the unintended consequence of causing another kind.

Even more worrisome than the unintended consequence of causing CHF by treatment with statin drugs in people with high blood cholesterol is a recent news report that portends a tremendous increase in such outcomes of iatric negligence. The U. S. Food and Drug Administration has approved the expanded use of the statin drug Crestor in people who do not have cardiovascular disease (CVD) or high blood cholesterol, a group previously considered not at risk of CVD. The justification for this decision was the "Jupiter" study claim that patients on Crestor had a 44 percent reduction in CVD-associated events (in a less than 2-year study) than did patients on a placebo (44).

Thus, Crestor, a statin drug, has now been approved as preventive treatment for CVD. This decision will substantially boost the 2008 Crestor sales of $3.8 billion by adding up to 6 million new recipients of the drug (45). The discouraging fact is that the baby-aspirin-a-day treatment has a safer and better CVD preventive record than any statin drug (46) and is second only to smoking cessation as the most effective use of CVD prevention resources (47).

THE DIET-DISEASE CONNECTION: Many of the cardiovascular diseases that have long been assumed to be afflictions of the aging process are, in fact, nutritional diseases produced by silent inflammation. If saturated fats and cholesterol are not to blame, what dietary components are? An examination of the dietary links to CVD shows that one or more nutritional imbalances, excesses, and/or deficiencies contribute to CVDs.

Numerous epidemiological studies reveal the importance of the balance between omega-6 and omega-3 EFAs for cardiovascular health. For example, a study of 1,300 men in Europe found that those with the highest levels of omega-3 fatty acids in their tissues had the lowest heart attack rates (48). A study of more than 43,000 men in the United States, aged 40 to 75, showed that the rate of myocardial infarction decreased with increasing intake of omega-3 alpha-linolenic acid (49). The latter study concluded that the data support a specific preventive effect against myocardial infarction by alpha-linolenic acid intake. Interestingly, the authors also concluded that their data did *not* support an association between dietary intake of saturated fat and coronary heart disease.

Excessive consumption of carbohydrates, primarily in the form of sugar and starch, is a major factor in the development of atherosclerotic diseases. As described in Chapter Nine, glucose released from food stimulates the secretion of the hormone insulin. In addition to sending acetyl CoA to body fat and cholesterol, insulin stimulates delta 5-desaturase, which directs DGLA to the biosynthesis of proinflammatory AA (Figure 9-1).

Finally, the fact that proinflammatory blood levels of homocysteine resulting from a deficiency of B-vitamins can cause arteriosclerosis (14) confirms the theory that a nutritional deficiency has the potential to create a proinflammatory environment and cause cardiovascular disease. The fact that homocysteine is capable of causing inflammation is supported by demonstration of its ability to release arachidonic acid, the precursor of proinflammatory eicosanoids, from cellular membranes (15).

CANCER

Cancer is a feared disease that is not well understood and in many cases seemingly impossible to cure. Cancer is a malignant process whereby an otherwise normal cell becomes deviant, grows unrestrainedly, and ultimately invades surrounding tissues. Because it can strike just about any organ or tissue, in any stage of its host's life cycle, cancer is often thought of as a collection of diseases. However, such is not the case. Cancers, once formed, all follow a similar course of unrestricted growth and invasiveness and are treated medically with the same therapeutic regime.

THE ROLE OF MUTATIONS: The conventional theory of cancer causation is that a cell somewhere in the body undergoes a mutation that causes that cell to become deviant. The kinds, number, and/or sequence of mutations required for initiation of cancer development is still a matter of speculation. Mutations are not rare events; they are caused by agents that damage cellular DNA. Commonly known examples are cosmic rays, sunlight, x-rays, other forms of ionizing radiation, and carcinogenic chemicals.

It is estimated that humans carry many thousands of mutated cells all of the time, but most are repaired or destroyed by the body's protective systems as soon as they are created. All living organisms have several levels of biochemical repair systems within them to detect and repair genetic damage (50; 51). Cancers are the result of failures in these protective systems.

THE ROLE OF INFLAMMATION: Modern medicine, which has long assumed that cancer is associated with inflammation, now accepts the fact that cancer is, in fact, the result of chronic inflammation. A major cause of chronic inflammation is unhealthful nutritional habits. Although numerous defects in the current official American nutrition policy can be cited as promoters of chronic inflammation, it would be simplistic to indict any one defect as the sole culprit. Rather, a lifetime of nutritional excesses, imbalances, and deficiencies must be charged with the responsibility for the current attack rates of cancer now being experienced by the public.

NORMAL VERSUS CANCER CELLS: In order to evaluate the role of nutrition in the conditions that promote cancer development, it would be instructive to look at what are the differences between normal cells and their malignant brethren who have lost their identity as kin.

In an excellent presentation of their theory that cancer development can best be understood as the microevolution of damaged cells (52), Hickey and Roberts describe the differences between normal and cancer cells: cancer cells grow uncontrollably, fail to breed true, and are long-lived; they are variable in size and shape with nuclei that are distorted, over-sized, and usually contain a greater number of chromosomes than normal; and they abandon the restrictions that controlled the growth of their parent cells. Probably the most important difference between normal and cancer cells is their metabolism, namely the sum of biochemical reactions that underlie all aspects of cellular growth, reproduction, and death.

Cellular Metabolism: Although oxygen is essential for cellular functioning, an excess can do oxidative damage by stealing electrons from vital biochemicals. Free radicals, which can be generated by a cell's own metabolic activity, also do oxidative damage. Healthy cells must constantly be protected against oxidative damage.

Cellular metabolism is governed by a cell's redox environment. The balance between reduction and oxidation in a cell is referred to as its redox environment. Normal, healthy cells have a reducing environment, whereas the environment in cancer cells is oxidizing. The redox environment is a measure of cellular health.

Healthy cells have a surplus of antioxidants. Antioxidants defend against injurious oxidations and provide cells with a reducing redox environment. The body's own metabolism provides some antioxidants (e.g. glutathione, coenzyme Q10, and alpha-lipoic acid) but the major source of antioxidants, including the essential vitamins C and E, must be provided in food. Healthy cells have enzymatic redox cycles that protect antioxidants against oxidative pressures.

Cancer cells, on the other hand, contain a high level of oxidants. The ability of cancer cells to defend themselves against oxidation is poor; their antioxidant defenses are deficient. As far as is known, no cancer has a full complement of defenses against free radical attack (52, p. 60). On the contrary, the redox cycle mechanism fails in cancer cells and as a result large amounts of oxidants are produced.

Glucose as the Energy Source: An oxidative redox state stimulates growth and cell division, which promotes and greatly increases a cancer's mass. As cancer cells multiply and the tumor becomes larger, their supply of oxygen is pushed father away from them and, of necessity, they rely more and more on anaerobic metabolism. The metabolic pathway known as glycolysis (see Figure 6-1) produces metabolic energy in a series of reactions from glucose to pyruvate without a need for oxygen. Although cancer cells can use oxygen they are more dependent than normal cells on glucose as a source of energy.

Ascorbic Acid: Ascorbic acid is an essential nutrient that serves as the major water-soluble antioxidant in the extra-cellular fluid of the body. In good health, it normally acts as an antioxidant, but cancer cells handle ascorbic acid differently from normal cells. The details of the behavior of ascorbic acid in cancer cells are intricate, but ultimately they depend on the ability of ascorbic acid to act as an oxidant (*not* as an antioxidant). The great therapeutic benefit of oxidized ascorbic acid is that it can kill cancer cells without harming normal cells (53).

In brief, the mechanism whereby ascorbic acid destroys cancer cells is that when it enters the oxidizing environment of a cancer, it is oxidized to dehydroascorbic acid. Because of structural similarity between dehydroascorbic acid and glucose (cancer's preferred energy source), cancer cells cannot distinguish between them. Thus, when dehydroascorbic acid is present in high concentrations it competes effectively with glucose for active transport into cancer cells by glucose pumps. Once inside, dehydroascorbic acid generates hydrogen peroxide and other oxidants that the cancer cells cannot counter. The very high levels of hydrogen peroxide cause either apoptosis (programmed cell death) or necrosis of cancer cells.

THE DIET-DISEASE CONNECTION: Although numerous defects in the current official American nutrition policy can be cited as promoters of chronic inflammation, it would be simplistic to indict any one as the sole culprit as a cause of cancer. Rather, a lifetime of nutritional excesses, imbalances, and deficiencies must be charged with the responsibility for the current attack rates of cancer now being experienced by the public.

Because of cancer's long latent period and the complexity of the dietary contributions to its development, the most intelligent – and only – answer to dealing with cancer is prevention. But, except for smoking cessation programs, modern medicine has no preventive programs for cancers. Current medical practice consists of early cancer detection and removal of the cancerous tissues with appropriate means such as surgery or destruction of these tissues with ionizing radiation and/or chemotherapy.

In recent years, the tremendous focus on discovering a cure for cancer has overwhelmed serious efforts to prevent cancer. America's only accomplishment in this direction has been a national smoking cessation program. It has been very effective in preventing both lung cancer and cardiovascular diseases. Importantly however, not all lung cancer or all cardiovascular diseases were prevented by smoking cessation – not all people stopped smoking. The lesson to be remembered when thinking about the possibility of cancer prevention working, is that a national voluntary educational smoking cessation program is preventing a large number lung cancers and cardiovascular diseases at very low cost.

CANCER PREVENTION: Today, it is known that many common cancers are caused by the modern American diet. This diet contains too much linoleic acid (LA) from vegetable fats and oils; a large excess of sugar and starch; an insufficiency of the essential fatty acids, EPA and DHA; and a deficiency of essential vitamins and minerals, particularly the antioxidants. Even minor dietary changes in this direction would help reduce national cancer attack rates.

ANTIOXIDANT INTAKE: The importance of a reducing environment within the body for cancer prevention is shown by the fact that just a moderate increase in the oxidative environment within cells can stimulate cell growth and division – an especially undesirable situation when defective cells are present. The redox environment is dependent on the antioxidant content of the diet. Dietary antioxidants are found primarily in fruits and vegetables. Probably the most important of the antioxidants is ascorbic acid. The daily intake should be 1000-2000 mg/day. A glass of orange juice may prevent scurvy, but it cannot provide sufficient antioxidant to have any impact on prevention of cancer.

Sugar/Starch Intake: A nutritional excess that bears a great deal of the responsibility for cancer causation is a chronic excess of high-glycemic carbohydrate foods, notably sugar and starch. The high and unstable blood glucose and insulin levels that accompany such a diet create a general proinflammatory milieu in the body by stimulating the delta-5-desaturase enzyme (see Figure 9-1).

Independent of its stimulation of proinflammatory eicosanoids, excess glucose interferes in the immune system's role in cancer prevention. It does so by competing with ascorbic acid for control of a secondary metabolic pathway known as the hexose monophosphate (HMP) shunt. As described in Chapter Six (Figure 6-2), the HMP shunt is a metabolic detour between glucose-6-phosphate and fructose-6-phosphate of the glycolytic pathway that it supports the immune system in its role of host defense.

Glucose inhibits the HMP shunt and ascorbic acid stimulates it. Because entry into the shunt has no preference for either glucose or ascorbic acid, it will follow the directive of whichever of the two is in excess. A great excess of glucose, a deficiency of ascorbic acid, or both seriously affect the body's immune function capabilities, which is a significant liability for cancer prevention. Fortunately, the body supports the large demand for ascorbic acid by immune system cells by actively transporting ascorbic acid to them against a plasma gradient (see Figure 6-2).

Excess sugar is not only detrimental in a cancer-prevention diet but also in a cancer-therapy diet. Glucose is the preferred food for cancer cells; therefore, any cancer patient would be wise to avoid foods that nourish cancer and promote its growth. An interesting added benefit from a short-term, low-carbohydrate, calorie-restricted ketogenic diet appears to be elevated blood antioxidative capacity with no increase in oxidative stress in healthy individuals (55).

MICRONUTRIENT DEFICIENCIES: Deficiencies of any one or more micronutrients have the potential to cause DNA damage, thereby setting the stage for cancer formation (56). For example, vitamin D has been shown to have potent anticancer properties (57). Data from a review of 63 epidemiological studies (1966-2004) suggest that supplementation to improve vitamin D status could reduce cancer incidence and mortality (58). Another example is vitamin B_6: The connection between low blood levels of vitamin B_6, inflammatory markers, and the occurrence of inflammatory diseases was confirmed by examination of over 4,000 participants of the NHANES (National Health and Nutrition Examination Survey) 2003-2004 annual survey (59).

A review of the scientific evidence supporting the benefits of a cancer-prevention diet contains a long list of micronutrients considered to be of especial benefit in cancer prevention. It also estimates that 30 to 40 percent of all cancer could be prevented by dietary and lifestyle changes alone. The review further proposes that a diet following the guidelines prescribed in the review could result in as much as a 60-70 percent decrease in incidence of certain cancers (60).

ESSENTIAL FATTY ACIDS: It is well established that the dietary omega-6 to omega-3 EFA ratio plays an important role in the carcinogenic process, tumor proliferation, signaling, and induction of apoptosis (61). The scientific literature is replete with epidemiological and clinical studies suggesting that omega-3 fatty acids inhibit and omega-6 fatty acids promote carcinogenesis. Potential mechanisms for explaining how intakes of omega-3 fatty acids modify the risks for development of breast, prostate, and other hormonal-related cancers are reviewed by Larson (62). The scientific literature offers great, unexploited opportunities to the nutrition and medical communities for dietary solutions that offer promise of success not only in the prevention but also in the treatment of cancers.

DISEASES OF THE EYE

Increasing numbers of older adults are suffering from impaired vision in the form of age-related macular degeneration (AMD), detached retina, and diabetic retinopathy. All three of these diseases are preventable.

AGE-RELATED MACULAR DEGENERATION (AMD): AMD is the leading cause of blindness in adults over 65 years old. It is estimated that more than 2 million residents of the United States have some form of AMD. Treatment is helpful, but often does not prevent some degree of blindness. Another 7 million individuals have diagnosable drusen, an early sign of AMD. Drusen are tiny white or yellow accumulations of extra-cellular material that build up under the retina (63). There are two forms of AMD, dry and a wet. The dry form is the most common. Vision is destroyed by slow degeneration of photo-receptors, which produces thinning of retinal layers and deposits of drusen. In the wet form, an inner retinal layer is damaged by invasive growth of new small blood vessels that lead to severe vision loss.

The cause of AMD is insufficient DHA to protect eye tissues caused by a combination of dietary deficiency of DHA and the oxidative destruction of DHA inside the body by dietary deficiency of antioxidants (63; 64).

DIABETIC RETINOPATHY: Diabetic retinopathy has become increasingly common because of the continually growing numbers of diabetes victims. About 45% of diabetics are found to have some stage of diabetic retinopathy at the time they are diagnosed as having diabetes. With this disease, vision loss occurs because blood vessels in the eyes are made increasingly more fragile by diabetes. These damaged blood vessels leak blood into the eye, blurring vision. Blood may also leak into the center of the eye where straight-ahead vision occurs; this results in swelling of the eye and blurred vision (65).

Diabetic retinopathy is completely preventable by avoiding type-2 diabetes (28; 31; 32). This is done by following the personal prevention program at the end of Chapter 11. Briefly, the personal prevention program entails minimizing dietary sugar and starches, controlling LA intake, and balancing essential fatty acids by increasing dietary intake of EPA and DHA. This solves the diabetic retinopathy problem.

DETACHED RETINA: Detached retina occurs when the retina peels away from its normal location at the back of the eye. Blindness always occurs unless there is prompt treatment. Detached retina occurs mostly in older adults and is believed to be the result of trauma or a family history of this disease (66). However, there is also evidence that retinal detachment can almost certainly be prevented by ample dietary DHA and anti-oxidants (64).

DIET-DISEASE CONNECTION: Photoreceptor cells are exposed to light, oxygen, and other stresses that create reactive oxygen free radicals capable of quickly destroying these delicate cells. In the absence of antioxidants, oxidative stress also destroys DHA (67).

The photoreceptor cells in the eyes contain more DHA than any other cells in the body (63). DHA deprivation in animals causes impairments of retinal and brain functions (64). In order to protect the eyes, DHA continually flows via the blood stream to the photoreceptor cells and other sensitive parts of the eyes (64). This DHA is converted via 15-lipoxygenase-1 into neuroprotectin NPD1. NPD1 is a potent lipid mediator that induces cell-protective, pro-survival, anti-inflammatory repair actions that prevent and/or halt progression of retinal degenerative diseases (66). In short, DHA via NPD1 protects and repairs damage due to retinal aging, inflammation, bright light, and oxidation.

IMPORTANCE OF ANTIOXIDANTS: The DHA molecule is easily oxidized and destroyed by normal oxidative stress in the sensitive tissues of the eyes. Hence, healthy eyes require antioxidants to protect the all-important DHA. Nature handles this problem by bringing a dietary anti-oxidant, lutein, into the eye. Research shows that lutein is concentrated in the macula, a small area of the retina that is responsible for central vision.

Lutein is a natural antioxidant that is abundant in the green leaves of plants. It is assumed that lutein is naturally concentrated in the eye to protect it from oxidative stress. This belief has been confirmed by studies showing that dietary lutein/zeaxanthin intake is independently associated with a decreased likelihood of macular degeneration (68).

MENTAL DISORDERS

Mental disorders take many forms, with a wide array of manifestations and intensity of symptoms. They occur unexpectedly in all age groups, independent of gender or economic status. The main diagnostic categories used by Abram Hoffer, the father of orthomolecular psychiatry are: 1) schizophrenias; 2) mood disorders, i.e. depression; 3) addictions; 4) children with learning or behavioral disorders; 5) adult personal or behavioral disorders; and 6) organic disorders, i.e. Alzheimer's disease, strokes (69).

Studies suggesting that unhealthful dietary habits could have a significant impact on psychiatric disorders have recently begun to appear in the scientific literature. Perhaps the least cynical explanation for rejecting a link between diet and disease is that of Hoffer.

… our findings violated several basic beliefs then common to psychiatry: [One] That schizophrenia was not a disease, it was a way of life resulting from conscious or subconscious psychosocial problems…The profession's opinion that since the disease had no biochemical basis, giving any vitamin, no matter the dose, would do no good…It followed that giving vitamins was useless, wasteful, and even dangerous because of hypothetical toxicities (69, p.161).

Orthomolecular psychiatry, if not modern psychiatry, accepts the premise that the brain is a physical organ that requires adequate and appropriate nutrition just as all the other organs and tissues of the body do to function properly. The imperative to consider nutrition as a key participant in causation of psychiatric disorders is found in paleobiology. Docosahexaenoic acid (DHA), a 22-carbon, 6-double bond, omega-3 fatty acid, and arachidonic acid (AA), a 20-carbon, 4-double bond, omega-6 fatty acid were determinants of evolution not only of life forms 3 billion years ago but also of the human brain with the appearance of the first hominid ancestors 4 million years ago (70).

The utilization of omega-6 fatty acids from the land-based food chain and omega-3 fatty acids from the marine-based food chain, in a ratio between 1:1 and 2:1, played a critical role throughout the eons in development of the brain of the modern-day human. The paleobiological record is compelling evidence for the absolute nutritional requirement for the essential fatty acids. Maternal omega-3 malnutrition occurring before and/or during pregnancy compromises fetal development. (71).

CHILDHOOD DISORDERS: The two most common of the mental, developmental, and behavioral disorders of childhood are attention deficit-hyperactivity disorder (ADHD) and autism spectrum disorder (ASD). There is ample evidence that both have had conspicuous increases in prevalence in recent years, but to date there seems to be no general consensus as to the etiology of either of these difficult and distressing afflictions. However, a close link between digestive disorders and children with ASD, ADHD, and other learning disabilities has been clinically demonstrated and successfully ministered to by English physician and nutritionist, Dr. Campbell-McBride (72).

Additionally, there is considerable interest in the role that nutrition, especially maternal nutrition, may play in the occurrence of ASD, ADHD, and other birth defects or dysfunctions. A review of the scientific literature on the relationship between maternal nutrition and low birth weight supports the conclusion that maternal malnutrition during pregnancy is the most powerful predictor of infant brain size, growth, and survival. Although socioeconomic status is an overriding circumstance, the specific etiologic nutrients associated with low birth weight and poor pregnancy outcomes appear to be deficiencies primarily of omega-3 essential fatty acids and B vitamins. About 7 percent of low birth weight infants are born prematurely. Low birth weight leads to impaired growth with attendant risk of mental retardation and chronic adult disease (73).

Numerous studies have shown that a significant fraction of very low birth weight preterm infants who survive infancy suffer lifelong motor, cognitive, and behavioral dysfunction. In one study of 91 preterm children, 26 percent had a positive result on M-CHAT, the Modified Checklist for Autism in Toddlers screening tool (74). In a series of approximately 1,000 two-year-old preterm children, 21 percent tested positive on M-CHAT. After eliminating children who had pre-existing mental or physical impairments, 10 percent of the remaining otherwise-normal children tested positive on M-CHAT, which is double the rate usual for normal-term children (75).

Dietary intake of omega-3 EFAs has been shown to increase gestational duration and decrease the incidence of premature birth in humans. Numerous studies of premature infants indicate that they have low levels of docosahexaenoic acid (DHA) in the blood, which correlates with abnormal eye and brain function. The addition of omega-3 EFAs to mother's milk fed to 37 premature infants for a six-month period resulted in a positive association with growth parameters and increase in head circumference (76).

DEPRESSION: Depression is not only the most common of the psychiatric disorders but also seems to be the least well characterized. It is a catch-all category for patients suffering from widely varying degrees of despair and dejection. This category of mental illness includes two types, reactive depression and endogenous depression (77). Reactive depression refers to the feelings of grief, such as that from the loss of a loved one, where the depression is appropriate to the personal life situation. Endogenous depression refers to depression for which there is no life situation that could account for the depression. The diagnosis of endogenous depression is dependent on the judgment of a psychiatrist.

Reactive depression is a condition that, unfortunately, is experienced by virtually everyone at some point in life, but with time healing occurs and the depression leaves, or at least diminishes to the point where normal activities can be resumed. Endogenous depression, on the other hand, appears to have a convincing nutritional component. For example, depressive patients show a significant depletion of total omega-3 EFAs in the membranes of their red blood cells as compared with controls (78).

In addition, many years of experience in medical management of patients with depression has shown that many of them respond well to a diet that restricts high-glycemic carbohydrates. There is a consistent association between depression, and saccharine disease (77). Saccharine disease is the long-forgotten name for the metabolic sequence of hypoglycemia/insulin resistance/type-2 diabetes, which is now known to be a consequence of a high-glycemic carbohydrate diet and an initiator of chronic inflammation.

The clue that chronic inflammation may be a cause of or contributor to depression suggests that anti-inflammatory omega-3 fatty acids could be therapeutic. That such is the case is supported by considerable epidemiological and clinical data. A study of the biochemicals in the brain that are involved in major depression show a similarity of action between the antidepressant Prozac and the omega-3 fatty acids EPA and DHA. The potential biochemical mechanisms for the antidepressive action of omega-3 EFAs are discussed by Stoll (79).

Bipolar Disorder: In 1993, Stoll began a search for chemicals that shared biochemical actions with mood stabilizers but had never before been tested in bipolar disorder. A well-designed, double-blind, nine-month-long study using 31 patients with unstable, difficult-to-treat bipolar disorder was initiated using 1,000 milligram fish oil capsules containing 70 percent omega-3 fatty acids. The dosage used in the study was 9.6 grams of omega-3 per day, which translates to 13 or 14 capsules per day (79). At four months, the omega-3 patients were doing remarkably well while those receiving placebos were failing to recover or relapsing. Because the treated group was doing so well, it was decided to terminate the study at that point and offer omega-3 therapy to all (80).

Postpartum Depression: Probably the most tragic of the depressions is one that affects new young mothers. The heartrending stories of maternal infanticide reported in the news media have brought knowledge of these sad episodes to public attention. Post partum depression is more common than recognized (81; 82). Although episodes of infanticide are rare, the illness is more appalling when one realizes that it is preventable.

There is considerable evidence that post partum depression is strongly linked to a nutritional deficiency of essential fatty acids (79). The heavy demand for DHA and AA by the fetus for its developing brain (70) depletes the EFA stores of the mother unless she obtains an adequate supply of them in her diet during pregnancy and postpartum.

SCHIZOPHRENIA: Schizophrenia is a spectrum of psychiatric conditions that have similar symptoms. The schizophrenic patient cannot discriminate between thought and perception and often has rapid and inexplicable mood swings. The split between thought and perception renders the patient unable to correctly judge the real world and distinguish it from illusions and hallucinations (83). The pattern of occurrence in families has led to the suggestion that schizophrenia is a genetic disease; the twin birth mate of a schizophrenic has a 48 percent chance of becoming schizophrenic, and the offspring of two schizophrenics has a 47 percent chance of developing the disorder (84).

Regardless of what the genetic involvement is in schizophrenia, it is apparent that nutrition plays more than an ancillary role. Interestingly, prior to the mid-1950s, one of the standard treatments for schizophrenia was insulin coma therapy, which caused blood glucose levels to plummet and coma to set in (69). It perhaps offered a portent of decades-later anecdotal reports by many recovered schizophrenics who had suffered with hypoglycemia and credited their recovery to a low carbohydrate diet (84).

More recent research studies have established that a substantial number of schizophrenics are deficient in omega-3 fatty acids and that dietary supplementation with EPA results in significant improvement in symptoms (79). In a double-blind, placebo-controlled, randomized trial, 231 young adult schizophrenic prisoners who received supplements of vitamins, minerals, and essential fatty acids for a minimum of two weeks committed 26 percent fewer disciplinary offences during the trial than did controls (84).

Perhaps the most direct evidence for a nutritional relationship comes from a biochemical pathway common to all schizophrenics, which accounts for the thought and perceptual symptoms. This is the formation of adrenochrome from the oxidation of adrenalin (69; 83; 84). Early in his psychiatric practice, Hoffer noticed that the urine of schizophrenic patients was always brown colored. Isolation of the brown pigment showed that it was adrenochrome (oxidized adrenaline). Later research revealed that adrenochrome produced the same psychotic symptomatology as mescaline and LSD (69).

Thus, schizophrenia is one of the few mental diseases in which the biochemistry responsible for the development of the disorder has been elucidated. Although a number of widely different circumstances can stimulate production of excess adrenochrome, its production is the final biochemical reaction that leads to the symptoms of schizophrenia.

The nutritional relationship with schizophrenia is its successful orthomolecular management with the vitamin niacin (vitamin B$_3$). Biochemically, niacin reduces the synthesis of adrenalin, which, in turn, reduces the amount of adrenochrome formed. It is interesting to note that the niacin deficiency disease, pellagra, produces schizophrenic-like symptoms and that, in their earliest stages, cases of pellagra cannot be differentiated from those with schizophrenia (83).

ORGANIC DISORDERS: The organic mental disorders, a preponderance of which are associated with aging, manifest themselves primarily as cognitive dysfunctions of varying degree. These disorders are commonly grouped together under the heading of senile mental disorders or senile dementias. Among these, only two have been traced to actual physical changes in the brain that can be seen and identified by pathologists. These disorders are Alzheimer's disease and dementias caused by small strokes, also known as multi-infarct dementias.

The other common dementias seen among older adults include depression, anxiety disorders, memory loss, and confusion. These ailments do not seem to have observable lesions in the brain, but can be diagnosed only by observing the behavioral patterns of the patient. In the early stages of all of these disorders, the victims show a range of nervous, psychiatric, behavioral, and personality problems that are difficult to diagnose accurately.

Symptoms, particularly at first, are vague and overlap one another. For example, slight memory loss, confusion, or other signs of mental deterioration may indicate the early stages of any one of the senile mental disorders, including Alzheimer's disease or mild, unrecognized strokes. As these disorders become more severe, changes in behavior, attitudes, and mental performance become sufficiently pronounced so that more specific diagnoses are made possible.

Alzheimer's Disease: Alzheimer's disease is the senile dementia that has been most studied and for which considerable epidemiological and clinical findings associated with nutritional practices are available. A number of studies suggest that dietary excesses of sugar and starch may be related to the ultimate occurrence of Alzheimer's disease. High cholesterol values (>240 mg/dl) (a prominent symptom of a high-glycemic diet) diagnosed in midlife represents a significant risk factor in development of Alzheimer's disease in old age. Even borderline cholesterol values (200-239 mg/dl) are associated with an increased risk (85).

Diabetes in 824 elderly participants, almost exclusively type-2, which is the consequence of insulin resistance from long-standing high-glycemic diet, was associated with a 65 percent increase in risk of developing Alzheimer's disease compared with elderly participants who were not diabetic (86).

An imbalance of omega-6 and omega-3 fatty acids is also implicated as a contributing factor for Alzheimer's disease. The incidence of Alzheimer's disease correlates positively with dietary intake of omega-6 fatty acids and negatively with omega-3 fatty acids (79; 87). A recent randomized, double-blind, placebo-controlled study of 485 participants over 55 years of age reports that intake of 900 mg per day of algal omega-3 docosahexaenoic acid for a six months period resulted in a significant improvement in performance on memory and learning tasks as compared with the placebo group (88).

Magnesium/Aluminum: Magnesium deficiency is strongly associated with Alzheimer's disease and other senile dementias (89). Magnesium is known to be essential for healthful brain metabolism and also for protection of the brain against the effects of adventitious trace metals in the diet. Magnesium serves as a coenzyme for a number of important enzyme systems in the brain.

When the brain is deficient in magnesium, other metals present in the diet take its place. When aluminum substitutes for magnesium, it disrupts the normal biochemistry of the brain and causes damage. It is interesting to speculate that the aluminum found at autopsy in brain tissue of Alzheimer's patients probably is the result of deposition of aluminum resulting from aborted attempts by the body to use aluminum as a coenzyme in the absence of magnesium. The metal the body most commonly uses as a replacement for magnesium is aluminum, a trace metal regularly found in the American diet.

B-vitamins: B-vitamin deficiencies also play a role in psychiatric disorders. A high prevalence of inadequate vitamin B status is commonly found in nutritional studies in the elderly. It has long been known that among the earliest symptoms of deficiencies of certain B vitamins, notably B_3 (niacin) and B_6 (pyridoxine), are changes in perception, including illusion and hallucinations (77). Deficiencies in vitamins B_{12}, folic acid, and B_6 have been shown to be responsible for nutritional hyperhomocysteinemia (14). A number of studies have shown that hyperhomocysteinemia is highly prevalent in the elderly (90) and that poor cognition in the elderly is a likely accompaniment of hyperhomocysteinemia (91).

Hostility, Violence, and Self-Harm: The epidemiological data associating nutritional deficiencies with violent and aggressive behavior has led to a number of clinical studies in which the association has been shown to be a contributing factor (92; 93). The evidence that criminal and other antisocial behaviors are due in part to nutritional deficiencies, particularly of omega-3 fatty acids, is strong (94). The current and ongoing research of Hibbeln and colleagues is providing a wealth of information on the relationship between nutrition and pathologies of the brain (95).

SUICIDE

In the last half century, suicide has grown to become the tenth leading cause of death in the United States. In the year 2011, 39,909 people died from this cause and about ten times as many people failed attempted suicides (96).

Depression is a major risk factor for suicide. Depression includes feelings of sadness or irritability, loss of interest in usual activities, inability to experience pleasure, feelings of guilt or worthlessness, and thoughts of death or suicide. Other symptoms include inability to concentrate, difficulty making decisions, fatigue, lack of energy, restlessness, and changes in sleep, appetite, and activity levels (97).

The increasing rates of suicide in America suggest that the prevention methods currently employed are not effective. Existing programs are based on psychotherapeutic interventions, community support, and antidepressant drugs. Logic based on the science reported in Part Two of this book suggests that a significant fraction of our current suicide epidemic is probably caused by nutritional deficiencies. A fact not considered by today's ineffective suicide prevention programs is that the brain is a part of the human body and, as all the other organs and parts of the body, the brain requires appropriate nutrition in order to function properly (69; 70).

The American public might still be unaware of the statistics that revealed the deplorable suicide epidemic in America if it were not for the fact that the American military services are also seeing record numbers of suicides. With a month left in the year 2012, suicides among active-duty forces reached 323, surpassing the previous high of 310 suicides set in 2009 (98). Suicide is now a serious national mental health problem that includes both civilians and military personnel.

The National Institute of Mental Health and other involved agencies, including the military, consider suicides to be psychiatric disorders. The National Institute of Mental Health and other involved agencies, including the American military, appear to have deemed that suicides are exclusively the type of mental disorders that need to be prevented and treated by psychiatrists and psychiatric methods. Thus, national suicide prevention programs consist of visits with psychiatrists, and "talk" that includes widespread community support, a national suicide prevention telephone life line, and extensive use of anti-depressant drugs.

Antidepressants are the third most common prescription drug taken by Americans of all ages. Over the period from 1988–2008, the rate of antidepressant use in the United States increased by 400 percent (99). In other words, the underlying causes of America's suicide epidemics are considered to be mental stresses and a deficiency of prescription drugs.

The idea that suicides might be systemic in nature and the result of a nutritional deficiency is not taken seriously. However, an independent study using military records (99) published in 2011, documents the value of omega-3 fatty acids for the prevention of suicides. Blood serum samples from eight hundred military suicides were compared with similar serum samples from a control group, namely veterans who had not committed suicide (blood serum samples reflect fatty acid dietary intakes). Almost all of the 800 controls (99.1%) had been in combat zones whereas only 495 of the 800 suicide cases had a record of being in combat zones.

The findings based on serum sample assays provided the following results: Low DHA status turned out to be a significant risk factor for suicide death in the American Military. Nearly all military personnel in all 1600 samples that comprised this study had low long chain omega-3 fatty acid, DHA and EPA, status compared to North American, Asian, Australian, and Mediterranean populations. Further, only the subjects with the highest levels of DHA were protected. The risk of suicide death was 62% greater among men with lower serum DHA levels. Two other fatty acids were associated with reduced risk of suicide, stearic acid (saturated fat) and DGLA, an omega-6 substrate for anti-inflammatory eicosanoids (100).

It has been known for many years that the omega-3 essential fatty acid, DHA, is required for construction and maintenance of brain, nerve, and eye tissues. And it is also known that DHA cannot be biosynthesized by the body and must be obtained from the diet. Studies done in civilian populations indicate that low fish consumption and low DHA tissue levels are associated with increased risk of suicides. Two grams per day of fish oil (EPA and DHA) decreased suicidal thinking, and depressive symptoms (100)

References

1.)   Taubes G. *Good Calories, Bad Calories*. New York, NY: Alfred Knopf, 2007.

2.)   Ottoboni A, Ottoboni, F. The Food Guide Pyramid: Will the defects be corrected. *Journal of American Physicians and Surgeons*. 2004; **9**(4): 109-113.

3.)   Porter R. *The Greatest Benefit to Mankind*. New York, NY: W. W. Norton & Company, Inc., 1997.

4.)   Golding J, et al. High levels of depressive symptoms in pregnancy with low omega-3 fatty acid intake from fish. *Epidemiology*. 2009;**29**(4): 598-603.

5.)   Monograph: Docosahexaenoic acid (DHA). *Alternative Medicine Review*. 2009; **14**(4): 391-399.

6.)   Sears B. *The Anti-inflammation Zone*. New York, NY: Regan Books/Harper Collins, 2005.

7.)   Serhan CN. Lipoxins and aspirin-triggered 15-epi-lipoxins are the first lipid mediators of endogenous anti-inflammation and resolution. *Prostaglandins, Leucotrienes and Essential Fatty Acids*. 2005; **73**: 141.

8.)   http://en.wikipedia.org/wiki/Inflammation#Cardinal_signs/ Accessed Sept. 30, 2012.

9.)   Simopoulos AP. The importance of the omega-6/omega-3 fatty acid ratio in cardiovascular and other chronic diseases. *Experimental Biology and Medicine*. 2008; **233**: 674-688.

10.)   Hibbeln JR, et al. Healthy intakes of n-3 and n-6 fatty acids: estimations considering world wide diversity. *American Journal of Clinical Nutrition*. 2006; **8**(3 supp.): 1483S-93S.

11.)   *Dietary Reference Intakes: The Essential Guide to Nutrient Requirements*. Washington, DC: The National Academies Press, 2006.

12.)   Fan Y-Y, Ramos KS, Chapkin RS. Importance of dietary g-linolenic acid in human health and nutrition. *Prostaglandins, Leukotrienes, and Essential Fatty Acids*. 1997; **54**: 101–107.

13.)   Merched AJ, et al. Nutragenic disruption of inflammation-resolution homeostasis and atherogenesis. *Journal of Nutrigenetics and Nutrigenomics*. 2011; **4**: 12-24.

14.)   McCully, K, McCully M. *The Heart Revolution*. New York, NY: HarperCollins, 1999.

15.)   Signorello MG, et al. Effect of homocysteine on arachidonic acid release in human platelets. *European Journal of Clinical Investigation*. 2002; **32**(4): 279-84.

16.)   Montuschi P, et al. Isoprostanes: markers and mediators of oxidative stress. FASEB Journal 2004; **18**: 1791-1800.

17.)   Reaven GM. The role of insulin resistance in human disease. Diabetes. 1988; **37**(12): 1595-1607.

18.)   Whitmer RA. The epidemiology of adiposity and dementia. Current Alzheimer Research. 2007; 4(2): 117-22.

19.)   Whitmer RA, et al. Central obesity and increased risk of dementia more than three decades later. Neurology. 2008; **71**(14): 1057-1064.

20.)   Luchsinger JA. Adiposity and Alzheimer's disease. Current Alzheimer Research. 2007; **4**(2): 127–134.

21.)   Pi-Sunyer FX. The Obesity Epidemic: Pathophysiology and Consequences. Obesity Research. 2002; **10**: 97S–104.

22.)   Murray MA. Encyclopedia of Nutritional Supplements. Rocklin, CA: Prima Publishing, 1996.

23.)   Rhoades RA, Tanner GA. *Medical Physiology*. Boston, MA: Little, Brown and Company, 1995.

24.)   Atkins RC. Dr. Atkins' New Diet Revolution. New York, NY: Avon Books, Inc. 1999.

25.)   Gittleman AL. Your Body Knows Best. New York, NY: Simon & Schuster, 1997.

26.)   Lipetz P. The Good Calorie Diet. New York, NY: Harper Paperbacks, 1996.

27.)   Aviva M, et al. The disease burden associated with overweight and obesity. Journal of the America Medical Association. 1999; **282**(16): 1523-1529.

28.) Fries F, Vickery DM. *Take Care of Yourself, Fourth Edition*. Reading, MA: Addison-Wesley Publishing Company, Inc., 1989.

29.) Williams RJ. *You Are Extraordinary*. New York, NY: Random House, Inc., 1967.

30.) Hensley S. Scientists Find Gene Variation in Adult Diabetes. *The Wall Street Journal*. September 27, 2000: B-1.

31.) Eades MR, Eades MD. *Protein Power, Paperback Edition*. New York, NY: Bantam Books, 1999.

32.) Sears, Barry. *The Anti-Aging Zone*. New York, NY: Regan Books, HarperCollins Publishers, 1999.

33.) Schwarzbein D, Deville N. The Schwarzbein Principle. Deerfield Beach, FL: Health Communications, Inc. 1999.

34.) http://www.diabetes.co.uk/global-diabetes/diabetes-in-india.html/ Accessed Sept. 30, 2012

35.) Raheja BS, et al. Significance of omega-6 to omega-3 ratio for insulin action in diabetics. *Annals of the New York Academy of Sciences*. 1993; **683**: 258-271.

36.) Ramsden CE, et al. Dietary fat quality and coronary heart disease: A unified theory based on evolutionary, historical, global, and modern perspectives. *Current Treatment Options in Cardiovascular Medicine*. 2009; **11**: 289-301.

37.) http://www.cnp.usda.govt/DGAsMeetings4.htm/ (09/30/12. Not available - unable to find substitute)

38.) Ravnskov U. *The Cholesterol Myth: Exposing the Fallacy that Saturated Fat and Cholesterol Cause Heart Disease*. Washington, DC: NewTrends Publishing Inc., 2000.

39.) Ravnskov U. *Fat and Cholesterol are Good for You!* Sweden: GB Publishing, 2009.

40.) http://www.mayoclinic.com/health/prehypertension/DS00788/ Accessed Sept. 30, 2012

41.) http://en.wikipedia.org/wiki/Blood_pressure/ Accessed Sept. 30, 2012

42.) Langsjoen, PH. Alleviating congestive heart failure with coenzyme Q10. *Life Extension Magazine*, February. 2008.

43.) Beltowski J, et al. Adverse effects of statins. *Current Drug Safety*. 2009; **4**(3): 1-19.

44.) http://www.nejm.org/doi/pdf/10.1056/NEJMoa0807646/ Accessed Sept. 30, 2012

45.) http://online.wsj.com/article/SB10001424052748703630404575053821708459574.html/ Accessed Sept. 30, 2012

46.) Metcalf E. Aspirin: The Miracle Drug. New York, NY: Avery: a member of the Penguin Group, 2005.

47.) Kahn R, et al. The Impact of Prevention on Reducing the Burden of Cardiovascular Disease. *Circulation*. 2008; **118**; 576-585.

48.) Guallar E. et al. Omega-3 fatty acids in adipose tissue and risk of myocardial infarction. *Arteriosclerosis, Thrombosis, and Vascular Biology* 1999; **19**(4): 1111-1118.

49.) Asherio A., et al. Dietary fat and risk of coronary heart disease in men; cohort follow up study in the United States. *British Medical Journal*. 1996; **313**(7049): 84-90.

50.) Walker GC. Inducible DNA repair systems. *Annual Review of Biochemistry*. 1985; **54**: 425-457.

51.) Ames BN, et al. DNA lesions, inducible DNA repair, and cell division. *Environmental Health Perspectives*. 1993; **101** (Suppl 5): 35-44.

52.) Hickey S, Roberts H. *Cancer: Nutrition and Survival*. 2005.

53.) Hickey S, Saul AW. *Vitamin C: The Real Story*. Laguna Beach, CA: Basic Health Publicat, Inc., 2008.

54.) Chen Q, et al. Pharmacologic ascorbic acid concentrations selectively kill cancer cells. *Proceedings of the National Academy of Sciences*. 2005; **102**(38): 13604-13609.

55.) Nazarewicz RR et al. Effect of short-term ketogenic diet on redox status of human blood. *Rejuvenation Research*. 2007; **10**(4):435-440.

56.) Ames BN. Are vitamin and mineral deficiencies a major cancer risk? *Nature Reviews Cancer*. 2002.

57.) Giovannucci E, et al. Prospective study of predictors of vitamin D status and cancer incidence and mortality in men. *Journal of the National Institute*. 2006; **98**(7): 451-459.

58.) Garland CF, et al. The role of vitamin D in cancer prevention. *American Journal of Public Health*. 2006; **96**(2): 252-261.

59.) Morris MS et al. Vitamin B6 intake is inversely related to, and the requirement is affected by, inflammation status. *The Journal of Nutrition*. 2010; **140**: 103-110.

60.) Donaldson MS. Nutrition and Cancer: A review of the evidence for an anti-cancer diet. *Nutrition Journal*. 2004; **3**: 19 (an online journal, 21 pages).

61.) Colquhoun A, et al. Fatty acids, eicosanoids and cancer. *Nutritional Therapy & Metabolism*. 2009; **27**(3):105-12.

62.) Larson SC et al. Dietary long-chain n-3 fatty acids for the prevention of cancer: a review of potential mechanisms. *American Journal of Clinical Nutrition*. 2004; **79**: 935-945.

63.) Bazan NG, et al. Rescue and repair during photoreceptor cell renewal mediated by docosahexaenoic acid-derived neuroprotectin D1. Thematic Review Series: Lipids and Lipid Metabolism in the Eye. *Journal of Lipid Research*. 2010; **51**. Available online. Accessed Sept. 30, 2012 http://www.jlr.org/search?author1=bazan&fulltext=&pubdate_year=&volume=&firstpage=&submit=yes/

64.) Zhang C, Bazan NG. Lipid-mediated cell signaling protects against injury and neurodegeneration. *Journal of Nutrition*. 2010; **140**(4): 858-53. Epub 2010 Feb 24.

65.) Diabetic Neuropathy. National Eye Institute, Bethesda, MD 29892. http://www.nei.nih.gov/ downloaded April 27, 2012/ Accessed Sept. 30, 2012

66.) Detached Retina. University of Michigan Kellogg Eye Center, Ann Arbor, MI 46106. downloaded April 28, 2012. http://www.kellogg.umich.edu/patientcare/conditions/detached.retina.html#clinic/ Accessed Sept. 30, 2012

67.) Bazan NG. Cellular and molecular events mediated by docosahexaenoic acid-derived neuroprotectin D1 signaling in photoreceptor cell survival and brain protection. *Prostaglandins, Leukotrienes, and Essential Fatty Acids*. 2009; **81**(2-3): 205-211. doi:10.1016/j.plefa.2009.05.024.

68.) AREDS Report No. 22. The relationship of dietary carotenoid and vitamin A, E, and C intake with age-related macular degeneration in a case-control study. *Arch Ophthalmol*. 2007; **125**(9): 1225-32.

69.) Hoffer A. *Adventures in Psychiatry*. Calderon, Ontario, Canada: KOS Publishing Inc., 2005.

70.) Crawford MA, et al. The role of docosahexaenoic and arachidonic acids as determinants of evolution and hominid brain development. in *Fisheries for Global Welfare and Environment, Fifth World Fisheries Congress 2008*. ed. Tsukamoto K, et al. © by TERRAPUB 2008.

71.) Ottoboni F, Ottoboni A. Can attention deficit-hyperactivity disorder result from nutritional deficiency? *Journal of American Physicians and Surgeons*. 2003; **8**(2): 58-60. 72.) Campbell-McBride N. Gut and Psychology: A Natural Treatment for Dyspraxia, Autism, ADD, Dyslexia, ADHD, Depression, Schizophrenia. Cambridge, UK: Medinform Publishing, 2004.

72.) Muthayya S. Maternal nutrition & low birth weight – what is really important? *Indian Journal of Medical Research*. 2009; **130**:600-608.

73.) Limperopoulos C, et al. Positive screening for autism in ex-preterm infants: prevalence and risk factors. *Pediatrics.* 2008; **121**(4):758-765.

74.) Kuban K, et al. Positive screening on modified-checklist for autism in toddlers (M-CHAT) in extremely low gestational age newborns. *Journal of Pediatrics.* 2009; **154**(4): 535-540.

75.) Barboza SM, et al. n-3 polyunsaturated fatty acids in milk is associated to weight gain and growth in premature infants. *Lipids in Health and Disease.* 2009; **8**:23-32.

76.) Hoffer A, Walker M. *Putting it All Together: The New Orthomolecular Nutrition.* New Canaan, CT: Keats Publishing, Inc. 1996.

77.) Peet M, et al. Depletion of omega-3 fatty acid levels in red blood cell membranes of depressive patients. *Biological Psychiatry.* 1998; **43**: 314-319.

78.) Stoll AL. *The Omega-3 Connection: The Groundbreaking Antidepression Diet and Brain Program.* New York, NY: A Fireside Book: Simon & Schuster. 2001.

79.) http://www.cdc.gov/search.do?q=postpartum+depression&spell=1&ie=utf8/ Accessed Sept. 30, 2012

80.) Prevalence of self-reported postpartum depressive symptoms. *Morbidity and Mortality Weekly Report.* 2008; **57**(14): 361-6.

81.) Stoll AL, et al. Omega-3 fatty acids in bipolar disorder: a preliminary double-blind, placebo-controlled trial. *Archives of General Psychiatry.* 1999; **56**: 415-416.

82.) Hoffer A. *Orthomolecular Treatment for Schizophrenia.* Lincolnwood, IL: Keats, NTC/Contemporary Publishing Group, 1999.

83.) Foster HD. *What Really Causes Schizophrenia.* Victoria, BC, Canada: Trafford Publishing, 2003.

84.) Solomon A, et al. Midlife serum cholesterol and increased risk of Alzheimer's and vascular dementia three decades later. *Dementia and Geriatric Cognitive Disorders.* 2009; **28**:75-80.

85.) Arvanitakis Z, et al. Diabetes Mellitus and risk of Alzheimer disease and decline in cognitive function. *Archives of Neurology.* 2004; **61**: 661-666.

86.) Gillette Guyonnet S, et al. IANA task force on nutrition and cognitive decline with aging. *Journal of Nutrition, Health Aging.* 2007; **11**(2): 132-152.

87.) Yurko-Mauro K, et al. Beneficial effects of docosahexaenoic acid on cognition in age related cognitive decline. *Alzheimer's & Dementia: The Journal of the Alzheimer's Association.* 2010; **6**(6): 456-464.

88.) Dean C. *The Miracle of Magnesium.* New Your, NY: Ballentine Books, 2003.

89.) Selhub J, et al. Vitamin status and intake as primary determinants of homocysteinemia in an elderly population. *Journal of the American Medical Association.* 1993; **270**: 2693-8.

90.) Johnson MA, et al. Hyperhomocysteinemia and vitamin B12 deficiency in the elderly using Title lllc nutrition services. *American Journal of Clinical Nutrition.* 2003; **77**: 211-20.

91.) Hibbeln JR, et al. Omega-3 fatty acid deficiencies in neurodevelopment, aggression, and autonomic dysregulation: Opportunities for intervention. *International Review of Psychiatry.* 2006; **18**(2): 107

92.) Hallahan B, et al. Omega-3 fatty acid supplementation in patients with recurrent self-harm. *British Journal of Psychiatry.* 2007; **190**: 118-122.

93.) Buydens-Branchey L, Branchey M, Hibbeln JR. Associations between increases in plasma n-3 polyunsaturated fatty acids following supplementation and decreases in anger and anxiety in substance abusers. *Progress in Neuro-Psychoparmacology and Biological Psychiatry.* 2008; **32**(2): 568-575.

94.) Hibbeln JR. National Institute on Alcohol Abuse and Alcoholism, 31 Center Drive (31/1B58), Bethesda, MD 20892. Email: pjhibbeln@niaaa.nih.gov/

95.) http://www.cdc.gov/nchs/fastats/mental.htm/. Accessed on November 24, 2012.

96.) *Diagnostic and statistical manual of mental disorders, fourth edition.* Washington, DC: American Psychiatric Association, 2000.

97.) http://www.usatoday.com/story/news/nation/2012/11/18/navy-suicides-army/1702403/

98.) Pratt LA, Brody DJ, Gu Q. Antidepressant use in persons aged 12 and over: United States, 2005–2008. NCHS data brief, no 76. Hyattsville, MD: National Center for Health Statistics. 2011.

99.) Lewis MD, et al. Suicide Deaths of Active Duty U.S. Military and Omega-3 Fatty Acid Status: A Case Control Comparison. Journal of Clinical Psychiatry. 2011; **72**(12): 1585–1590.

Chapter Eleven

Disease Prevention – the Shunned Science

Diseases do not just happen. Every disease has a cause, and once this cause is known, prevention is often the next most reasonable and cost-effective step. **Anon.**

The United States is in the midst of enormous epidemics of chronic debilitating diseases, the most important of which are cardiovascular diseases, type-2 diabetes, mental disorders, and cancer. Attack rates of these diseases began increasing in the mid-20th century and have grown steadily since that time. They are major causes of death in older adults, and, in recent years, their numbers have been rising in younger age groups. Overall, these diseases are, by far, the major causes of disability and death in the United States.

Currently, medical care costs for these diseases, both public and private, add up to about one trillion dollars annually. Expenditures on health care in the United States rose from $714 billion in 1990 to over $2.3 trillion in 2008. Absent reform, health care costs are expected to continue to rise significantly in the foreseeable future (1). The reasons are that the population at most risk for these diseases (those over 65 years old) is increasing and the cost of medical care is rising because of the growing use of more costly medical, diagnostic, and treatment methods.

America faces this enormously costly health care crisis today because national health policy is focused almost exclusively on diagnosing and treating rather than preventing the growing epidemics of chronic diseases. Under the current diagnose-and-treat scenario, chronic diseases are allowed to occur and progress until they reach the stage where they can be diagnosed medically. At this point, these diseases are, for the most part, not curable, only treatable. Very importantly, each new diagnosis represents a new patient and a new recurring medical care cost.

The Current System

The nation's current medical care system cannot cure these diseases. It can treat symptoms and extend life somewhat with drugs and surgery but it cannot maintain wellness by treating these diseases. And medical treatments are not benign. In the year 2000, Starfield reported that deaths from errors in hospitals due to unnecessary surgery, medication errors, harmful effects of medications, and nosocomial infections caused 225,000 deaths per year and constituted the third leading cause of death in the U.S. after heart disease and cancer (2).

A similar review done by the National Institute of Medicine in 2006, found that at least 1.5 million patients are sickened, injured, or killed each year by errors in prescribing, dispensing, and taking medications. At least 400,000 of these incidents happened in hospitals, 800,000 in nursing homes and facilities for the elderly, and 530,000 in Medicare recipients treated in outpatient clinics (3).

This does not imply, in any way, that medical diagnosis and treatment are not competent or not important. To the contrary, diagnosis and treatment and other medical programs are required to care for victims of accidents, illnesses, diseases, and other problems that inevitably occur in all population groups.

However, attempting to use the nation's overworked diagnose-and -treat system to cope with large and growing epidemics of chronic diseases that are largely preventable is clearly ineffective and economically unsustainable. The reasonable answer to this dilemma is to utilize science-based prevention (public health) programs to prevent disease and significantly reduce the numbers of new cases.

Various investigations have charged that incompetence, abuse of mandate, and dishonesty contribute to the high costs of these programs. This is true. According to Peterson, fraud and incompetence may amount to 10% of total costs and includes over-billing, lack of generic drug emphasis, unlimited treatment without regard to cost, and the absence of a way of measuring comparative costs and outcomes of various treatments (4, p. 205ff).

But solving these problems alone will not stop the relentlessly growing costs of medical care. The real cost problem is that early diagnosis and treatment, otherwise known as preventive medicine, no matter how carefully and honestly done, is the most expensive and inefficient way of dealing with epidemics of any kind.

Engineers would describe the use of a diagnose-and-treat medical care system for handling of large and growing epidemics as a positive feedback system that will self-destruct eventually because it creates conditions that encourage steadily escalating costs. What happens is that each newly diagnosed case represents a new and predictable profit stream. This growing stream stimulates innovation in better diagnostic and treatment methods.

Better diagnostic and treatment methods are usually more costly per individual patient and, at the same time, enable earlier detection of existing diseases and the discovery of previously unrecognized new diseases. Both generate more profits that stimulate more innovation. The result is a vicious circle that grows stronger with time.

Such conditions predict that the cost of providing medical care for the current chronic disease epidemics will be limited only by the total amount of money available. A former editor of a major journal has written that...

> American health care has become a vast profit-oriented industry. The revenue of this industry constitutes the country's health-care costs. As in any other industry, providers constantly strive to increase their profitable sales, but unlike other industries, consumers exercise little control over their consumption of products and services. It should not be surprising that such a system is afflicted not only with relentless inflation, but also with neglect of the needs of the uninsured and with failure to promote the use of valuable but unprofitable health services (5).

American policymakers have been concerned about the growing costs of medical care for a number of years. Proposed solutions have ranged from creation of a government-operated national medical care system to simply tinkering with the existing system by restricting eligibility, controlling prices, limiting provider liability, increasing taxes, and increasing patient fees.

All of these solutions are destined to fail because policymakers have ignored primary prevention and focused almost exclusively on the impossible task of fixing the ravenous diagnose-and-treat system. What is clear from long experience with all types of epidemics is that scientifically sound primary prevention programs are the only approach proven to be effective and low in cost.

WHAT IS DISEASE PREVENTION?

The phrase "disease prevention" simply means "to preclude or stop a disease from occurring." When a disease is prevented, no illness occurs and no medical care is required. In precise terms, this type of prevention is called primary prevention. Its methods are clear-cut: It uses sound science and strict logic, not pseudo science or the consensus opinion of a group of experts, to identify the true cause of a disease; and it eliminates that disease by eliminating its cause using the best practical means available. Although simple, these steps, when diligently followed, have proven to work; they are a sure-fire recipe for reliable disease prevention.

Few people today realize the importance of disease prevention. Preventive programs protect whole communities, rich and poor, at low cost, and are effective against both infectious and non-infectious diseases.

THE CONTRIBUTION OF DR. SNOW

The science of disease prevention was nonexistent before a London physician, John Snow, discovered the key to ending the cholera epidemics that were common in nineteenth century England and in many other countries. In 1836, more than 50,000 people died of cholera in England. It was then that Snow began to suspect that filth was somehow connected with cholera; however, there was no general agreement about the cause, and there was no cure (6, p. 402).

The prevalent theory was that cholera was caused by the foul smells that emanated from the uncontrolled filth in the streets. At the time, there were no sanitation systems. Each household threw its human waste and garbage out into the streets to drain away in putrid ditches and pools. Polluted drinking water was not suspected as a cause of disease, and there was no effort to provide clean drinking water. Scientists of the time, with their primitive microscopes, had seen very tiny organisms in such polluted water, but microbiology was yet to be discovered and the tiny organisms that these scientists observed in their microscopes were not believed to be a possible cause of any disease.

Dr. Snow, unable to help his patients who were dying from cholera, decided to interview the 93 families in his neighborhood that had been hit by cholera and compare the details of their eating and living habits with the eating and living habits of families in the same neighborhood that had no cholera. He made careful notes about each family.

Studying these notes, he found no common link with the type of food eaten or the ages of the cholera victims. But he did find that, unlike the general population, workers at a local brewery and inmates housed in a nearby jail had no cholera at all. Both of these establishments used their own wells for drinking water. Very importantly, he noticed that cholera occurred only in families that got their drinking water from one well; this well had a hand pump set up over an open community well on Broad Street.

Dr. Snow took the time to walk around and look carefully at this well. He saw that human waste was draining from a filthy ditch in the street into the well. Remembering the awful diarrhea suffered by cholera victims, he thought that maybe the human waste from the sick cholera victims draining into the Broad Street well was somehow connected with the spread of cholera. To prove or disprove his idea, he asked city officials to remove the handle from the Broad Street Pump so that local people would have to use a different source of water. In a short time, new cases of cholera stopped occurring among people who used the Broad Street Pump. He had rightly concluded that the water from this well was the cause of the disease (6, p. 412).

THE LESSONS FROM DR. SNOW: Three powerful lessons have come from Snow's work. The first lesson is that common sense and good judgment are as important as highly sophisticated methodology in discovering the cause of a disease. The second lesson is that the suspected cause must be proven by some valid means to be labeled as the actual cause. For Snow this was removing the pump handle, preventing use of the water from the Broad Street well, and observing that new cases of cholera stopped occurring. The third lesson is that when the cause or the source is accurately known, the disease can be prevented absolutely by eliminating the cause or by cutting the connection between the source of the infection and the human population.

Snow's work encouraged the City of London and many other cities to eliminate cholera by constructing systems to provide clean drinking water uncontaminated by sewage. This required the design and construction of municipal sewage collection systems and separate fresh water pumping and purification plants. These systems are common today. Such plants prevent cholera as well as a wide range of other serious diseases that are spread by water contaminated by human and animal waste products.

Primary Prevention versus Secondary Prevention

Until about 1970, prevention meant to preclude or stop a disease from occurring. Today, if you were to ask a physician for advice on how to prevent heart disease, diabetes, or any other chronic disease, it is almost certain that you would be told to get regular medical checkups so that any potential health problem can be diagnosed early and treated without delay. This is not primary prevention, and it does not prevent disease. Unfortunately, the term prevention is now used as a synonym for what might be called secondary prevention, which is the province of preventive medicine or preventive care. Secondary prevention actually means early diagnosis and treatment.

Early diagnosis and treatment is an important and necessary part of a comprehensive health care system because its mission is to discover disease early so that treatment can begin without delay. Its objective is to control pain, minimize disability, and prolong the life of the patient. However, costs are high because it does not prevent disease. Secondary prevention requires individual attention to patients by medical professionals in a continuing series of office visits, laboratory tests, drugs, surgery, and hospital services.

The fact that most periodic medical checkups are virtually without value was demonstrated by a study at Kaiser Hospital in Oakland, California (7, p. 883). Between 1964 and 1973, a group of about 5,000 patients was encouraged to have frequent checkups and a comparable group of about 5,000 patients was not encouraged to do so. Members of the first group had far more frequent examinations than the second group, but physicians who evaluated the health status of all participants during the seven year period found no significant difference between the two groups in incidence of disease, disability, or death.

Primary prevention seldom deals with individual patients. The work of prevention is ordinarily done by public health agencies where objectives are to discover the underlying causes of diseases and then to take steps to eliminate the cause or cut the route of transmission of the disease. As a result, relatively few public health professionals today are medical doctors. Most are engineers, scientists, laboratory personnel, and technicians. Historical experience indicates that the most beneficial and efficient health care system includes both medical care and primary prevention.

The Saga of Public Health

Few people today realize that one of mankind's great gifts is the science and practice of disease prevention. Roy Porter, a respected medical historian, pointed out that:

> …facts indicate how little the practice of medicine weighs in the balance of health. Late stage crisis [medical] management of victims is very costly and of little benefit compared to preventive programs (6, p. 714).

The idea of preventing illnesses is deep-rooted; it probably originated in prehistoric times when humans learned that it was not safe to eat certain plants because they caused illness or death. All societies throughout time have been concerned about the causes and cures of illnesses. The most primitive of peoples had notions of why ill-health occurred and how to deal with it. The practice of prevention possibly predated the practice of healing:

> Prevention lies in living in accord with nature, in harmony with the seasons and elements and the supernatural powers that haunt the landscape… Another preventive is a good diet. Foods should be consumed which give strength and assimilate natural products which, resembling the body, are beneficial to it (6, p. 39).

THE EARLY DAYS

But it was not until the advent of Dr. Snow and his remove-the-pump-handle method of proving cause and effect that the science of disease prevention had its beginning. The development was furthered by an interest in vital statistics that was pioneered by the Prussian army chaplain Johann Peter Süssmilch in the 18th century (6, p. 293). In the early 1800's, questions began to be asked about numbers of death, causes of death, ages of death, and life expectancies according to possible causes, such as the influence of neighborhoods and income levels.

The idea of tabulating and analyzing death rates and disease rates surfaced in France and England in the 19th century. This work led to the realization that disease rates were different in different population groups. Poor neighborhoods had more sickness and death than rich neighborhoods. Foul smelling, dirty areas were more prone to diseases like dysentery and cholera than clean ones. People living and working around seaports were shown to have many outbreaks of strange and dangerous diseases. Laws requiring quarantine of incoming ships probably came from such statistics.

The profession, practice, and organizational structure that ultimately resulted from centuries-long efforts to prevent disease became the discipline known today as public health. Public health is not an ideology, a religion, or a political belief, but rather a practical method for preventing epidemics of disease along with their associated human and economic costs. It is silent and inconspicuous.

When at its best, nothing happens: there are no epidemics, food and water are safe to consume, citizens are well informed concerning personal habits that affect their health, children are immunized, the air is breathable, factories obey worker safety standards, there is little class-based disparity in disease or life expectancy, and few members of the citizenry go untreated when they develop addictions to alcohol or narcotic substances (8, p. 7).

But the road to a functioning public health system was not easy, with human behavior being the biggest enemy to its establishment. Slavery, religious and racial biases, gross wealth disparities, profound ignorance, squalor, political corruption, and medical corruption all contributed at one time or another to the distressing obstacles that had to be overcome (8). The charge of the many small departments of public health that were launched throughout the country was merely prevention of infectious diseases.

The science and practice of disease prevention was the accepted and in many cases the only approach to disease control for the first half of the 20th century. For hundreds of years prior to that time, infectious diseases, often in epidemic proportions, were major causes of death because they were usually impossible to cure and, as a rule, affected large population groups.

Yet long before antibiotics and reasonably good medical science were available, some infectious diseases, such as cholera, were controlled by effective preventive programs that remain in place today. Such programs include purification of domestic water supplies, sewage treatment, mosquito and rodent abatement, pasteurization of milk, food sanitation, communicable disease monitoring, and immunization programs. Today, people and policymakers tend to forget that these programs literally have saved millions of lives over the past several hundred years.

THE HIGH POINT

Disease prevention finally achieved serious public support a little over a hundred years ago. It was growing and had a clear purpose – to discover and eliminate the cause of disease so that new cases of that disease simply did not occur again. At the turn of the 19th century, the U.S. Public Health Service Commissioned Corps headed by a Surgeon General was created. Shortly after its creation, the Corps faced a major test with the outbreak of a major epidemic of pellagra across the southern United States (9).

THE PELLAGRA EPIDEMIC: The pellagra epidemic marked an important milestone in the mission of the Public Health Service; it widened its purview from prevention of infectious diseases to prevention of any disease, regardless of etiology, that threatened the well being of members of the general public. The pellagra epidemic also forced the acceptance by the medical community and general public that serious, even lethal, disease could be caused by a nutritional deficiency.

Pellagra was an old disease, known for over two hundred years in southern Europe by its classic symptoms of red rash, schizoid-like dementia, and its association with poverty. The first recorded case of pellagra in the United States occurred in 1902. The disease spread rapidly throughout the southern states and soon reached epidemic proportions. It was assumed that the disease was an infectious one, a conviction that lasted for decades despite the fact that it was not communicable and that all efforts to isolate its microorganism or vector failed.

The underlying cause of pellagra was found to be high consumption of maize (corn). Because of its low cost, good taste, and easy availability, corn, became the staple food in poor countries and displaced traditional diets that included sufficient amounts of meat, eggs, and dairy products. The high-corn diet was deficient in niacin, a B-vitamin. The result was pellagra, a malady characterized by an itchy rash, no appetite, sore tongue, depression, dementia, diarrhea, headaches, dizziness, weight loss, and eventual death.

Over its course, the epidemic produced more than 3 million cases and caused 100,000 deaths in 15 southern states. By 1908, the epidemic had become a matter of great concern to the medical establishment, the news media, politicians, and the general public. The public became panicked, and the Surgeon General reported that pellagra threatened to become a national calamity. Southern pride was offended at the suggestion that the disease was associated with poverty and malnutrition. Southern legislators and organizations demanded that the infectious agent be identified. Pellagra was a social stigma and, thus, it was more acceptable for it to be considered infectious rather than due to poverty.

Bollet tells the fascinating story of the social and political forces that seriously interfered with medical research and its investigation of the epidemic and its causes (9). By 1914, the epidemiological and clinical studies of Dr. Joseph Goldberger, an officer in the Public Health Service, showed that social and economic factors were responsible for pellagra and that the disease could be reversed and prevented by dietary means.

These scientific data had no calming effect on the controversy. Dissenting voices did not begin to quiet until yeast, which was found to contain a powerful antipellagra substance, began being used in the mid-1920s to treat pellagra patients. The demonstration at this time that pellagra was caused by a deficiency of vitamin B_3 (niacin) finally settled the argument, but the outbreak lasted until 1940.

AN ADDED RESPONSIBILITY: Although the demonstration that a deficiency of the B-vitamin niacin could cause a dreadful and deadly epidemic did not have a major impact on the view that epidemics could only be caused by infectious organisms, it did mark the beginning of a new responsibility for the Public Health Service - noninfectious diseases. A number of maladies that affected large numbers of people but were apparently noninfectious now came under their purview.

These maladies are now largely nonexistent because their causes were exposed and eliminated. They are no longer remembered because they were old preventive programs directed at the epidemics of noninfectious chronic diseases. Although these old programs are largely ignored and forgotten, they are still in operation today and remain effective in preventing disease.

Goiter and cretinism, crippling chronic diseases of the thyroid gland, were virtually eliminated in the United States many years ago by the addition of iodine to table salt. The fortification of grain products with the B-vitamins, niacin and thiamin, eliminated two fatal debilitating diseases, pellagra, and beriberi. Fortification of milk with vitamin D has greatly reduced the incidence of rickets, the crippling childhood disease. And the recent, but long-delayed, fortification of foods with folic acid is reducing the number of neural tube birth defects.

Until about 1950, America had the best public health prevention system in the world. It was comprised of local, state, and federal public health agencies with academic support from schools of public health in major universities. Over the years, particularly in the first half of the 20th century, this public health system had identified the causes of many diseases and promoted projects to eliminate the causes. Many of these projects involved building sanitary sewage systems and water treatment plants that are still serving the public today. These early efforts have prevented untold millions of illnesses and deaths.

THE DEMISE

It took centuries to build a public health system and less than two decades to bring it down. America's public health infrastructure, once the envy of the world, was in a shambles by the end of the 20th century (8, p. 282). It is essential to understand what caused the collapse in order to prevent reliving it. In addition to the causes of the collapse, the changes in public attitudes and activities that have occurred since the collapse as they relate to the mission of public health must be examined. It is important to learn not only from past mistakes but also from past successes.

It is now obvious that politicians and other policymakers, beginning in about 1955, methodically destroyed the best public health disease prevention system in the world. Even today, they have no understanding of scientific disease prevention or the enormous value of maintaining a high level of wellness in the American population (8).

What Went Wrong?

How did this misfortune happen? From the beginning, politicians, social advocates, and private citizens attempted to influence the activities of public health professionals – and they often succeeded, as happened in the pellagra epidemic (9). Another difficulty for public health was that from the very start the medical profession held a guarded skepticism toward the aims and approaches of public health.

This wariness is a natural outcome of the differences in goals between the two professions, which often are at variance with each other. Physicians treat individuals and have the utmost concern for their privacy and protection. Public health experts treat groups of people and consider that, if an individual poses a health threat to the community, the needs of the individual are subordinate to those of the community. This is the basic difference between curative medicine and preventive medicine – the difference between unrestricted freedom and compulsory constraint.

These difficulties were ever-present challenges that public health had to overcome to achieve the accomplishments it did at the peak of its success. Although annoying, the difficulties were manageable problems that might have made some small contribution to the demise, but other more significant issues that did have major impacts entered the picture in the mid-20th century.

THE PENICILLIN EFFECT

A literal revolution in medical treatment of infectious diseases occurred with the introduction of the sulfa drugs just prior to World War II. This was followed shortly by the advent of penicillin. The dreaded, almost-always-lethal streptococcal infections suddenly became of little more consequence than a bad cold. And cases of formerly untreatable gonorrhea were dispensed with in a matter of days. Epidemics of infectious diseases were averted along with the panic they engendered. The public became less concerned about the threat of plagues and ultimately forgot that they had ever existed.

What grew out of this revolution was a national obsession with diagnosis and treatment, a large medical care system, and growing prescription drug sales. The medical and pharmaceutical industries became highly profitable and gained tremendous political influence, to the detriment of primary prevention. What emerged after a half century were relentlessly increasing medical care costs, growing chronic disease epidemics, resistance to employ the valuable but unprofitable disease prevention know-how, and the demise of public health's efforts insofar as chronic disease prevention was concerned.

SOCIETAL CHANGES

Garrett skillfully documents the relationship between the changes that occurred in the 20th century to an array of economic, cultural, political, social forces and the fate and fortunes of public health during that period (8). Sometime during the 20th century, a slow transformation from the moral responsibility and discipline of America's founders to a more self-absorbed, self-interested permissiveness began to be observed. The most rapid changes occurred between the time of the Great Depression of the 1930s, with its culture of survival, and the 1960s era of the flower children, with its culture of happiness.

Individual Rights: Irrespective of what drove the changes, post-WWII America saw an unprecedented increase in individual rights and freedoms and diminution of individual concerns for the opinions of society. The rights revolution, which was spurred during the 1960s, embraced labor rights, student rights, racial rights and sexual rights. The rights revolution brought much good and much detrimental to the health and well being of society. The good was civil rights and benefits; the detrimental was societal ills and epidemics of disease.

The right to display sexuality openly, though very liberating and satisfying for some, led to a tremendous increase in the incidence of sexually transmitted diseases (STDs). It also ushered in the age of teenage pregnancies and unwed motherhood. The right to indulge in mind-altering drugs brought an explosion in the production and use of marijuana, which is theorized to be a gateway to drug addiction. The rise in heroin use, primarily "among fifteen to twenty-nine year old males," led to spread of hepatitis and HIV infections among users through shared needles and syringes (8, p. 341).

Television: Shortly after the end of WWII, the United States suddenly became a TV nation. People exchanged social interaction with their families for lives glued to what became known as the "boob tube," further eroding the cultural importance of the family unit. People became captives of the newly energized advertising industry. From long hours watching TV, their caloric intake rose and their exercise level dropped (8, p. 340).

Poison Paranoia: Dread of man-made chemicals and anxiety about their carcinogenicity were implanted into the public psyche in 1962 with the publication of Rachel Carson's provocative book *Silent Spring*. Carson's description of the damage done by pesticides to the environment and wildlife invigorated the environmental movement. Health and environmental concerns generated volumes of new legislation and stirred political activism. Public cynicism and dismay gave rise to a strong anti-industry, anti-pesticide bias

With every passing 1970s day, another chemical was implicated, another pollutant named. Public panic rose and, in the end, that would leave public health vulnerable to a large, and often effective, assault on its credibility (8, p. 355).

Antigovernment Attitudes: President Reagan gave voice to public concern about the creeping overreach of government regulations with his famous remark that government does not cause the problem, but rather that government is the problem. A general lack of respect for government programs plus a heightened sense of importance of the individual as opposed to that of the community that developed during the Reagan years did not enhance approval of the principles of public health.

PUBLIC HEALTH EDUCATION

During latter half of the 20th century, university schools of public health appear to have lost much of their traditional interest in scientific disease prevention. After about 1970, these schools became involved with research into the relationships between wealth, poverty, and disease. Findings based on statistical studies of population groups showed that prosperous people were generally healthier than poor people and that this difference was to some extent related to access to good medical care. Many public health researchers concluded that these findings proved that best and simplest way to prevent disease was to discover methods that would convert poor people into prosperous people.

Thus, the mission of the major schools of public health has been redirected largely from training of professionals in the science and skills of identification and prevention of diseases of public health consequence to study and research of societal issues that relate to poverty and its eradication. The scientific data describing the role of nutrition in the etiology of diseases of major public health consequence are virtually ignored.

Relative to the acknowledged diet-disease connection, a review of the pertinent literature fails to reveal recognition by any American school of public health of the existence of considerable scientific data that challenge the validity of the current official heart-healthy dietary guidelines. To the contrary, the Department of Nutrition at the Harvard School of Public Health, the foremost school of public health in the United States, is a major supporter and recognized authority for the official low-fat, high carbohydrate diet (10).

MEDICARE AND MEDICAID

In the debates that preceded enactment of Medicare and Medicaid, numerous questions were asked about what were their goals. The questions, though debated, were never answered. Political leaders merely assumed that everyone wanted and needed more medical care (8, p. 346). Public health advocates argued for a more balanced program that included primary prevention as a basic component, but the demand for medical care services won over the need for prevention.

Thus, the Medicare and Medicaid programs were created without any provision for a disease prevention capability. Also, funding for the previously established federal, state, and local public health disease prevention programs was curtailed. Medicare and Medicaid completely reshaped American healthcare and had a profound, diminishing effect on public health.

The Medicare and Medicaid programs were able to change national health policy because they appealed to virtually every member of the electorate. Federal monetary support shifted away from disease prevention and towards more medical care, prescription drug research, and cures for cancers and AIDS. Capital-intensive medicine, such as heart surgery, use of more sophisticated drugs, and genetic research grew steadily. At the same time, due to the ever-weakening preventive programs, attack rates of major chronic diseases and psychosomatic disorders also grew steadily.

Peterson suggests that the enormous cost of Medicare and other politically popular entitlement programs crowded out traditional budget items within the federal budget, such as disease prevention research and public health programs that were aimed at future-oriented governmental activities (4, p. 46). There is also reason to believe that the enormous political power of pharmaceutical companies helped foster this trend.

According to Angell for example, the pharmaceutical industry was employing 675 lobbyists in Washington, DC in 2002, more than one for each member of Congress. They donated 85 million dollars to politicians and allied political groups in the 1999 -2000 election cycle. And in the period 1980 - 2000, drug sales tripled, and the industry became, by far, the most profitable business in the country (5).

The pharmaceutical industry likewise influences doctors. In 2001, for example, drug companies employed 88,000 sales representatives to regularly visit doctors' offices to tout drugs and to give away 11 billion dollars worth of free drugs, golf balls, books, free lunches, and tickets to sporting events. Drug companies also provide doctors with free educational programs to satisfy requirements for continuing medical education.

Such programs promote drug-intensive medical practice and, of great significance, they comprise over half of the continuing education available to doctors (5). In the context of their unchallenged national lobbying power, it is worth recognizing that public health programs that study and promote prevention of diseases rather than diagnosis and treatment of diseases are a threat to the profit-making objectives of this industry.

SCIENCE BY LEGISLATION

A number of decades ago, politicians discovered a useful method for bypassing inopportune scientific facts. Often, in the course of legislative proceedings, an underlying scientific truth is found that runs counter to some proposed legislation designed to satisfy a public demand or some political self-interest. The matter is easily solved by holding committee hearings, which are promoted as objective fact-finding sessions by soliciting testimony from all interested parties. The statements of participants are recorded and drawn from by committee staff to form a consensus opinion that the committee deems to be honest – and is in concert with the needs of the proposed legislation.

The creation of a consensus, an essential element in providing validation for legislators, is, in effect, creation of bogus scientific truth by legislation. Such legislative slight-of-hand can have, and has had, a profound negative impact on public health.

The Banning of DDT: The banning of the pesticide DDT is an example of the adverse impact that politically-derived scientific facts, justifiably termed "junk" science, has had on public health. Other examples can be found in Wildavsky's in-depth analyses of major environmental issues in which journalists and environmentalists have promoted junk science to obtain favorable political action (11) and in Lehr's collection of essays on the abuse of science in matters of environmental importance (12).

In 1948, Dr. Paul Müller won the Nobel Prize in Medicine and Physiology in recognition for his discovery of dichloro-diphenyl-trichloroethane (DDT) and its life-saving properties by virtue of its phenomenal control of vector-borne diseases. During WWII, many millions of people in Europe and the Pacific theater were literally dusted with DDT to kill the vectors of deadly diseases such as typhus. Also in the Pacific theater, barrels of drinking water that served the troops were laced with DDT to kill mosquito larvae. DDT never caused a human death but saved millions if lives. DDT was hailed as a miraculous life-saving chemical (13).

The Turning of the Tide: After the wartime need was over, the use of DDT against food crop pests began. The resistance of DDT to degradation, which made it very valuable as a pesticide, became the basis for its undoing – it was detectable on crops for long periods of time after application. Thus, DDT residues were found associated with some untoward occurrences after its application and assumed to be the cause. From the time that DDT became the malevolent star of Rachel Carson's *Silent Spring* in 1962 until it was finally banned by the Environmental Protection Agency (EPA) in 1972, it was decried as the scourge of the planet.

The panic and public outcry against DDT clouded objective discussions of the toxicology of DDT – it was not politically correct to explain that the science of toxicology demonstrated that DDT was of very low toxicity to humans and other animal forms (13). After lengthy hearings, including testimony from toxicologists concerning the true risks from use of DDT, a consensus was achieved and the DDT ban was mandated by Congress.

The effect of the ban was immediately felt in the agricultural industry. In California, during decades of use of DDT, other than a rare case of dermatitis, there were no occupational illnesses attributable to its use. Of greater importance, DDT had never caused a single death among farm workers. With the ban, organophosphate pesticides were substituted for DDT, and their use increased greatly, accompanied by epidemics of farm-worker poisonings and an occasional death or two each year (13). Human lives were traded for a questionable environmental benefit.

The Current Status: In the longer term, the DDT ban resulted in the preventable deaths in Africa of tens of millions of pregnant women and of children less than five years of age (14). The loss of DDT to third-world mosquito abatement programs continues to this day and is charged with millions of deaths each year from malaria. An historical record of the DDT controversy, including notes from 1972 EPA report on DDT, can be found in a series of papers in *21st Century Science and Technology* (15).

EMASCULATION OF THE SURGEON GENERAL

The U. S. Marine Hospital Service, the forerunner of the U.S. Public Health Service, was created in 1798 to care for sick or injured merchant seamen. However, it was not until 1889 that it became the U.S. Public Health Service when the United States Congress authorized a fully staffed Commission Corp, organized along military lines, with a centralized administration under a medical officer with the title of Surgeon General.

For the many decades prior to 1968, the Surgeon General had broad public health responsibilities and powers and reported directly to the Secretary of Health, Education, and Welfare. In 1968, a major reorganization took place that abolished the independent Office of the Surgeon General. The approximately 2000 public health scientists that constituted the Surgeon General's staff were dispersed among other government agencies. The Surgeon General became a deputy to the Assistant Secretary of Health.

The Surgeon General thereby became a political appointee with no authority or responsibility. This eliminated independent leadership and assistance to primary prevention programs in public health agencies. The people of America no longer had an independent Surgeon General who was both professionally competent and free from political manipulation; there was no longer a government agency with knowledge and standing to push governmental policies in the direction of good science in the areas of disease prevention and public health (8).

The question of why the Office of the Surgeon General was emasculated abruptly in 1968 has never been answered publicly. But coincidentally, a few years earlier, the landmark report issued by Surgeon General Luther Terry's Advisory Committee on Smoking and Health (16), created a public, and political storm. Despite the furor, the data were unassailable; it was an example of superbly-developed epidemiologic research. The Surgeon General report on smoking and health marked the beginning of fundamental change in the economics of the tobacco industry and a significant modification in the smoking habits of the American public that continues to the present day:

> The antismoking campaign is a major public health success with few parallels in the history of public health. It is being accomplished despite the addictive nature of tobacco and the powerful economic forces promoting its use (17).

What a formidable motivation for political retaliation!

THE CORRUPTION OF EPIDEMIOLOGY

Probably one of the most significant impediments to the solution of today's fiscal crisis in health care is the misuse, either inadvertent or deliberate, of the major tool for investigation of chronic disease causation. That tool is the science of epidemiology.

DR. SNOW FORGOTTEN? The lessons of Dr. Snow, mentioned above, illustrate the basic approach to disease investigation and prevention. Today, Snow's approach is called epidemiology. Its essence is: First, use available science to see if there is an association between two situations; Second, if there is a statistical association, prove the association is causal using sound scientific methodology.

In Snow's case the available science was data tabulated from interviews of both the sick and the healthy, plus common sense to identify the possible source. He saw that his tabulated data showed a clear association between the ill people and the Broad Street Well. But he also had the good sense to know that associations do not prove cause and effect. He proved the association by removing the pump handle. When new cases of cholera failed to appear, he knew that the well was the true cause of his cholera cases. Modern epidemiologists frequently assume that association proves cause and effect and neglect to "remove the pump handle." Curiously, they tend to forget that associations do not prove cause and effect. They seem to have forgotten Snow's second lesson.

IGNORANCE OF KOCH'S POSTULATES? Modern epidemiology, literally the science of epidemics, refers to the study of the incidence, prevalence, and movement of diseases that attack many people in a population at the same time. It is based on an old statistical methodology that was designed decades earlier to record and analyze disease incidence. After discovery that microorganisms were the cause of infections, the methods of epidemiology were adapted for use in the investigation of epidemics of infectious diseases.

The model for a sound epidemiological study was established in 1876 by German physician Robert Koch (13). In essence, Koch's postulates set the criteria for determining whether there was an association between an organism and a disease and, if there was association, what specific steps were required to establish whether the association was causal. Thus, Koch's postulates had the two essential parts of epidemiology: one, association (might the organism have caused the disease?) and two, causation (did the organism actually trigger the disease?). Part two is proof that is analogous to Dr. Snow's removal of the pump handle. Koch's postulates became a requirement in the study of epidemics of infectious diseases. Had Koch's postulates not been ignored during the pellagra epidemic, the fact that the disease was not of infectious origin would have been accepted much sooner.

EPIDEMIOLOGIC INCOMPETENCE: The epidemics at issue in this book are, to a great extent, the result of the failure of almost all of the epidemiologists who studied diet versus disease to learn from Snow's work. A reading of a variety of papers that were representative of the huge number that sprung forth from early inquiries into the relationship between diet and heart disease makes it obvious that most looked only for associations, and incompletely at that.

Influenced by the popularity at the time of Ancel Keys' lipid hypothesis, only the fat component of the diet was considered in most of the studies. The carbohydrate component was largely ignored. In no case was there any attempt to "remove the pump handle" to prove the association was causal. Chapter Three provides a detailed description of the flaws in the epidemiology on which the early research that led to the so-called heart-healthy diet was based.

The failure of the official nutrition policy to slow the epidemics of chronic disease has fostered another false proposition, namely that regular exercise is required for good health. Rather than concede that the low-fat diet plan itself may be the problem, some other reason had to be found for its ineffectiveness. A very convenient excuse for the lack of effect of the official nutrition policy was an alleged laziness of the general public. It was obvious that people got fat because they did not exercise enough!

The faulty epidemiology showing that exercise makes people healthy provided the justification needed to create the MyPyramid icon with exercise as a third dimension (18). The defect in the many studies on which this decision was made is that no study is capable of distinguishing between people who are healthy because they exercise and people who exercise because they are healthy. The new icon will have no impact on preventing diseases but will delay exposure of the heart-healthy diet as being not heart healthy.

Public Health Today

By the late 1990s the role of public health had pretty much been settled. Funding for public health agencies to support primary prevention activities had been curtailed. Today, the United States no longer has a serious, scientifically-based chronic disease prevention program. Federal public health funds have largely shifted toward medical care and research and away from disease prevention. There is no Surgeon General to provide nonpartisan, scientifically valid investigation of matters of critical importance to the health of the entire nation, such as occurred with the report on cigarette smoking.

No Federal agency, including Medicare and Medicaid, seems to have any interest in utilizing old fashioned public health-type investigative programs aimed at discovering the causes and learning how to prevent effectively our current large and growing epidemics of chronic diseases. The use of impartial scientific facts in the diagnosis of and remedial action for the current epidemics of chronic diseases is shunned and replaced by the opinions of so-called experts.

CURRENT PUBLIC HEALTH ACTIVITIES

Fortunately, the practice of collection, tabulation, and analysis of vital statistics is still an active function of governmental and private agencies, which appears to have been unaffected by the misfortunes of public health system. Vital statistics serve as the central data bank for public health that provides signals when disease prevention activities are needed and guides their progress. Weekly reports are compiled by the Center for Disease Control and published by the Massachusetts Medical Society (19).

Traditional public health services established many decades ago – sewage treatment, water treatment, mosquito and other vector abatement, food fortification, and immunizations – are still in existence and functioning. These basic services are largely taken for granted by modern societies; their proper functioning and maintenance is primarily the responsibility of local municipalities.

It is worth reflecting on the fact that, even today, drinking water is not safe to drink in many parts of the world, but it is safe in the United States. This important reality did not happen by accident. It was done many years ago by professional public health programs, supported by the voting public. Good minds utilized the sciences of disease prevention to justify the extent and costs of municipal water treatment systems, and professional engineers designed and constructed these systems. These systems are a legacy from more than a century ago when the public understood the miracle of disease prevention.

Traditional public health programs have consistently exhibited several unique and tremendously valuable features that are worth pointing out: Once put into place, they operate reliably and steadily, usually under local control, as part of the national infrastructure; They require little or no effort on the part of the average person and usually enjoy popular support; Costs per individual served are very low and the targeted diseases are effectively and reliably prevented; Finally, they protect everyone within their jurisdictions regardless of income or social status.

PRESENT DAY FOLLY

World history tells us that governmental behavior that is antithetical to the best interests of its citizens is common to all ages. The political factors that led to the demise of the public health system in the United States plus the corruption of epidemiology and of sound science itself are antithetical to the public good and have caused it untold damage. Barbara Tuchman, in her book *The March of Folly* (20), describes such large scale deceit as folly, namely the pursuit of policies based on false premises and fallacious reasoning.

Tuchman suggests that these activities have their roots in various combinations of greed, self-interest, incompetence, moral failure, corruption, and inability to admit error. Such governmental activities, in one form or another, persist for long periods, are extremely costly, and usually end in national disaster. Tuchman points out that large scale folly has become dangerously common in our time. Tuchman is correct. The governmental activities that have led to the current epidemics of modern nutritional diseases are neatly explained by Tuchman's *March of Folly*.

Political decisions have painted America into a nearly impossible corner. The only viable answer is to reduce patient loads by rebuilding the American public health system with the clear mission to prevent the modern nutritional diseases. The most telling need for rebuilding the public health system is that the escalating costs of medical care in the United States are not being matched by improvements in the health status of its citizens.

Quite the contrary, a three-decade long, in-depth analysis of data from twelve comparison industrial countries revealed that as relative spending on health care has increased the United States has fallen behind with respect to fifteen-year survival rates of adult men and women. Of the twelve comparison countries, the United States was among the highest in spending for medical care and among the lowest in fifteen-year survival rates. It was suggested that, investments in public health may be more efficient in increasing survival than any further investments in medical care (21).

Effective maintenance of wellness in any population group requires a preventive component as well as a medical care component. The history of medicine shows that it is unrealistic to believe that epidemics of any kind, infectious or noninfectious, can be controlled by early detection and treatment. Funding for research and medical advances alone will alleviate neither the cost nor the suffering of individuals faced with a chronic disease. Without concomitant investments in public health prevention and control efforts to implement the prevention research results we already have, rising health care costs and preventable deaths will continue. Americans deserve a national commitment to translating critically important research findings into practical public health solutions (22).

Rebuilding the Public Health System

Americans have serious work ahead. The task is not to begin from the beginning, but to build on the existing knowledge of disease prevention and on existing local public health organizations. The initial charge should be prevention of chronic nutritional diseases that are threatening to bankrupt the health care system. It is beyond the scope of this book to do more than outline a few thoughts on requirements for this extremely important issue.

REQUIREMENTS

It appears that a successful public health program requires active public interest, a valid and honest plan, and competent management and leadership. As David Walker, former comptroller general of the United States, pointed out relative to current governmental fiscal irresponsibility and the burgeoning costs of health care legislation (23): "...the American people are absolutely starved for two things: the truth, and leadership."

NEED FOR PUBLIC SUPPORT: It is difficult to find any public endeavor that survives and thrives if it fails to provide something of value to at least some segment of the public. Usually, the greater the public involvement, the more successful the endeavor becomes. In the history of the public health movement, there were times when active involvement, positive or negative, by the public resulted in some sort of change in direction of public health activities. Among these happenings, there were two that were remarkable in bringing about sweeping changes in public health administration.

Outrage: In New York City, the incident involved citizen outrage. In the latter half of the 19th century, the city's Board of Health was in a shambles, the local political machine, Tammany Hall, controlled all services, inspectors blackmailed their clients, preventive services were nonexistent, and the public was angered and exasperated. Finally, when a cholera epidemic broke out in Europe, New Yorkers were concerned that the deplorable sanitary conditions put them at risk. They took matters into their own hands, bypassed Tammany, and created their own new Metropolitan Board of Health. It is recorded that New York escaped the cholera epidemic with few deaths (8, p. 289ff).

Approval: The second notable event occurred in the mid-1960s in response to the Surgeon General's report on smoking and health, mentioned above. However, this time the public mood was not one of anger but of acceptance. For decades there had been a general recognition that smoking was not a healthful habit.

The Surgeon General's report motivated a receptive public. It became actively engaged in antismoking campaigns. Demands for smoking cessation programs became overwhelming. Despite the tremendous political and economic forces operating against their efforts, public health groups convinced the general public that smoking was not a healthful habit. Over the years, there has been slow but persistent success that continues to this day.

Current Attitude: Current public interest in public health appears to be essentially nonexistent, despite the facts that tell us the need is great. The public is abundantly aware that obesity has become a very serious health problem. There is little recognition by the general public that most obesity is merely an indicator of an inflammatory diet and that inflammation lies at the core of all of the chronic nutritional diseases. Even so, people are very concerned as they grow older about the epidemics of these diseases that are taking a toll among them.

The public is also abundantly aware of the high cost of medical care and the need for remedial action. But as with their concerns for their personal health, they do not know what to do about it. The public is not aware that a competent and honest public health program could help on both accounts. It could reveal the actual dietary cause and prevention of the modern nutritional diseases, and in preventing them, it could greatly relieve the financial burden that is devastating the United States economy.

NEED FOR TRUTH AND SOUND SCIENCE: First, it must be acknowledged that reconstituting a public health system directed at preventing chronic nutritional diseases requires that the dogma of the *Dietary Guidelines for Americans,* which holds that the major determinants of chronic diseases are dietary fats and cholesterol, must be relinquished. Nutritional scientists, as with all unbiased scientists, must have their minds open to the totality of scientific literature relating to the relationship of nutrients to health and disease.

The fact is that the wealth of biochemical and clinical literature, which, in simplest terms, point to dietary excesses of sugar and excesses of dietary omega-6 over omega-3 EFAs as causes of the chronic inflammatory processes that, in turn, cause obesity, type-2 diabetes, cardiovascular diseases and dementias, is completely ignored by the nutrition experts responsible for official policy. If they are to provide the public with honest, sound nutrition information, the medical and nutrition establishments must free themselves of whatever hold it is that makes them support the folly of current nutrition policy.

It is urgent that the existing centrally-planned nutrition policy be replaced by freely available, factual, scientifically-sound dietary information that people can use to plan their own diets. There is no need for the nutrition autocrats who assemble periodically to review selected data and then rubber-stamp present dogma.

Presently, the only hope for a public that wants the truth about how to avoid the so-called diseases of aging comes from the few scientists and physicians not bound by the dogma of the nutrition establishment who have been speaking out for over a decade about the harmful effects of the official nutrition policy (24; 25; 26; 27; 28). These pioneers have been joined in recent years by a host of other scientists, many of whom come from rapidly advancing fields, such as nutritional and molecular biochemistry, that explain the scientific basis for diet-induced inflammation. The voices of these scientists are beginning to be heard and their story beginning to be told.

NEED FOR LEADERSHIP: Since the abolition of the Office of the Surgeon General, central leadership in the public health movement has been nonexistent. The tremendous success of the last nonpartisan Surgeon General was that he was a highly respected scientist/physician whose science was accurate and his efforts sincere.

At the present time, the only leadership that exists is local and comes from local health departments, which vary tremendously in funding and capability. With proper financial and scientific support they would be ideal vehicles for rekindling public interest in public health. Their staffs are the public health professionals who are at the interface between people and government. They usually have significant public contact with services they provide and clinics they offer.

National leadership is required. The Federal public health service must be reinstituted along with a scientifically qualified, independent, nonpartisan Surgeon General and a staff of professional field officers to assist local health agencies to apply the sciences of disease prevention.

A Model for Public Action?

In the early days of the public health movement, great improvements in public health services were achieved by very vocal public demands for action. As mentioned above, in the late 1800s, an epidemic of cholera, an often fatal disease at the time, broke out in Europe. The deplorable sanitary conditions that existed in New York City in the late 1800s put its citizens at great risk of cholera from European visitors. Unable to get the attention of the Board of Health, New Yorkers took matters into their own hands; they created their own independent Board of Health that was able to successfully promote enough city-wide sanitary measures to prevent a cholera epidemic.

Today, the cholera threat faced by the residents of New York City many decades ago was minimal when compared to the damage currently being done to the citizens of the United States who are following the official dietary guidelines of their government. The science presented in this book indicates that the noninfectious chronic disease that are now epidemic in this country are preventable. However, this scientific information is ignored. Other than smoking cessation, there are no prevention programs for the chronic inflammatory diseases. In fact, it appears that no one is even thinking about one.

Will the burden of the chronic inflammatory diseases finally become sufficiently onerous for the public to demand or perhaps even undertake privately a prevention program? Could the current tragedy of breast cancer serve as a model for a preventive program that would avert future tragedy not only of breast cancer but all cancers?

THE TRAGEDY OF BREAST CANCER: The tragedy of breast cancer is that many of its victims are young women in the prime of life. If they are unmarried, they may never marry or may never have children. If they are young mothers, their husbands and children may never know a normal family life. If they survive through pain and suffering, there is usually difficult-to-bear deformity.

Breast cancer is not a rare illness. The American people know that we are in the midst of a terrible epidemic of breast cancer. It would be difficult to find a person who does not know at least one person who has been devastated by breast cancer. And the American people are willing to do something about it. Every year there are massive fundraising drives to fund research for a cure. There are times set aside when everyone wears pink, the color symbolic of the plight of breast cancer victims. Local volunteer groups throughout the United States donate their time going door to door to remind their neighbors of the need to be aware, to learn how to check for lumps, to obtain mammograms, and to raise money to help breast cancer victims.

The public is most willing and empathetic, but they are faced with a national policy that says breast cancer is not preventable. It states that the only hope for cancer victims is early detection and medical treatment that is painful, not certain, and may or may not cure. With regard to prevention, it says that the only way to prevent cancer is to avoid saturated fats and pig out on grains. Science knows better; the mechanism whereby linoleic acid, the major component of vegetable fats and oils, causes breast cancer has been described in the scientific literature (29: 30; 31, see also Chapter Nine).

In view of the great national interest in breast cancer, the time has come for a few breast-cancer-prevention-activists, somewhere in this great nation, to read and learn a few scientific facts and then set up their own local breast cancer prevention program. Every citizen can take part: Walk around; Talk to your neighbors; Put together a brochure; Tell people the American diet is the cause of breast cancer; Tell them what to eat and what not to eat (it is really quite simple). When you prevent disease, there is no disease; people are healthy and stay healthy. A self-help nutrition plan effective against all chronic inflammatory diseases, including breast cancer, is outlined at the end of this chapter.

If All Else Fails

The prospects for repudiation of the proscription against dietary saturated fats and cholesterol by the nutrition establishment are essentially zero. There was a vague hope prior to the 2005 revision of the guidelines that, after twenty-five years of implementation, the continued worsening of the epidemics of chronic diseases would suggest that the recommended diet was not working. Instead, it was decided that it was not the diet but lack of exercise that was the problem, and a whole new process and pictograph incorporating exercise were designed (18).

The 2010 revision of the *Dietary Guidelines* makes essentially no change in the prior recommendations. Moreover, the addition of exercise to the guidelines will delay any recognition that the diet is to blame for at least another twenty-five years. Meanwhile the human toll from bad nutritional advice will continue.

Therefore, it is urgent that individuals become responsible for their own health. They must learn the basics of healthful nutrition from authors that present sound science rather than flawed dogma and take steps to incorporate the simple basics of good nutrition into their daily fare. If all else fails: You are on your own! You must take care of yourself.

CONSIDER PERSONAL PREVENTION: Any disease can be prevented by removing its cause or causes. The biochemistry presented earlier makes clear that the broad underlying cause of chronic inflammatory diseases is chronic inflammation. More specifically, it is known that excess consumption of high glycemic carbohydrates (sugar and starch) and linoleic acid (LA), are major causes of this chronic inflammation. It is known how to replace these particular offending dietary components with other components that are anti-inflammatory. And finally it is also known that secondary influences, such as dietary anti-oxidants and magnesium, will be required for effective prevention.

It is reasonable to ask how a single prevention program can put a stop to a range of different diseases that include obesity, cardiovascular diseases, Alzheimer's disease, type-2 diabetes, cancer, arthritis, and others. First, all of these diseases have one underlying cause; long-term, low-level inflammation brought about primarily by diet. Different diseases occur because, individuals differ in many aspects.

Examples of these differences are dietary patterns, eating habits, ages, genetic backgrounds, oxidative stress, occupational environments, and harmful habits such as smoking. Various combinations of these differences influence individual biochemistry and physiology that, in turn, determine the actual disease outcome.

In setting up a home prevention program, understand that primary prevention is not designed to cure disease. The objective is to protect healthy people so that no disease occurs. Reversal may be possible with a few of the inflammatory diseases. Arthritic pain, type-2 diabetes, obesity, and cardiovascular diseases are likely to be reversible, particularly in the early stages. Diseases with tissue damage such as seen in Alzheimer's disease may not be reversible. The ideal option for individuals who already have symptoms is to coordinate dietary change with medical supervision.

The most interesting way to show individuals how to carry out their own prevention programs is to use a practical example. Alzheimer's disease is used here as the example because every person and every family will benefit enormously by prevention. Importantly, a prevention program for Alzheimer's disease will also prevent all of the inflammatory diseases including macular degeneration, heart disease, stroke, type-2 diabetes, obesity, arthritis, arthritic pains, and many cancers.

A Personal Prevention Program: The following is a list of nutritional problems that contribute to chronic inflammation. Each problem is accompanied by a proposed remedy. A nutritional program that incorporates these remedies is based on the most current scientific information available for design of a chronic disease prevention program.

Problem #1: Excess dietary sugar and starch (high glycemic carbohydrates) and inadequate protein and fat.

Do Your Own Prevention: Follow the recommendations in Chapter Twelve to design a healthful basic diet plan. Eliminate high glycemic carbohydrates. Start with your protein requirement, and then plan the balance of your fat and carbohydrate intakes around this. You will find that this diet will be comprised of 30% animal protein calories, at least 30% animal fat calories and, and not more than 40% low glycemic carbohydrate calories.

Problem #2: Too much dietary linoleic acid (LA).

Do Your Own Prevention: Reduce consumption of vegetable fats and oils to a minimum. Even though food labels do not mention LA content, reading labels will help. Labels that list vegetable fats, oils, trans-fats, or polyunsaturated fats are very likely to contain high LA.

Problem #3: Dietary deficiency of DHA and EPA.

Do Your Own Prevention: Take DHA and EPA every day. Take one teaspoon of cod liver oil and 3 teaspoons of fish oil per day. This combination will provide necessary vitamins A and D, and in addition, will satisfy average needs for DHA and EPA.

Problem #4: Anti-oxidant deficiency causes oxidative stress that produces inflammation.

Do Your Own Prevention: Anti-oxidants are available in fruits and vegetables, but most adults need to take extra anti-oxidants, such as ascorbic acid (vitamin C), beta carotene, vitamin E (mixed tocopherols), and lycopene. Green tea is a good source of antioxidants.

Problem #5: High blood homocysteine levels are inflammatory.

Do Your Own Prevention: Ensure safe homocysteine levels. Take three vitamins daily, B-6, B-12, and folic acid (now available in one capsule).

Problem #6: Deficiency of magnesium causes constipation and malfunction of a wide variety of enzyme systems including those in the brain.

Do Your Own Prevention: Daily magnesium requirement is about 700 to 800 milligrams. The average dietary intake of magnesium is about 200 milligrams per day. Take magnesium pills or use milk of magnesia (MOM). MOM is a convenient and inexpensive method of magnesium supplementation. Each teaspoon of MOM contains approximately 150 milligrams of magnesium. One or two teaspoons of MOM at bedtime is an excellent way to supplement your magnesium intake.

Problem #7: D6D enzyme malfunction can occur and no medical test is available to check for this problem.

Do Your Own Prevention: Your D6D may be malfunctioning if the above dietary adjustments seem not to work. Consider the following after discussing the matter with your doctor: Cut all possible LA from diet; Take four, 200 milligram capsules of DHA and three borage oil (240 milligrams of GLA) capsules daily; Take one with each meal and take the fourth DHA at bedtime.

A daily aspirin tablet taken as currently recommended by the medical profession will promote the biosynthesis of aspirin-triggered lipid mediators.

References

1.)   Centers for Medicare and Medicaid Services, Office of the Actuary, National Health Statistics Group, National Health Care Expenditure Data. January 2010.

2.)   Starfield B. Is US Health Really the Best in the World? *Journal of the American Medical Association.* 2000; **284**(4): 483-485.

3.)   http://www.iom.edu/~/media/Files/Report%20Files/2006/Preventing-Medication-Errors-Quality-Chasm-Series/medicationerrorsnew.pdf/ Accessed Oct. 01, 2012.

4.)   Peterson PG. *Running on Empty.* New York, NY: Farrar, Straus, and Giroux, 2004.

5.)   Angell M. *The Truth About the Drug Companies.* New York, NY: Random House, Inc., 2004.

6.)   Porter R. *The Greatest Benefit to Mankind.* New York, NY: W.W. Norton & Company, Inc., 1997.

7.)   Heiby WA. *The Reverse Effect: How vitamins and Minerals Promote Health and Cause Disease.* Deerfield, IL: MediScience Publishers, 1988.

8.)   Garrett L. *Betrayal of Trust: The Global Collapse of Public Health.* New York, NY: Hyperion, 2000.

9.)   Bollet AJ. Politics and pellagra: The epidemic of pellagra in the U.S. in the early 20th century. *The Yale Journal of Biology and Medicine.* 1992; **65**: 211-221.

10.)   Willett WC. (Co-Developed with the Harvard School of Public Health). *Eat, Drink, and Be Healthy: the Harvard Medical School Guide to Healthy Eating.* New York, NY: Free Press, 2001.

11.)   Wildavsky A. *But Is It True: A Citizen's Guide to Environmental Health and Safety Issues.* Cambridge, MA: Harvard University Press, 1995.

12.)   Rational Readings on Environmental Concerns. Lehr JH ed. New York, NY: John Wiley &Sons, 1992.

13.)   Frank P, Ottoboni MA. *The Dose Makes the Poison: A Plain Language Guide to Toxicology, 3rd ed.* New York, NY: John Wiley & Sons, 2011.

14.)   Malloy S. *Green Hell: How Environmentalists Plan to Control Your Life and What You Can Do to Stop Them.* Washington, DC: Regnery Publishing, 2009.

15.)   https://www.21stcenturysciencetech.com/DDT.html/ Accessed Oct. 01, 2012.

16.) http://en.wikipedia.org/wiki/Smoking_and_Health:_Report_of_the_Advisory_Committee_to_the_Surgeon_General_of_the_United_States/ Accessed Oct. 01, 2012.

17.) http://www.cdc.gov/tobacco/data_statistics/sgr/history/index.htm/ Accessed Oct. 01, 2012.

18.) http://www.choosemyplate.gov/food-groups/downloads/MyPyramid_Getting_Started.pdf/ Accessed Oct. 01, 2012.

19.) *Morbidity and Mortality Weekly Report.* Massachusetts Medical Society, P.O. Box 9120, Waltham, MA 02454.

20.) Tuchman BW. *The March of Folly.* New York, NY: Ballantine Books, 1984.

21.) Muennig PA, Giled SA. What changes in survival rates tell us about US health care. *Health Affairs.* 2010; **29**(11). (*Health Affairs* Web First, October 7, 2010).

22.) Hardy GE Jr. The burden of chronic disease: the future is prevention. *Preventing Chronic Disease.* 2004; **1**(2). http://www.cdc.gov/pcd/issues/2004/apr/04_0006.htm/ Accessed Oct. 01, 2012.

23.) ftp://www.marl.iastate.edu/Warren/Reading/GAO%20predictions.pdf/ Accessed Oct. 01, 2012.

24.) Atkins RC. *Dr. Atkins' New Diet Revolution.* New York, NY: Avon Books, Inc. 1999.

25.) Eades MR, Eades MD. *Protein Power, Paperback Edition.* New York, NY: Bantam Books, 1999.

26.) Enig MG. *Know Your Fats.* Silver Springs, MD: Bethesda Press, 2000.

27.) Sears B. *The Anti-Inflammation Zone.* New York, NY: Regan Books, HarperCollins Publishers, 2005.

28.) Simopoulos AP, Robinson J. *The Omega Diet.* New York, NY: HarperCollins Publishers, 1999.

29.) Colquhoun A, Miyake JA, Benadiba M. Fatty acids, eicosanoids, and cancer. *Nutritional Therapy and Metabolism.* 2009; **37**(3): 105-112.

30.) Spindler SA, et al. Production of 13-hydroxyoctadecadienoic acid (13-HODE) by prostate tumors and cell lines. *Biochemical and Biophysical Research Communications.* 1997; **239**(3):775-81.

31.) Sauer LA, et al. Eicosapentaenoic acid suppresses cell proliferation in MCF-7 human breast cancer xenografts in nude rats via a pertussis toxin-sensitive signal transduction pathway. *Journal of Nutrition,* 2005; **135**: 2124-2129.)

Chapter Twelve

What Do You Do Now?

However much you read in theory, if you do not put it into practice, you are uninformed. Anon. - It is not the going out of the port, but the coming in, that determines the success of a voyage **Henry Ward Beecher. Proverbs from Plymouth Pulpit (1887).**

Two relentless campaigns sponsored by the federal government, one to convert the entire American population to the so-called heart-healthy, high-carbohydrate diet and the other to treat rather than prevent chronic diseases, are folly. At best, the heart-healthy diet is not effective in preventing chronic diseases, including heart disease, and at worst, is causing the very diseases that it was designed to prevent. Similarly, the policy that supports early detection and treatment (secondary prevention) rather than primary prevention, as described in Chapter Eleven, is also flawed.

Secondary prevention seldom cures, but rather it attempts to control symptoms using drugs and surgery. This approach frequently has serious side effects and is so costly that it threatens the national budget. More importantly, secondary prevention is not capable of dealing with nutritional diseases because the only cure for a nutritional disease is correction of the nutritional defect that caused it. Nutritional diseases are controllable only by proper nutrition.

The sole proven method for prevention of the chronic inflammatory diseases is to follow dietary and lifestyle plans that will neither initiate nor sustain such diseases. The scientific evidence cited and discussed in Part Two of this book provides ample evidence that the modern nutritional diseases can be prevented, or at least delayed, by serious dietary change. At this juncture, the question is "What do you do now?" The question is not new. Over the decades many diet plans have been proposed and implemented, but most have failed. Those that have been effective have been based on solid science.

Take Action

The first step is to determine your Body Mass Index (BMI). The Body Mass Index is the official measure of overweight and obesity. It is an excellent tool in the planning of a healthful diet and lifestyle. As explained in Chapter Two, overweight and obesity are growing public health problems affecting approximately 100 million American adults. It is important that you know your BMI because obesity and overweight are powerful risk factors for hypertension, lipid disorders (high blood cholesterol and triglycerides), adult onset diabetes, coronary heart disease, stroke, gallbladder disease, osteoarthritis, sleep apnea and other respiratory problems, and certain cancers.

CALCULATE YOUR BODY MASS INDEX (BMI)

The number you obtain for your BMI will tell you whether you are of normal weight, overweight, or obese. Calculating a BMI can be confusing because the formula uses meters for height and kilograms for weight; most Americans are not familiar with meter and kilogram scales. Because it is important for everyone should know their own BMI, a simplified version using the more familiar inches and pounds in place of meters and kilograms is presented below.

The BMI calculated by using inches and pounds is exactly the same as that calculated from weight in kilograms and height in meters, except that inches and pounds are more familiar quantities: Multiply body weight in pounds by 704.5, and divide this product by height in inches squared. As an example, assume a person weighs 140 pounds and is 68 inches tall. To determine his/her BMI on a calculator (or by hand), multiply his body weight, 140 pounds, by 704.5. The product is 98630. Then, calculate his/her height squared (68 x 68), which gives the number 4624. Now, divide 98630 by 4624. The result, 21.33, is his/her BMI. Normal weight is a BMI under 25; overweight is a BMI between 25 and 29.9; and obesity is a BMI of more of than 30.

WORK WITH YOUR DOCTOR

If you are an older adult, or are taking prescription drugs, or have any kind of medical condition, including obesity, talk to your doctor before you make any changes in your diet, eating habits, or nutritional supplements. Explain to your doctor that this diet is aimed at preventing diseases, not curing them. Tell your doctor that you want to improve your health, by improving your nutrition. Offer to show him this book. If you are taking prescription drugs, be aware that in the first weeks of this diet, your need for certain prescription drugs probably will decline and the doctor may need to reduce your daily doses of prescription drugs. Weight loss on this diet is gradual, so do not expect quick results.

LOOK AT YOUR LIFESTYLE

Examine your lifestyle with the view toward eliminating unhealthful habits. Your habits and daily routines are very important determinants of the quality of your life in older age. Reflect on your use of tobacco and alcohol. The harmful effects of smoking are well known. If you smoke, you can reduce your risks of cardiovascular disease, lung disease, and cancer enormously by stopping, plus, you will save money and reduce the fire hazard in your home. With regard to alcohol, one or two drinks per day are not harmful and may be healthful. But as a rule, excessive alcohol use costs money, damages family life, increases the chances of accidents, and may result in a chronic disease.

A New Approach

Diet plans based on an approximately 40 percent or less of low-glycemic carbohydrate, 30 percent protein, and 30 percent fat or more are nutritionally sound and have proven beneficial to individuals who have followed them faithfully (1; 2). The major difficulty with these diet plans is that they contradict the recommendations of the U.S. government-sponsored nutrition policy (3) as described in Chapter One and, as a result, instill a sense of doubt in the minds of many people.

In addition, the word diet has come to have an unpleasant connotation for many people. For some the word diet brings thoughts of food deprivation and a restricted menu. To others, it stirs up visions of unappetizing and unpalatable food. To almost everyone, diet means a lack of the pleasant, satisfying feeling that comes from a good meal. It is appropriate to say that the diet recommended here will be appetizing, satisfying, and healthful.

A NEW WAY OF THINKING

To avoid the problem of disagreeable associations with what should be a pleasure of life, do not equate "planning a new diet" with "going on a diet." Rather, look at it as embarking on a journey that will bring you to a whole new way of thinking about nutrition. The journey will be of value in helping you understand the difference between a diet that fosters and supports optimum health and normal weight and your former diet that perhaps brought you into the overweight, suboptimal health category. Using nutrition to prevent chronic diseases is not "going on a diet" but rather an activity that is appropriately referred to as primary disease prevention.

A NEW WAY OF PLANNING

A major obstacle to the planning of any menu is the calorie conundrum. The problem is the same, regardless of whether you are planning a healthful diet or simply following MyPyramid (4 - Note that recently MyPyramid's name has been changed to My Plate). A recent survey by the International Food Information Council Foundation found that only one of eight adults knows how many and what kinds of calories to eat each day (5). Calories confusion is common, and a real deterrent to menu planning.

If calories intimidate you, do not be concerned. Calorie counts are not necessary for planning a healthful, disease prevention diet. You do not go to the grocery store to buy a bag of calories; you buy potatoes, meat, and butter. What is important to know is which foods are carbohydrates, which are proteins, and which are fats.

Another confusing issue is that menus have always been based on identifiable dishes, such as an omelet with cheese, a green salad with tuna, or spaghetti and meatballs. The daily chore of having to thumb through recipe books and decide on what to cook and how much to eat is so frustrating that most people give up the whole idea of trying to follow a healthful eating plan and just eat ad libitum.

A far easier and quicker way to plan your meals and snacks is to base your menus on your own specific needs, for protein, fats, and carbohydrates. As an example, it is much simpler to decide to have a piece of steak to provide the protein, some butter to provide the fat, and some fresh asparagus as the carbohydrate. Given this general approach, depending on your body's needs, your personal wishes, and what happens to be in the refrigerator, you can substitute in each category. For example, other meat, fish, cheese, or eggs can take the place of the protein in the steak. The following is a simple way of designing a healthful menu that is not only calorie-silent but also quick and easy.

START WITH YOUR PROTEIN REQUIREMENT (CHAPTER SEVEN)

Proteins are of critical importance for every life function. Therefore, the first task in planning a healthful nutritional regime is to determine your requirement for protein. Go to Table 7-3 to calculate your protein requirement in grams; assume a sedentary life style unless you regularly engage in active exercise. This will give you your absolute minimum protein requirement. It is a simple and easy calculation because it will be half of your lean body weight if you are not overweight. For example, if you weigh 140 pounds, your daily protein need is half of 140 pounds or 70 grams per day. Spread this quantity of protein over the number of meals and snacks you eat in a day.

PROTEIN CHOICES: Next, know your protein choices. These are meats, fish, eggs, and full-fat cheeses. Whole milk and whole milk products, such as cottage cheese and yogurt contain good protein. Note they are accompanied by adequate amounts of carbohydrates, thus be sure to account for these in planning your carbohydrate intake. Consider milk and milk products as being already balanced with carbohydrates. Do not use non-fat milk, reduced-fat milk, or such milk products. Soy milk, soy protein and soy products, are not healthful and should not be used at all (6).

PROTEIN PORTIONS: Once you know your protein requirement in grams, figuring food portions in grams is not difficult. All food labels show protein content in grams for given serving sizes. They also show protein, fat, and carbohydrate contents in grams. Study and use these labels to guide you in determining protein, fat, and carbohydrate levels in packaged foods like tuna fish, milk, sardines, canned meats, and cheese. For fresh foods like meat and fish that usually have no labels, the following equivalents that were worked out by Sears (1), can be very helpful:

1 egg contains 7 grams of protein
1 ounce of fresh meat contains 7 grams of protein.
1.5 ounces of fresh fish contains 7 grams of protein.
1 ounce slice of cheese contains 7 grams of protein.

Egg Units: A quick and easy way for a busy person to assure getting the minimum amount of protein every day is to translate his/her protein requirement into egg units and then keep track of the daily consumption of egg units. Think of one egg as a unit that provides 7 grams of protein. Therefore, if you have a lean body weight of 140 pounds, your need for 70 grams of protein per day would be satisfied by ten egg units (7grams per egg x 10). In terms of protein, two eggs for breakfast, a quarter pound (4 ounces) of ground meat for lunch, and a six ounce salmon filet for dinner would equal 10 egg units.

The major effort required in using the egg unit method is remembering that there are 7 grams (one egg unit) in 1 ounce of meat, 1.5 ounces of fish, and 1 ounce of cheese. This is much less formidable than trying to plan how much meat, fish, cheese, and eggs to eat a day to satisfy a requirement for 30 percent of the calories as protein.

ADD YOUR FAT REQUIREMENT (CHAPTER EIGHT)

Once an individual's daily protein need is known, as described above, aim for at least 4 grams of fat for every 7 grams of protein; plan for about 4 grams fat to go along with one egg unit (or 7 grams) of protein. Much of the time, this will be automatic because full-fat dairy products, meat, fish, eggs, and full fat cheese already contain the minimum amounts of fat required. Extra fat is not a problem and can be used to fit your appetite for fat. So feel free to use butter, cream, bacon, and olives and to eat the extra fat on meat and roasts. High-fat hamburger is the healthy choice, compared to the lower fat variety.

Do not use vegetable seed oils and fats, including margarine. The only healthful fats come from animals and fruits. The animal fats are in meat, fish, eggs, and dairy products. The fruit fats are primarily olive oil and coconut oil. Be sure that your daily fat allotment includes adequate amounts of the omega-3 essential fatty acids (Chapter Nine).

It is important to avoid vegetable seed oils including peanut oil, peanut butter, and peanuts. All are rich in omega-6 linoleic acid, which is excessively high in the American diet. Unfortunately, the famous peanut butter and jelly sandwich contains too much linoleic acid and sugar and should be avoided.

ADD YOUR CARBOHYDRATES (CHAPTER SIX)

Avoid high glycemic carbohydrates. These are sugar, sweets of all kinds, starches, pasta, bread, and grain products such as cold and hot cereals. These foods are mostly glucose, which rapidly enters the bloodstream and raises insulin levels. Some of this glucose goes to providing energy, but most, under the influence of the high insulin levels, is converted to body fat and cholesterol. When carbohydrates of the high-glycemic variety are absent from the diet, fats are used naturally by your body for energy and will not cause weight gain or high cholesterol. Low glycemic carbohydrates are green vegetables, summer squashes, salad greens, berries, non-tropical fruits, and beans.

Carbohydrates should never be eaten alone, but with protein and fat as described above. Aim for no more than 9 grams of low glycemic carbohydrates for every 7 grams of protein. There is no limit on green vegetables. Fresh fruit should be restricted to nontropical fruits; apples, peaches, plums, pears, apricots, nectarines, berries, and melons. Fresh fruit portions the size of a half of an apple contains about 9 grams of low glycemic carbohydrates. For instance, three quarters of an apple and three ounces of steak make a perfect lunch. If you are still hungry, eat another ounce of steak plus a quarter of an apple.

HIDDEN SUGAR AND ARTIFICIAL SWEETENERS: Read labels carefully to exclude products that contain hidden sugar, such as high fructose corn syrup, dextrose, grape juice, sugar, dehydrated sugar cane juice, and even artificial sweeteners. Artificial sweeteners may be a long-term health problem because they stimulate insulin release even though they do not raise blood glucose levels. This is an unnatural physiological state. And there are reports in the literature that artificial sweeteners can cause unusual excitability in children.

EXEMPTIONS FOR PHYSICALLY ACTIVE CHILDREN: Because children tend to burn a lot of energy, some higher glycemic carbohydrates in the form of brown rice or potatoes may be included in their daily diet. These carbohydrates can be used in amounts up to two or three tablespoons as part of a meal that contains ample protein, fat and green vegetables. Cooked dry beans may be used instead of potatoes, rice, and green vegetables because beans are not high-glycemic and their fiber content makes them a good substitute for green vegetables. It is important to recognize that unless the use of the extra carbohydrates is accompanied by adequate physical activity, unwanted weight gain can occur.

HUNGER: Once the sugar and starch have been removed from the diet, hunger will become a more accurate and reliable guide to an individual's true food needs. On this new diet, it is normal and usual for an average individual's daily calorie intake to decline significantly and for body weight to drop gradually to normal. If you are hungry with this diet, increase daily protein intake and both fat and carbohydrates proportionately. If you are too full on this diet, do the opposite; cut all three components, protein, fat, and carbohydrates proportionately. You will soon learn that you will eat more due to hunger when you are physically active than when you are sedentary.

A QUICK SUM UP

Aim for balanced meals. First estimate your daily protein need in grams. Then split the daily protein need up into three meals. Then for every 7 grams of protein, include at least 4 grams of fat and not more than 9 grams of low glycemic carbohydrate. This is not as complicated as it sounds.

A BALANCED SNACK: As an example, use cheese as the protein. Look at the label. Most cheese has 7 grams of protein in a one ounce slice. One ounce of cheese also has about 8 grams of fat and near zero carbohydrate. The amount of fat in the cheese is good because it is more than 4 grams and there is no limit on fats. And according to the rules, zero carbohydrate is also acceptable so a slice of cheese, by itself, is a good snack. It can be made tastier by adding a quarter of an apple, which contains about 9 grams of carbohydrate.

A STEAK LUNCH: Pick a steak about the size of the palm of your hand. It will weigh 3 to 4 ounces and will contain 21 to 28 grams of protein. This is about the right amount of protein for lunch or dinner. Add a green salad, a glass of whole milk or water. A chunk of butter to melt on the steak will add to the nutritive value.

BREAKFAST: Depending on your protein needs, prepare two or three eggs fried in butter, or any way you like. Add bacon if you wish. A quarter of an apple per egg or vegetables in an omelet can be used for carbohydrate, but these are optional. Note that probably the worst breakfast that you can possibly eat is dry cereal, a banana, skim milk, and orange juice. It contains no protein or fat, but lots of high glycemic carbohydrates. Such meals eventually result in both chronic inflammation and loss of muscle mass.

WHAT TO DO ABOUT NUTMEATS?

Nutmeats are difficult to categorize. Some people consider them as protein foods and some as carbohydrate foods. Sears places them in the fat category (7). In general, nuts are made of about 50 to 70 percent true fats, with the balance divided approximately evenly between protein and carbohydrate. Thus, they are most logically classed as fats. However, these fats are predominantly omega-6 linoleic acid.

Unless part of a recipe, nutmeats are usually eaten as snack foods. They are a good source of essential micronutrients. However, if they are counted in a nutritional regime as part of the fat component, their intake should be restricted. Unlike animal fats, their consumption in excess may not be harmless. Because their sources are plants, almost without exception they have very high omega-6 concentrations with little or no omega-3 EFAs. Thus in large quantities, they tend to promote a proinflammatory environment in the body. This is often results in symptoms of allergy.

Peanuts are an extreme example of this proinflammatory property. Although generally thought of as nuts by the general public, peanuts are actually legumes. Their omega-6 linoleic acid content is approximately twice that of the true nuts. This could account for peanut's action as a potent allergen, especially among children addicted to peanut butter and jelly sandwiches.

Supplements

Whether to include supplements routinely in a nutritional plan is a subject of debate within the health care profession. In an ideal world, food would provide all of the essential nutrients, in the appropriate amounts, that are required for optimum health. With careful study and planning, adequate quantities of many essential nutrients can be provided by food. However, there are a few vitamins and minerals that are either difficult or impossible to obtain from food alone. If you are young, active, and have a good appetite, the chances are that your food intake will be satisfying most of your essential nutrient requirements. If you take prescription drugs, talk to your doctor before taking any other supplements or herbs. If you decide to include supplements in your regimen, at a minimum take a daily multivitamin/mineral supplement. After reviewing Chapter Five, think about adding the following.

VITAMINS

B-VITAMINS: Consider a daily B-complex supplement that contains at least 10 milligrams of B6, 400 micrograms of B12, and 400 micrograms of folic acid. If you cannot find a combination product, take them as individual supplements. The combination will help protect against cardiovascular damage caused by excessive blood homocysteine levels, as described by Kilmer McCully in The Heart Revolution (8). Individuals worried about cardiovascular damage and high cholesterol levels should also read Ravnskov's The Cholesterol Myths (9).

VITAMIN C: Consider taking 1,000-3,000 milligrams of vitamin C daily. Take it in divided doses as ascorbic acid either as capsules or as crystals dissolved in a glass of water. One quarter of a teaspoon of crystals equals approximately 1,000 milligrams. In addition to Chapter Five, read the section on cancer in Chapter Ten.

VITAMIN D: Consider taking a minimum of 1,000 IU of vitamin D_3 a day, particularly in the winter months. People taking statin drugs should be especially concerned about their vitamin D status (10).

MINERALS

CALCIUM/MAGNESIUM: For bone health, drink at least a quart of whole milk (not skim) a day. A quart provides about 1,200 milligrams of calcium and 130 milligrams of magnesium. Because dietary magnesium should be at least a half to three quarters that of calcium (for good heart health and function), supplement your intake of magnesium to make a total of 600- 750 milligrams per day. If for any reason you do not drink milk, take daily supplements that total about 1,200 milligrams of calcium and 600 to 750 milligrams of magnesium. An easy, inexpensive method of taking magnesium is as milk of magnesia (MOM). A teaspoon of MOM contains about 160 milligrams of magnesium. One or two teaspoons of MOM are well below the laxative dose of two tablespoons.

Constipation: Constipation is a common complaint whenever a major dietary change is made. This may be due to the fact that a large fraction of the Americans public is deficient in magnesium and an important symptom of magnesium deficiency is constipation. Milk of magnesia will resolve the problem because it is a good source of magnesium; magnesium is what the body uses to regulate the fluidity in the bowel. The daily magnesium requirement for the average adult is about 700 to 800 milligrams. Adjust your magnesium dose a teaspoon at a time at bedtime. A teaspoon of milk of magnesia contains about 150 milligrams of magnesium. If your need is less than two teaspoons, choose your comfort dose and keep using the milk of magnesia. If it is more than two teaspoons (300 milligrams), add magnesium capsules to your diet.

SULFUR - METHYLSULFONYLMETHANE (MSM): Organic sulfur is the only sulfur the body can use to make skin, hair, connective tissue, hormones, enzymes, and helper biochemicals of all kinds. Organic sulfur in the diet is provided primarily by the two sulfur amino acids in protein, cysteine and methionine. Thus, low-protein diets are deficient or, at best, only marginal in organic sulfur. If your diet is low in animal protein, take 750-1,000 milligrams of MSM (organic sulfur) a day.

SELENIUM: Because of extensive evidence that selenium has anticarcinogenic properties, especially against prostate cancer, consider a selenium supplement. However, use caution in using this mineral. The margin of safety between the amount that is essential and the amount that is toxic is very narrow. Check the label of any vitamin and mineral supplements you are taking to make sure you are getting at least 50 micrograms and no more than 200 micrograms a day.

BIOCHEMICAL INTERMEDIATES

Biochemical intermediates are synthesized by the body, but they are also supplied in small amounts by the diet. With illness, aging, or in the case of drug-induced nutrient depletion, supplements may be indicated for some intermediates of special importance. The intermediates listed below are just two of many dozens of valuable biochemicals available to the public. The only caveat is study before buying.

ALPHA-LIPOIC ACID (LIPOIC ACID): Alpha-lipoic acid is a valuable antioxidant and necessary coenzyme that participates in many biochemical reactions. It plays a special role in protecting the activity of other antioxidants. Although the body can make alpha-lipoic acid, its biosynthesis declines with age while the need for it increases.

COENZYME Q10 (COQ): Like many biochemicals, the body synthesizes what it needs. The aging process increases the need for CoQ but reduces the ability of the body to synthesize it. CoQ is of vital importance in the utilization of oxygen by all cells and tissues of the body. The heart, with the greatest oxygen demand of any tissue, needs a greater supply of CoQ to prevent congestive heart failure. Perhaps more important, many drugs, including the commonly prescribed statins for high cholesterol, cause deficiencies of CoQ. A symptom of CoQ deficiency is great fatigue. A deficiency of CoQ can lead to congestive heart failure as a result of a weakened heart muscle (11). Consult your doctor for dosage of CoQ if you are taking statin drugs.

Final Thoughts

The experience of writing this book has raised thoughts of the past and worries about the future of the human family. The American diet over the last hundred years seems to be a story of the triumph of junk science over real science. This is the situation today despite the fact that the biochemical pathways that nutrients follow in the body are reasonably well known and competent studies relating diet to human health have scientifically validated the detrimental effects of high-glycemic diets and essential fatty acid imbalances.

Is it possible that, after surviving all of the wars and misery of recorded human history, the future of man may ultimately be determined by something as simple as a series of low cost, nonpatentable, readily available biochemicals derived from long-chain polyunsaturated fatty acids with their first double bond in the omega-3 position?

References

1.)   Sears B. *Enter the Zone*. New York, NY: Regan Books, HarperCollins Publishers, 1995.

2.)   Eades MR, Eades MD. *Protein Power LifePlan*. New York, NY: Wellness Central: Hachette Book Group, 2000.

3.)   *Dietary Reference Intakes: The Essential Guide to Nutrient Requirements.* Washington, DC: The National Academies Press, 2006.

4.)   http://www.mypyramid.gov/ Accessed Sept. 26, 2012.

5.)   http://www.physiquespeak.com/2010/07/15/majority-of-americans-can't-count-calories/ Accessed Sept. 26, 2012.

6.)   Fallon SA, Enig MG. Tragedy and Hype: The Third International Soy Symposium. *Nexus Magazine*. 2000; **7**(3). (from: http://www.westonaprice.org/).

7.)   Sears B. Zone Food Blocks. New York, NY: Regan Books, Harper Collins Publishers, 1998.

8.)   McCully K, McCully M. *The Heart Revolution:* New York, NY: HarperCollins Publishers, 1999.

9.)   Ravnskov U. *The Cholesterol Myths*. Washington, DC: New Trends Publishing, Inc., 2000.

10.)   Kaufmann JM. Benefits of vitamin D supplementation. *Journal of American Physicians and Surgeons.* 2009; 14(2): 38-45.

11.)   Langsjoen PH, Langsjoen A. Coenzyme Q10 in cardiovascular disease with an emphasis on heart failure and myocardial ischemia. *Asia Pacific Heart Journal.* 1998; **7**(3): 160-168.

Ω

INDEX

Made in the USA
Middletown, DE
20 June 2015